AF449253

Progress in Pediatric Neurology III

PROGRESS IN
PEDIATRIC NEUROLOGY III

Editor

J. GORDON MILLICHAP, M.D., F.R.C.P.

Professor Emeritus of Pediatrics and Neurology,
Northwestern University Medical School;
Pediatric Neurologist,
Children's Memorial Hospital,
Chicago, Illinois

Formerly, Pediatric Neurologist,
Mayo Clinic

P N B • Publishers
Chicago

Published and Distributed Throughout the World by
PNB • Publishers
P.O. Box 11391
Chicago, Illinois 60611, U.S.A.

Printed in the U.S.A.

ISBN 0-9629115-6-9
Library of Congress Catalog Card Number: SN-94-1233
International Standard Serial Number: 1076-2728

Dedicated to the memory of
Nancy M. Millichap
who contributed to the
progress in pediatric neurology
by her efforts on behalf of the Auxiliary to the
American Academy of Neurology
and the annual scientific awards.

PREFACE

The material included in this book is based on a review of the literature published during the three year period, January 1994 through December 1996. The abstracts and editorial comments have appeared in monthly issues of *Pediatric Neurology Briefs* ©, Volumes VIII, IX and X. They have been compiled under subject heading and in chronological order of appearance in order to provide an update and overview of current PROGRESS IN PEDIATRIC NEUROLOGY. A comprehensive index is supplied so that the reader may have ready access to the material reviewed and the subject matter included in the editorial comments.

PROGRESS IN PEDIATRIC NEUROLOGY 1997 is the third book compiled from *Pediatric Neurology Briefs*©. The previous compendia in this series were published in 1991 and 1994, and included articles from the literature of 1987 through December 1993. In the current volume, I have invited colleagues who are authorities in the subject to join me in providing an introduction to chapters with their opinion and overview of the most important advances. Their most valued contributions and assistance are gratefully acknowledged.

Epilepsy, headache, attention deficit and learning disorders, neuromuscular disorders, neuro-cutaneous syndromes, brain neoplasms, and congenital and degenerative diseases are some of the topics covered. The literature on antiepileptic drugs is reviewed in detail, and reports of newer anticonvulsants, notably gabapentin (Neurontin®), are included. The impact of advances in chromosomal and molecular genetics on our understanding of the pathogenesis, prevention, and treatment of the epilepsies and other neurological disorders is emphasized.

The specialty of pediatric neurology bridges not only pediatrics and neurology but also psychology and the education of learning disabled children. Environmental toxins and prenatal drug abuse, especially lead and cocaine, have received increased attention from our colleagues in public health and pharmacology, and the literature on neurotoxicology, nutrition, and diet-related illness has been reviewed. Original articles have been selected from the medical world literature and journals of pediatrics, neurology, developmental medicine, neurosurgery, psychology, psychiatry, epilepsy and other specialties. The editorial comments draw on both recent and past publications on each subject. The institutions and country of origin of the reports are provided in addition to full references.

PROGRESS IN PEDIATRIC NEUROLOGY is intended to provide pediatric neurologists, pediatricians, neurologists, neurosurgeons, psychiatrists, psychologists, geneticists, educators and other interested professionals with an update of the diagnosis, etiology, pathology, treatment and prognosis of nervous diseases of infants, children and adolescents.

J. GORDON MILLICHAP, M.D., F.R.C.P.

CONTRIBUTORS

ISRAEL ALFONSO, M.D.

Associate Professor of Neurology and Pediatrics, University of Miami; Head, Section of Neonatal Neurology, Department of Neurology, Miami Children's Hospital, Miami, FL.

JOEL CHARROW, M.D.

Associate Professor of Pediatrics, Northwestern University Medical School; Acting Head, Section of Clinical Genetics, Department of Pediatrics, Children's Memorial Hospital, Chicago, IL.

PAUL RICHARD DYKEN, M.D.

Director, Institute for Research in Childhood Neurodegenerative Diseases; Formerly, Professor and Chairman, Department of Neurology, University of Alabama; Mobile, AL.

JOSEPH MAYTAL, M.D.

Associate Professor of Neurology and Pediatrics, Albert Einstein College of Medicine; Division of Neurology, Schneider Children's Hospital, New Hyde Park, NY.

JOHN H. MENKES, M.D.

Professor Emeritus of Neurology and Pediatrics, University of California, Los Angeles; Director, Pediatric Neurology, Cedars-Sinai Medical Center, Los Angeles, CA.

HARVEY B. SARNAT, M.D., F.R.C.P.C

Professor of Neurology, Pediatrics and Pathology (Neuropathology), University of Washington; Head, Division of Pediatric Neurology, Children's Hospital and Medical Center, Seattle, WA.

CONTRIBUTORS (continued)

CYNTHIA V. STACK, M.D.
  Associate Professor of Pediatrics and Neurology, Northwestern
University Medical School; Section of Neurophysiology and
Electroencephalography, Division of Neurology, Children's
Memorial Hospital, Chicago, IL.
CHARLES N. SWISHER, M.D.
  Associate Professor of Pediatrics and Neurology, Northwestern
University Medical School; Acting Head, Division of Neurology,
Children's Memorial Hospital, Chicago, IL.
JOHN WILSON, Ph.D., F.R.C.P.
  Formerly Senior Consultant Neurologist, Great Ormond Street
Hospital for Children, and the Institute of Child Health, London.

TABLE OF CONTENTS

Progress in Pediatric Neurology III

CHAPTER **1**

EPILEPSY AND RELATED DISORDERS

INTRODUCTION

Articles on pediatric epilepsy account for approximately thirty per cent of the total number of publications selected from the literature for review and commentary in Volume III of **Progress in Pediatric Neurology.** Side effects of antiepileptic drugs (AEDs) have been the subject of more than 30 original publications in the literature related to pediatric neurology during the years 1994 through 1996, the three year period covered in this volume of the series. The emphasis on toxicity of the drugs used in epilepsy, comprising 16 per cent of the pages devoted to this chapter, has prompted the research and development of newer effective remedies with less risk of serious side effects, especially those reactions involving the blood and liver.

Gabapentin (Neurontin®) has been approved for patients 12 years of age and older who have partial and secondarily generalized seizures. Placebo-controlled, multicenter clinical trials of gabapentin in adult patients have demonstrated efficacy and safety of this new AED. The absence of interactions between gabapentin and other AEDs and the rarity of serious adverse effects has encouraged the expansion of clinical trials to include children with epilepsy. Two studies of gabapentin in children with epilepsy were reported at the December 1996 meeting of the American Epilepsy Society (AES). One, a multicenter, open-label study of gabapentin monotherapy in pediatric patients, aged 4 to 13 years, demonstrated satisfactory seizure control and safety in 93 per cent of children with benign epilepsy with centrotemporal spikes (BECTS). A second study of 74 children, ages 2 to 12 years, with refractory epilepsy found that gabapentin was well tolerated and seizures were reduced in one third. Gabapentin should prove to be a valuable therapy for pediatric epilepsy.

Lamotrigine (Lamictal®) is another new AED approved in the US for the treatment of refractory partial seizures in adults. Seven reports of the use of lamotrigine in children with epilepsy, presented at the recent meeting of the AES, demonstrated efficacy against a wide variety of seizure types, even in neonatal seizures, but a relatively high incidence of skin rash and movement disorders, including tremors, tics and choreoathetosis. Unlike drugs with more serious hepatotoxic effects, the lamotrigine-induced side effects were all reversible on withdrawal or reduction of the dose, although skin rash may sometimes cause concern.

Additional newer AEDs with infrequent trials in children include topiramate, tiagabine, and zonisamide. One remarkable report at the AES meeting had shown control of juvenile myoclonic epilepsy with methylphenidate, a novel new use for a widely used stimulant in the management of ADHD.

Fosphenytoin (Cerebyx®) is a new injectable

preparation that will replace injectable phenytoin sodium as of Jan 1997. Unlike phenytoin, fosphenytoin is water soluble and may be infused with dextrose or saline. Safety in pediatric patients has not yet been established but fosphenytoin should prove of value in the treatment of status epilepticus in children and is free of tissue damaging effects in neonates.

The ketogenic diet has been reintroduced with some enthusiasm from the Johns Hopkins devotees. Eleven studies from various centers reported beneficial effects of the diet in refractory childhood epilepsies at the 1996 AES meeting, but with some practical limitations and side effects. Many could not tolerate the diet or method of administration, and seizure-control was frequently short-lived. The original Mayo Clinic method of introduction of the diet without an initial period of starvation is, in my opinion, superior to the Johns Hopkins method, and does not require hospitalization of the child. Parental noncompliance or misunderstanding and inadequate dietary supervision in some centers may explain treatment failures. The recent attempts to disseminate information about the diet on the Internet should help physicians and other health care providers to provide the optimal support for patients and parents who are willing to endure this rigid and often unpalatable regimen. The ketogenic diet has a place in the treatment of children with seizures refractory to medications or with hypersensitivity reactions to various drugs.

Future research in pediatric epilepsy should emphasize molecular biology and seizure mechanisms and etiologies. The search for metabolic causes and specific treatments, such as pyridoxine, as demonstrated in a series of reports reviewed in this chapter, should always be intensively pursued. The cooperation of colleagues in genetics is important in the management of seizures in infants and young children in selected cases. This introduction and the overview of recent advances by my colleague, Dr Cynthia Stack, will supplement the abstracted articles that follow and provide some opinions on the direction of future research.   *J. Gordon Millichap, M.D.,* Editor.

OVERVIEW OF RECENT ADVANCES

Cynthia V. Stack, M.D.
Section of Neurophysiology and
Electroencephalography, Division of Neurology,
Childrens Memorial Hospital,
Northwestern University Medical School, Chicago, IL.

Areas of progress in pediatric neurology that benefit the child with epilepsy include 1) *advocacy* and the passage of the Health Insurance Portability and Accountability Act of 1996; 2) *communication* and the creation of the EFA web site on the Internet; 3) *diagnosis* by highly sophisticated, structural and functional imaging techniques and EEG studies; and 4) *treatment* by diet and novel hormonal methods in addition to newer anticonvulsant medications.

The new law, sponsored by Senators Nancy L. Kasselbaum and Edward M. Kennedy, will limit the ability of insurers to refuse coverage because of pre-existing condition. Persons with epilepsy will not be denied health coverage, but with limitations. A condition treated or diagnosed in the six months before enrollment in a group insurance plan may be subject to exclusion or limitation of benefits for one year. Genetic information about a condition would not be considered exclusionary in the absence of a diagnosis of the condition. The new law will provide continuation of insurance coverage and lessen the discrimination against patients with epilepsy and their families when they change jobs. The EFA in a Commentary (J Epilepsy 1996;9:298-299) applauds the law as a significant advance but remains vigilant to ensure that federal programs which benefit people with epilepsy are not threatened by budget pressures and cost cutting.

The creation of the EFA web site on the Internet (post-master @ efa. org) facilitates communication between physicians, and should permit immediate transmission of information to lay people (i.e. education of patients, families, organizations, affiliates, and donors), and the notification of health professionals regarding available research grants, opportunities, symposia, meetings, newsletters, clinical trials, and affiliate web sites. As an example of the value of the web site, in early 1996, a neurologist's statement on the Child Neurology list server alerted physicians that ACTH was no longer being manufactured and that it would soon be unobtainable for the treatment of infantile spasms. Within hours, not days or weeks, e-mail messages were alerting the entire epilepsy community, including the FDA, and a crisis was avoided. (EFA Commentary. J. Epilepsy 1996;9:146-147).

Diagnosis of focal cortical dysgenesis as a cause of epilepsies, previously regarded as "cryptogenic," is now possible because of the development of improved imaging techniques and EEG studies (J Clin Neurophysiol 1996;13:467-506). The recognition and localization of a structural cerebral lesion has sometimes explained the refractory nature of the seizures and has led to early surgical intervention and more satisfactory treatment methods.

Advances in treatment have included the further investigation and trial of diet and hormonal approaches, in addition to the introduction of novel anticonvulsant medications. Renewed interest in the ketogenic diet, resurrected by the Johns Hopkins Group, prompted presentation of five abstracts at the 1996 Child Neurology Society Annual Meeting. Subjects discussed included results of a multicenter study of the efficacy of the diet, its use in resistant epilepsy, organic disorders and the diet, EEG analysis of effects, and its complications. Also presented at the CNS 1996 Meeting, a most noteworthy advance in the pathophysiology and treatment of childhood epilepsy has been conducted by Tallie Z Baram and her colleagues at the University of California, Irvine, and Los Angeles, CA. The diligent, painstaking evaluation of the role of corticotropin releasing hormone (CRH) in the pathogenesis of infantile spasms culminated in a phase I trial of a CRH-antagonist as a new anticonvulsant treatment. *Cythia V. Stack, M.D.*

NEONATAL SEIZURES

BENIGN INFANTILE CONVULSIONS

Results of linkage analysis between benign infantile familial convulsions (BIFC) and two linked DNA markers, D20S19 and D20S20, in 52 members from eight BIFC pedigrees are reported from centers in Montpellier and Paris, France, and Rome and Treviso, Italy. The gene responsible for benign familial neonatal convulsions (BFNC) has been mapped to chromosome 20q in the close vicinity of these two DNA markers. Several recombinants were observed betweeen the BIFC locus and D20S19-D20S20 markers, whereas none appeared between the BFNC locus and the markers in 11 BFNC families. The gene responsible for BFNC is not implicated in BIFC. (Malafosse A et al. Benign infantile familial convulsions are not an allelic form of the benign familial neonatal convulsions gene. <u>Ann Neurol</u> April 1994;<u>35</u>:479-482). (Respond: Dr Malafosse, Laboratoire de Medicine Experimentale, CNRS UPR 9008-INSERM U249, Institut de Biologie, Bvd Henri IV, 34060 Montpellier, France).

COMMENT. The authors distinguish BFNC and BIFC by clinical and genetic markers, as follows: 1) onset of BFNC is before 3 months and BIFC, after 3 months of age; 2) seizures, generalized in BFNC and partial in BIFC; and 3) genetic heterogeneity.

Seizure patterns cannot be used to differentiate these benign familial convulsions without documentation by ictal EEG recordings. In a report of a neonate with BFNC who presented with seizures at 50 hours, at the Prince of Wales Children's Hospital, Randwick, Australia, ictal EEGs demonstrated a seizure of right frontal onset with secondary generalization and one of right frontal onset which remained focal. (Bye AME. Neonate with benign familial neonatal convulsions: Recorded generalized and focal seizures. <u>Pediatr Neurol</u> March 1994;<u>10</u>:164-165). BFNC is heterogeneous in clinical and EEG features and cannot be distinguished from BIFC on the basis of clinical seizure patterns. -Editor. *Ped Neur Briefs* May 1994.

SAFETY OF PHENOBARBITAL IN NEONATES WITH HIE

Phenobarbital treatment (20 mg/kg iv) had no significant effect on cerebral blood flow or blood pressure and heart rate, measured 60 min after a loading dose, in 7 term newborn infants with mild to moderate hypoxic ischemic encephalopathy examined in the Dept of Paediatrics, Alborg Hospital, Denmark. Phenobarbital imposed no risk of cerebrovascular damage in newborns with fetal distress. (Andersen K et al. The effect of phenobarbital on cerebral blood flow in newborn infants with foetal distress. <u>Eur J Pediatr</u> Aug 1994:153:584-587).

COMMENT. Phenobarbital is the most commonly used anticonvulsant in neonates and has been advocated in the prevention of periventricular hemorrhage in preterm infants. This demonstration of the safety of phenobarbital in neonates with HIE is encouraging and should offset in part the poor rating the drug has received in some febrile seizure studies. -Editor. *Ped Neur Briefs* Sept 1994.

IV PHENYTOIN AND SOFT TISSUE REACTION IN A NEONATE

A blue discoloration in the hand following an iv infusion of phenytoin in a term baby with neonatal convulsions is reported from Basildon Hospital, Essex, UK. A dose of 10 mg/kg was inadvertently diluted with sterile water rather than the recommended saline. The phenytoin infusion via a cannula was aborted after 2 ml/10 min when an intense blue discoloration appeared round the iv site at the dorsum of the hand. Capillary return and radial pulse were normal. On removal of the cannula, blood oozed freely, and the discoloration spread to the rest of the hand. Improvement occurred after 20 hrs and a blister appeared at the iv site. The lesion resolved within one week. A second iv phenytoin, diluted in saline, and given via a cannula in the foot was aborted when a similar reaction occurred. No systemic side effects were noted. Two possible factors are postulated for the injury: 1) precipitation of phenytoin with alteration in pH on contact with blood or infusing fluid and direct vascular injury and vasospasm; or 2) infiltration of drug with tissue reaction from alkaline solution. (Sharief N, Goonasekera C. Soft tissue injury associated with intravenous phenytoin in a neonate. Acta Paediatr Nov 1994;83:1218-1219). (Respond: Dr N Sharief, Basildon General Hospital, Nether Mayne, Basildon, Essex SS16 5NL, UK).

COMMENT. The authors refer to similar reports in the literature occurring in adults but none in infants and children. This type of tissue reaction to phenytoin in neonates appears to be a rare occurrence. Although slow iv injection of undiluted phenytoin parenteral solution (1-3 mg/kg/min) is recommended by some, most neonatologists and neurologists advocate dilution with normal saline prior to iv injection, infusion at a rate of no more than 0.75 mg/kg/min (Ramsay RE. Epilepsia 1993;34 (Suppl 1):S71), and followed by a normal saline flush. Avoidance of the hand and an in-line filter are additional precautions cited in the literature. Phenytoin should not be mixed in glucose solutions since the drug precipitates out in microcrystals.(Ramsay RE, 1993). Intramuscular injection of PHT should be avoided because of local discomfort, muscle necrosis, and slow and erratic absorption. -Editor. *Ped Neur Briefs* Dec 1994.

Cerebyx© (Fosphenytoin). As of Jan 1, 1997, Parke-Davis, manufacturer of Dilantin, will replace injectable Dilantin (phenytoin sodium injection) 50 mg/mL with injectable Cerebyx (fosphenytoin sodium injection) 50 mg phenytoin equivalents/mL. Cerebyx is rapidly and completely converted to phenytoin following administration, with superior infusion-site tolerability and a faster rate of administration. Unlike Dilantin, Cerebyx is water soluble and may be infused with dextrose or saline. Safety in pediatric patients has not yet been established. *Parke-Davis.*

EARLY AED WITHDRAWAL IN NEONATES WITH SEIZURES

The risk of seizure recurrence within the first year of life was evaluated in 31 surviving neonates whose antiepileptic treatment was discontinued after one to 65 days (median 4.5 days) in a study at the Neonatal Intensive Care Unit, University Hospital, Lund, Sweden. Seizures recurred in only 3 cases (8.3%): in 1 infant receiving prophylaxis, 1 treated for 65 days, and in 1 treated for 6 days. Seizure recurrence was not significantly related to structural brain changes, nor to epileptiform activity in the EEG during the 30 days after the first seizure. No infant with a normal neonatal EEG had seizure recurrence. In infants with a few neonatal seizures and a normal EEG, AEDs can be withdrawn soon after seizures are controlled. In infants with >10 seizures, AEDs can be withdrawn when the EEG is normal and before discharge. In infants with frequent seizures and abnormal EEG, longterm prophylactic antiepileptic treatment may still be preferable. The use of prophylactic treatment is not justified in most cases of neonatal seizures. (Hellstrom-Westas L et al. Low risk of seizure recurrence after early withdrawal of antiepileptic treatment in the neonatal period. <u>Arch Dis Child</u> March 1995;72:F97-F101). (Respond: Dr Lena Hellstrom-Westas, Department of Paediatrics, University Hospital, S-221 85 Lund, Sweden).

COMMENT. The goals of treatment with AEDs in this study were 1) to abolish both clinical and electrographic seizures, and 2) to keep treatment as short as possible. Controversies in the management of neonatal seizures are addressed in <u>Progress in Pediatric Neurology II</u>, 1994, pp14-15; and <u>Vol I</u>, 1991, pp10-11. Most authorities agree that seizures should be determined electrographically before long-term therapy is instituted. -Editor. *Ped Neur Briefs*   April 1995.

SERUM PROLACTIN AND NEONATAL SEIZURES

Serum prolactin (PRL) levels were studied in 28 newborn infants with acute encephalopathy (6 with seizures and 22 without) at the Children's Hospital of Philadelphia and St Christopher's Hospital for Children, Philadelphia, PA. Serum PRL was significantly higher at baseline and 15 min postictally in patients with seizures than in the nonictal group, but postictal levels were not different from baseline values. In both groups, patients with abnormal EEG backgrounds had higher PRL levels than those with normal EEG background. (Legido A et al. Serum prolactin in neonates with seizures. <u>Epilepsia</u> July 1995;36:682-686). (Reprints: Dr A Legido, Section of Neurology, St Christopher's Hospital for Children, Erie Ave at Front St, Philadelphia, PA 19134).

COMMENT. Newborns with EEG confirmed seizures, but without clinical manifestations, have high base-line serum PRL levels that do not increase postictally. These findings were contrary to those recently reported by Morales et al (1995) who found that only newborns with electroclinical seizures, not those with subclinical EEG seizures, had a significant postictal increase in PRL. Serum PRL levels correlate with the severity of the acute neonatal encephalopathy, as determined by the EEG background changes. -Editor. *Ped Neur Briefs*   July 1995.

CAUSES OF NEONATAL ENCEPHALOPATHY

Adverse factors in the family and maternal history, pregnancy, and birth related to the occurrence of neonatal encephalopathy (NE) in full term newborn infants were evaluated in a matched case-control study at the Institute for Child Health Research, West Perth, and the Department of Neonatology, Princess Margaret Hospital for Children, Subiacco, Western Australia. Of 89 cases studied, 42 met criteria for moderate or severe neonatal encephalopathy: *severe* NE -mechanical ventilation required for >24 hours, multiple anticonvulsants, coma, or death; *moderate* NE: -neurologic abnormalities or seizures requiring anticonvulsants, but resolving before discharge. The estimated incidence of NE in the first week of life was 3.75 per 1000 full term live births, and a case fatality of 8%. Intrapartum hypoxia was the cause of NE in only 5 cases, and antepartum factors were more significant and frequent. Maternal vaginal bleeding in pregnancy, physical trauma during pregnancy, maternal thyroxine treatment, and congenital abnormalities were significantly more frequent in NE patients than in controls. Maternal alcohol consumption, smoking during pregnancy, and gestational diabetes were not related to NE. (Adamson SJ et al. Predictors of neonatal encephalopathy in full term infants. BMJ 2 September 1995;311:598-602). (Respond: Professor Fiona Stanley, Institute for Child Health Research, PO Box 855, West Perth 6872, Western Australia, Australia).

COMMENT. Antepartum factors and preexisting neurologic abnormalities are important in the cause of neonatal encephalopathy occurring in full term infants. Intrapartum hypoxia is significant in only 6% of cases.

Problems with definitions and classifications of newborn encephalopathy are reviewed in Progress in Pediatric Neurology II, 1994, pp321-2. The clinical features of hypoxic-ischemic encephalopathy are not specific, and similar symptoms may be caused by metabolic disorders, infection or cerebral malformations. -Editor. *Ped Neur Briefs* Oct 1995.

NEONATAL SEIZURE CHARACTERISTICS

Seizure characteristics in 32 neonates were studied prospectively using prolonged video/EEG recording at the Prince of Wales Children's Hospital, Sydney, Australia. Seizures were generally frequent with limited electrographic spread. Of 1420 seizures recorded, 85% had no clinical manifestations. Clinical observations underestimated electrographic seizures in 54% of neonates. The use of portable EEG machines with only 4 electrodes underestimated seizures in 19 neonates and failed to recognize seizures present in 2. Seizures were generally recorded in both hemispheres, but restricted spread of the seizure discharge necessitated full electrode placements for identification. Some neonates had long interictal periods, and recordings >60 min were often required for diagnosis. (Bye AME, Flanagan D. Spatial and temporal characteristics of neonatal seizures. <u>Epilepsia</u> October 1995;36:1009-1016). (Reprints: Dr AME Bye, Department of Paediatric Neurology, Prince of Wales Children's Hospital, High Street, Randwick, 2031, NSW, Australia).

COMMENT. This study confirms that clinical features are unreliable markers of seizures in neonates, especially in those receiving antiepileptic drugs. Prolonged video/EEG monitoring is essential for confirmation of seizure control. -Editor. *Ped Neur Briefs* Oct 1995.

MINT TEA (PENNYROYAL) EPILEPTIC ENCEPHALOPATHY

Severe epileptic encephalopathy and fulminant liver failure with cerebral edema in two infants given tea brewed from home-grown mint plant leaves are reported from the Departments of Pediatrics and Neurology, University of California, Davis Medical Ceneter, Sacramento. The 1st case, an 8-week-old Hispanic boy failed to awaken the morning after developing fever and mild respiratory symptoms on the day before admission. His eyes were rolled back and he was hypotonic and hypoglycemic. He had hepatomegaly, gastrointestinal bleeding, and multiple organ failure. Generalized seizures developed on the 2nd day, and he died on the 4th day after admission. Tea brewed from a mint plant had been given by the mother for colic and congestion. Autopsy findings revealed hepatocellular necrosis, hemorrhagic renal necrosis, adrenal hemorrhage, cerebral edema, and necrosis and vacuolation of midbrain. The 2nd case, a 6-month-old Hispanic boy had a generalized tonic-clonic seizure following a 1 day illness with fever and vomiting. On admission, his serum glucose was 7 mg/dL. pupils were dilated and minimally reactive, and he had a coagulopathy and metabolic acidosis, gastrointestinal bleeding, and petechiae over the lower limbs. The liver was enlarged and liver function tests markedly abnormal. CT showed a straight sinus hemorrhage. Generalized seizures recurred on the 7th day, the EEG showed persistent epileptiform activity, and he developed a spastic rigidity. At discharge 2 months later, liver enzymes remained elevated, and a muscle biopsy showed myopathic changes. Tests for an infectious cause were negative. Serum collected at admission contained 25 ng/ml of pulegone and 41 ng/ml menthofuran. (Bakerink JA, Gospe SM Jr, Dimand RJ, Eldridge MW. Multiple organ failure after ingestion of pennyroyal oil from herbal tea in two infants. <u>Pediatrics</u> Nov 1996;98:944-947). (Reprints: Dr Marlowe W Eldridge, Section of Critical Care Medicine, Department of Pediatrics, University of California, Davis Medical Center, 2516 Stockton Blvd, Sacramento, CA 96817).

COMMENT. Most mint teas are nontoxic, but some home-grown mint plants used to brew home-made teas may contain pennyroyal oil, a highly neurotoxic and hepatotoxic agent. When mistakenly given to infants as a remedy for colic and other minor ailments, the chemical metabolites of the oil, pulegone and menthofuran, can deplete tissue enzymes and lead to multiorgan failure. The liver and brain are particularly vulnerable, and symptoms of mint tea poisoning include coma and convulsions. Other manifestations are cerebral edema, metabolic acidosis, hypoglycemia, gastrointestinal bleeding, and intravascular coagulopathy. Treatment consists of gastric lavage, activated charcoal, and N-acetylcysteine to replace hepatic glutathione depleted by the toxin. Hispanic parents especially, who frequently treat infants with home-grown herbs, should be warned of the hazards of certain mint plants. This report alerts physicians to the potential toxicity of mint teas and the inclusion of herbal remedies in the differential diagnosis of infantile epileptic encephalopathy. -Editor. *Ped Neur Briefs* Dec 1996.

EPILEPSY AND NON-EPILEPTIC EVENTS IN THE FIRST YEAR

The natural history of non-epileptic paroxysmal events (NEPE) in the first year of life was investigated in 22 babies referred for evaluation of suspected epileptic seizures at the Children's Medical Centre of Israel, Petah Tiqva, Israel. Of 9 diagnosed with epilepsy, 4 had infantile spasms and hypsarrhythmia, 2 had focal seizures and focal spikes, 2 had generalized seizures and diffuse spikes, and 1 had benign myoclonic epilepsy with EEG spike and wave. NEPEs in 13 consisted of the following movement patterns: 1) episodes of rapid eye blinking; 2) episodes of side to side head shaking; 3) body posturing and stretching; 4) masturbation-like activity; and 5) recurrent head flexion. Interictal EEGs were normal. NEPEs continued for periods of 2 weeks to 7 months and then resolved without antiepileptic treatment. Development was normal without relapse during follow up periods of 28 to 38 months. (Shuper A, Mimouni M. Problems of differentiation between epilepsy and non-epileptic paroxysmal events in the first year of life. <u>Arch Dis Child</u> 1995;73:342-344). (Respond: Dr Shuper, Children's Medical Centre of Israel, Beilinson Medical Campus, Petah Tiqva 49202, Israel).

COMMENT. In this study, almost 60% of infants referred for suspected epilepsy were presumed to have non-epileptic paroxysmal events that resolved relatively quickly without treatment. A maturational phenomenon was postulated. Prolonged EEG monitoring may have uncovered evidence of seizure discharges in some, but relatively long follow up without relapse was supportive of the NEPE diagnosis. The differential diagnosis includes benign myoclonus of early infancy, as described by Lombroso and Fejerman. -Editor. *Ped Neur Briefs* Dec 1995.

EEG MONITORING OF NEONATAL SEIZURES

Sixty-three neonates were investigated using prolonged video/EEG monitoring to identify seizures and determine the diagnostic efficiency of clinical observation and short duration EEGs at the Department of Paediatric Neurology, Prince of Wales Children's Hospital, Sydney, NSW, Australia. Thirty-two patients had seizures confirmed. Clinical observations after anticonvulsant treatment identified seizures in 66%, and a 60 min EEG revealed electrographic seizures in 76%, after phenobarbital treatment, and in 50% after addition of phenytoin. Short duration EEG avoids misdiagnoses in most patients with ambiguous clinical signs and aids substantially in the identification of neonatal seizures. (Bye A, Flanagan D. Electroencephalograms, clinical observations and the monitoring of neonatal seizures. <u>J Paediatr Child Health</u> December 1995;31:503-507). (Respond: Dr A Bye, Prince of Wales Children's Hospital, High St, Randwick, NSW 2031, Australia).

COMMENT. When clinical signs of seizures are controlled by anticonvulsants, a 60 min EEG is required to uncover subclinical neonatal seizures, and in some cases, especially when phenytoin has been given in addition to phenobarbital, prolonged video/EEG monitoring may be necessary in diagnosis. An EEG after infusion of anticonvulsant does not gaurantee seizure identification, but the probability of diagnosis increases in relation to the length of the recording. In a study at the Magee-Womens Hospital, Pittsburgh, PA, more than 50% of 92 neonates with seizures had only electrographic expression of seizures, and 16% exhibited electroclinical dissociation. (see <u>Progress in Pediatric Neurology II</u>, PNB Publishers, 1994, pp 11-16). -Editor. *Ped Neur Briefs* Jan 1996.

BENIGN PARTIAL EPILEPSY IN INFANCY

The frequency of occurrence of benign partial epilepsy in infancy (BPEI) in a first line general hospital was determined among 75 patients presenting with epilepsy in the first 2 years of age and evaluated between 1987 and 1993 at the Departments of Paediatrics, Anjo Kosei Hospital, Anjo Aichi, and Nagoya University School of Medicine, Nagoya, Japan. Twenty two (29%) fulfilled the definition of BPEI: partial or secondary generalized seizures, clusters of seizures in 17, normal development, normal EEG, and good response to treatment. Average age at onset was 5.9 months. Average seizure persistence was 3 months. (Okumura A et al. Benign partial epilepsy in infancy. <u>Arch Dis Child</u> Jan 1996;74:19-21). (Respond: Dr Okumura, Dept Paediat, Anjo Kosei Hospital, 12-38 Miyukihonmachi, Anjo Aichi 446, Japan).

COMMENT. Contrary to previous reports BPEI in this study was not rare. When cases of West's syndrome were excluded from the group, nearly half the patients presenting with epilepsy in the first two years of life fulfilled the criteria for BPEI. The initial manifestations of the BPEI observed at this center were impaired consciousness, decreased responsiveness, and cyanosis. -Editor. *Ped Neur Briefs* Feb 1996.

HIGH-RISK MARKERS FOR ASPHYXIAL NEONATAL SEIZURES

The value of clinical high-risk markers in detecting neonates having seizures within the first hour of life following intrapartum asphyxia was evaluated in term infants admitted to the neonatal intensive care unit at the University of Texas Southwestern Medical Center, Dallas, TX. Seizures developed in 5 (5.2%) of 96 infants with hypoxia ischemia or asphyxia. High-risk markers included fetal heart rate (FHRT) abnormalities only (36), FHRT abnormalities and meconium-stained amniotic fluid (MSAF) (20), MSAF only (23), 5 or less 5 min Apgar scores (21), umbilical cord arterial pH of 7 or less (21), and base deficits of -14 mEq/L (19). Significant relationships with seizures occurred with a combination of low 5-min Apgar scores, and the need for intubation in the delivery room in association with severe fetal acidemia. (Perlman JM, Risser R. Can asphyziated infants at risk for neonatal seizures be rapidly identified by current high-risk markers? <u>Pediatrics</u> April 1996;97:456-462). (Reprints: Dr JM Perlman, University of Texas Southwestern Medical Center at Dallas, 5323 Harry Hines Blvd, Dallas, TX 75235).

COMMENT. The combination of postnatal high-risk markers, 1) low 5-min Apgar score, and 2) severe fetal acidemia and intubation in the delivery room, will identify within the first hour after birth those infants at high risk for seizures resulting from perinatal asphyxia. Infants with subclinical seizures may have been overlooked since EEGs were not done routinely.

Neonatal seizures caused by asphyxia carry a poor prognosis; 43% had a poor outcome in a Dublin Collaborative study reported by Curtis PD et al, 1988. See <u>Progress in Pediatric Neurology I & II,</u> PNB Publ, 1991, 1994, for further articles concerning risk factors, prognosis, and the value of the EEG in prediction of continued seizure activity beyond the neonatal period. -Editor. *Ped Neur Briefs* April 1996.

FEBRILE SEIZURES

FEBRILE SEIZURES AND TEMPORAL LOBE EPILEPSY

The histories of 67 patients with medial temporal lobe seizures controlled by temporal lobectomy at a mean age of 27 years were evaluated at Yale University and Epilepsy Center, West Haven CT; Graduate Hospital, Philadelphia; Dartmouth-Hitchcock Medical Center; and VA Center, White River Junction, VT. Forty-five (67%) had histories of febrile seizures without CNS infection before 5 years of age, and of these, 33 had complex febrile seizures which lasted longer than 30 minutes. Other risk factors included head trauma (10%), and birth trauma (3%). Mean age at onset of complex partial epilepsy was 9 years. Seizures had become progressively worse over time in 22 patients before surgery. (French JA et al. Characteristics of medial temporal lobe epilepsy: I. Results of history and physical examination. <u>Ann Neurol</u> Dec 1993;<u>34</u>:774-780). (Respond: PD Williamson MD, Section of Neurology, Dartmouth-Hitchcock Medical Center, Lebanon, NH 03756).

COMMENT. Complex febrile seizures during infancy or early childhood are frequent antecedents of medial temporal lobe epilepsy developing in later childhood. An excellent response to surgery may be expected in adult patients with a temporal lobe epilepsy syndrome associated with a history of prolonged febrile seizures. These results confirm those reported recently from the Montreal Neurological Institute (see <u>Ped Neur Briefs</u> Nov 1993;<u>7</u>:87) and support Falconer's original suggestion of a causal relation between febrile seizures and medial temporal sclerosis (<u>Epilepsia</u> 1971;<u>12</u>:13).

Of 41 patients with adequate pathological examination and a history of febrile seizures, in the Dartmouth and Yale temporal lobe epilepsy study, 38 (93%) had mesial temporal sclerosis (Williamson PD et al. Characteristics of medial temporal lobe epilepsy: II. Interictal and ictal scalp electroencephalography, neuropsychological testing, neuroimaging, surgical results, and pathology. <u>Ann Neurol</u> Dec 1993;<u>34</u>:781-787). -Editor. *Ped Neur Briefs* Jan 1994.

SHIGELLOSIS FEBRILE STATUS EPILEPTICUS

A 4-year-old boy who became blind, deaf and mute after status epilepticus caused by hyperpyrexia from shigellosis is reported from the Sophia Children's Hospital, Rotterdam, The Netherlands. Hyperpyrexia and diarrhea developed 2 days after eating tainted Chinese food at a family feast. Stool cultures grew *Shigella flexneri.* CT showed cerebral swelling. He had several generalized tonic clonic seizures followed by status and prolonged coma. On day 9 he opened his eyes and localized painful stimuli. He was blind, deaf and mute. Vision and hearing recovered within 6 months but expressive language impairment was more persistent. At 4 year follow-up he could repeat simple sentences and speech was more fluent. A "disconnection syndrome" was proposed to explain the language deficit. (van Dongen HR et al. Blind, deaf and mute after a status epilepticus caused by hyperpyrexia from shigellosis - a case report with a four-year follow-up. <u>Neuropediatrics</u> Dec 1993;<u>24</u>:343-345). (Respond: Dr HR van Dongen, Dept of Child Neurology, Sophia Children's Hospital, 40 Dr Molewaterplein, 3015 GD Rotterdam, The Netherlands).

COMMENT. A reversible case of Kluver-Bucy syndrome in a 7-year-old child suffering from *Shigella flexneri* encephalopathy is reported from the Hebrew Univ of Jerusalem, Israel. (Guedalia JSB et al. <u>J Child Neurol</u> 1993;<u>8</u>:313-315). He was apathetic, his affect was dull, he did not recognize common objects or his relatives, he touched and placed objects in his mouth impulsively, and he exhibited an insatiable appetite and signs of bulimia. Hypermetamorphosis, a tendency to be distracted by minute visual stimuli, was questionable, and abnormal sexual behavior was absent. The patient showed 4 of the 6 classical signs of the K-B syndrome, a rare occurrence in children, and recovery was previously unreported.

Shigellae are chiefly waterborne, and foods were incriminated in only 8 of 366 outbreaks in one report, the organism spread by fecal contamination and improper food handling. (<u>Environmental Poisons in Our Food.</u> PNB Publishers, 1993). Children under 10 years of age are at greatest risk, and a neurotoxin produced by *Shigella shiga* has been implicated as a possible convulsive agent. The incidence of febrile convulsions with shigellosis is as high as 45% in some reports whereas shigella-negative diarrheas caused convulsions in less than 2%. The incidence was independent of the species of Shigella, that included

Flexner and Sonne, dysenteries not associated with neurotoxin formation. (Millichap JG. <u>Febrile Convulsions.</u> New York, Macmillan, 1968). -Editor. *Ped Neur Briefs* Feb 1994.

RISK FACTORS FOR FEBRILE SEIZURE RECURRENCE

The relation between postulated risk factors and seizure recurrence after a first febrile seizure (FS) was assessed by reanalysis of pooled data from five centers and follow-up studies and reported from the Sophia Children's Hospital, Rotterdam, The Netherlands. Of 2496 children with 1410 episodes of recurrent seizures, 32% had one, 15% had two, and 7% had three or more recurrent seizures after a first FS; 7% had a complex FS. The risk of FS recurrence was increased at ages 12 to 24 months, after a first and second recurrence, with a family history of seizures, and following FSs with a relatively low temperature ($<40^{\circ}$C). The risk of complex FS was increased if onset of FS was <12 months, if family history was positive for unprovoked seizures, and if the initial FS was focal or partial. (Offringa M et al. Risk factors for seizure recurrence in children with febrile seizures: A pooled analysis of individual patient data from five studies. <u>J Pediatr</u> April 1994;<u>124</u>:574-84). (Reprints: Martin Offringa MD, Room EE 2091, Erasmus University, PO Box 1738, 3000 DR, Rotterdam, The Netherlands).

COMMENT. In a previous report of a follow-up study of 155 Dutch children the principal author had concluded that the predictive value of combined risk factors (age at onset, family history, height of fever) was superior to that of single variables (see <u>Ped Neur Briefs</u> March 1992;<u>6</u>:17). Similar risk factors have been identified previously by a metaanalysis study (Berg AT et al. <u>J Pediatr</u> 1990;<u>116</u>:329-37) and a prospective study (Berg AT et al. <u>N Engl J Med</u> 1992;<u>327</u>:1122-7).

A threshold to febrile seizures based on the height of body temperature was first established in animals with seizures induced by microwave diathermy (Millichap JG. <u>Pediatrics</u> Jan 1959;<u>23</u>:76-85), and has been confirmed clinically (<u>Febrile Convulsions,</u> New York, Macmillan, 1968).

None of the patients in the pooled analysis study had received monitored prophylactic treatment, continuous or intermittent. Having established that 54% of children had one or more recurrences of febrile seizures, the authors may be encouraged to conduct trials of intermittent oral diazepam in their patient population at increased risk, especially in those between the ages of 12 and 24 months, with a positive family history, and whose first FS occurred with a temperature <40°C. -Editor. *Ped Neur Briefs* May 1994.

FIRST FEBRILE SEIZURE CHARACTERISTICS

Clinical characteristics of 910 first febrile seizures in children aged 8 to 34 months, evaluated by telephone interview of parents, are reported from the University of Washington School of Medicine, Seattle, WA. A male preponderance of 57% and a family history of febrile seizures in 29% were elicited. Focal seizures, including only eye deviation in the definition of some, were reported in 18%; Todd's paresis in 4%. Infections associated with fever included otitis media 32%, tonsillitis or URI 12%, viral exanthem 12%, and immunizations 2%. The average temperature recorded at the time of the seizure was 103.7°F. Prolonged seizures and recurrence in the same illness, factors related to increased risk of subsequent nonfebrile seizures, were significantly more frequent in children aged 8-11 months , when compared to those older than 12 months. (Farwell JR et al. First febrile seizure. Characteristics of the child, the seizure, and the illness. <u>Clin Pediatr</u> May 1994;33:263-267). (Respond: Jacqueline R Farwell MD, Division of Neurology, Children's Hospital, 4800 Sand Point Way NE, Seattle, WA 98105).

COMMENT. Notwithstanding the limitations of the method of data collection, some of the Seattle findings are of interest as they compare with numerous previous reports of similar clinical febrile seizure studies.

Between 1924 and 1965, 51 articles involving approximately 10,000 febrile seizure patients were published in the world literature. (Millichap JG. <u>Febrile Convulsions</u>, New York, Macmillan, 1968). A male preponderance was established in 29 series, with a mean sex ratio of 1.4 to 1, a family history of febrile seizures was found in 30%, and the mean threshold convulsive temperature was 104.0°F. In contrast to the Seattle findings, otitis media accounted for only 2.9% of associated fevers, and tonsillitis or pharyngitis was by far the most frequent illness, occurring in 59% of febrile episodes. Focal seizures were reported in a mean of 11%, and 14% in one prospective study.The incidence of Todd's paresis was 3.7% and similar to that observed in Seattle. Of prognostic importance is the confirmation of age at onset (< 1 year) as a risk factor for complex febrile seizures in this study.-Editor. *Ped Neur Briefs* June 1994.

HERPESVIRUS-6 INFECTION AND FEBRILE SEIZURES

Human herpesvirus-6 (HHV-6) infection, incidence, course, complications, and its potential for persistence or reactivation, was studied in infants and children under 3 years of age seen in the ER over a three-year period at the University of Rochester School of Medicine, NY. Of 1653 presenting with acute febrile illnesses, 160 (10%) had primary HHV-6 infection, documented by viremia and seroconversion, and of these, 21 (13%) had seizures, many appearing late and prolonged or recurrent. The risk of seizures among children 12-18 months old with HHV-6 infection was 29%. HHV-6 infections accounted for one third of all first-time febrile seizures in children up to 2 years of age. Among 1394 children under 2 years with fever not due to HHV-6, seizures occurred in 9%. The HHV-6 genome persisted in blood mononuclear cells in 66% of 56 children followed for 1 to 2 years after primary infection. Reactivation was suggested by subsequent increases in antibody titers and PCR in 16% and 6%, respectively. Presence of HHV-6 genome in 29% of 41 healthy neonates' mononuclear cells indicates intrauterine or perinatal transmission of the virus. Among children with HHV-6 illness, roseola was diagnosed in 17%. (Hall CB, Epstein LG et al. Human herpesvirus-6 infection in children. A prospective study of complications and reactivation. <u>N Engl J Med</u> Aug 18, 1994;331:432-8).

COMMENT. Human herpesvirus-6 infection in relation to febrile seizures is discussed in two previous issues of <u>Ped Neur Briefs</u> (April 1992; June 1993). These reports concerned a total of 23 infants with CNS complications of roseola (exanthem subitum) caused by HHV-6. The seizures were often prolonged, some were focal, and the csf showed a pleocytosis in 5.

The present report and findings suggest that HHV-6 infection may account for a much larger percentage of seizures with fever in children than previously recognized. In addition to roseola, HHV-6 infection presented as otitis or fever of undetermined cause. Febrile children with HHV-6 had significantly higher temperatures than HHV-negative children, the factor generally proposed to explain the frequency of seizures with roseola.

The study corroborates the suggestion that seizures with roseola, HHV-6, and fever are not always simple in type. They are frequently prolonged, recurrent, and complex, and sometimes a manifestation of encephalitis or encephalopathy. (<u>Progress in Pediatric Neurology II</u>, Millichap JG, Ed, PNB Publ, 1994, pp 410, 415). These findings further weaken the hypothesis of the so-called *simple febrile seizure* as a distinct disease entity.

For abstracts from the 16th annual conference on febrile convulsions held in Tokyo, Dec 18, 1993, see Fukuyama Y. <u>Brain Dev</u> July/Aug 1994;16:339-346. Papers included neurochemical aspects, EEG studies, and clinical, epidemiological, and treatment reports. The reputed safety and effectiveness of intermittent oral diazepam (0.4 mg/kg, 3 doses) at times of fever for prevention of recurrence of febrile seizures was supported in 23 children treated at Shimane Medical University and Central Hospital, Japan. -Editor. *Ped Neur Briefs* Sept 1994.

HERPESVIRUS-6 INFECTION AND FIRST FEBRILE SEIZURES

The association between acute human herpesvirus-6 (HHV-6) infection and first febrile convulsions was investigated prospectively in 42 children evaluated by virologic and serologic methods at the North Shore University Hospital-Cornell University Medical College, Manhasset, New York. Primary HHV-6 infection was documented by viral culture in 8 (19%), and fourfold rises in HHV-6 titer were present in 9 (26%) of 34 children whose blood was analyzed for acute and convalescent HHV-6 titers. The majority (10 of 11) HHV-6 cases were less than 24 months of age, and 3/11 had roseola. Viral isolation in CSF, attempted in 29, including 7 with evidence of HHV-6 illness, was negative. (Barone SR et al. Human herpesvirus-6 infection in children with first febrile seizures. <u>J Pediatr</u> July 1995;127:95-97). (Reprints: Stephen R Barone MD, North Shore University Hospital, 300 Community Drive, Manhasset, NY 11030).

COMMENT. Acute HHV-6 infection is a significant factor in the etiology of fever and convulsions in young children. Seizures associated with exanthem subitum and HHV-6 infection are not always simple in type, however. They are occasionally prolonged and complex and a manifestation of encephalitis or encephalopathy. See <u>Progress in Pediatric Neurology II</u>, 1994, Chicago, PNB Publishers, for a report and comment on HHV-6 infection, exanthem subitum, and encephalitis/encephalopathy. HHV-6 virus DNA was detected in the cerebrospinal fluid of 6 infants with exanthem subitum, 3 having a pleocytosis and elevated protein in the CSF. (Suga S et al. <u>Ann Neurol</u> 1993;33:597-603). Editor. *Ped Neur Briefs* Aug 1995.

HERPESVIRUS 6 INFECTION AND FEBRILE SEIZURES

The link between human herpesvirus-6 (HHV-6) and other viruses and febrile convulsions (FC) in 65 children (mean age 18 months) with a first episode of simple FC (Group 1) compared to 24 children (mean age 19 months) with a febrile syndrome without FC (Group 2), was examined at the University of Modena, and the Civil Hospital of Sassuolo, Italy. HHV-6 was found in 23/65 of group 1 patients and 12/24 of group 2; adenoviruses in 9/65 of group 1 and in 0/24 of group 2. Of 35% FC cases testing positive for HHV-6 only 17% had the typical exanthema. In the HHV-6 infected group, children who developed FC had lower total immunoglobulins, especially IgM. Children with FC were more likely to have a family history of FC and circulating granulocytes. Of 57 patients followed for 2 years, 9 (15%) had a second FC, and HHV-6 reactivations were three times more frequent in this group. (Bertolani MF, Portolani M, Marotti F et al. A study of childhood febrile convulsions with particular reference to HHV-6 infection: pathogenic considerations. <u>Child's Nerv Syst</u> Sept 1996;12:534-539). (Respond: Dr Maria F Bertolani, Section of Pediatrics, University of Modena, Largo del Pozzo, 71, I-41100 Modena, Italy).

COMMENT. The authors speculate that several viruses, especially HHV-6, may be implicated in causation of febrile convulsions in two thirds of cases, and may be reactivated to induce recurrences. The heredity factor is also important, involving a reduced immune response to viral infection in susceptible children. Those who develop FC with HHV-6 infection have a marked granulocytosis and reduced immunoglobulins, IgA and IgM. The influence of enhanced cytokine production in FC is unproven.

Febrile seizures caused by fever induced by HHV-

6 infection and roseola are not always simple in type. They are frequently prolonged, recurrent, and complex, and sometimes a manifestation of encephalitis or encephalopathy. For additional reports of HHV-6 infection and febrile seizures, see <u>Ped Neur Briefs</u> Sept 1994, and <u>Progress in Pediatric Neurology II</u>, 1994:410-411.

Iron deficiency anemia and febrile convulsions are linked in a study from the University of Naples, Italy. (Pisacane A, Sansone R, Impagliazzo N et al. <u>BMJ</u> 10 Aug 1996;313:343). Anemia (Hgb <105 g/l, serum iron <5.4 mcmol/l) occurred in 30% of FC cases compared to 10% in the non-FC control population. Iron deficiency anemia has also been associated with a case of reversible focal neurologic deficits, and with breath-holding spells. (Progress in Pediatric Neurology I, 1991:397-398). -Editor. *Ped Neur Briefs* Nov 1996.

HEIGHT OF TEMPERATURE: A FEBRILE SEIZURE RISK FACTOR

Risk factors were identified in 69 children with a first febrile seizure compared to 99 matched controls seen in a three year period at the Bronx Municipal Hospital Center, Montifiore Medical Center, and North Central Bronx Hospital, and Albert Einstein College of Medicine, New York. Multivariable analysis of data obtained from medical records and parent interviews showed that the height of body temperature and family history of febrile seizures were significant independent risk factors. The risk of having a febrile seizure almost doubled for each ^{0}F above 101. An association between otitis media and seizure frequency was related to the higher fevers with this infection. Gastroenteritis was not a factor and may have had a protective effect, although none had *Shigella*. A history of febrile seizures in at least one first-degree relative was obtained in 17 (25%) cases compared to 5 (5%) controls. Maternal smoking during pregnancy showed a significant predisposing trend. (Berg AT, Shinnar S et al. Risk factors for a first febrile seizure: A matched case-control study. <u>Epilepsia</u> April 1995;36:334-341). (Respond: Dr AT Berg, School of Allied Health Professions, Williston Hall, Northern Illinois University, DeKalb, IL 60115; Dr Shlomo Shinnar, Albert Einstein College of Medicine and Bronx Munic Hosp Ctr, Bronx, New York).

COMMENT. A previous study of 110 patients with febrile seizures examined between 1956 and 1958, almost forty years ago, at the Bronx Municipal Hospital Center, and laboratory investigations involving four animal species, reported in a series of five articles from the Albert Einstein College of Medicine, had established the height of the body temperature as a measure of febrile seizure threshold and the important determinant of occurrence or induction of fever-induced convulsions. In individual patients and in the group as a whole, seizures occurred when the degree of fever reached or surpassed the threshold convulsive temperature. Contrary to previous reports, the rapidity of rise of temperature was not a predisposing factor. (Millichap JG. Studies in febrile seizures I. Height of body temperature as a measure of the febrile seizure threshold. <u>Pediatrics</u> Jan 1959;23:76-85).

Age and maturity, changes in the balance of water and electrolytes in the brain, and various drugs were factors found to modify the threshold convulsive temperature in young animals. An antihistamine, diphenhydramine and the anticonvulsant, phenytoin lowered the threshold convulsive temperature and exacerbated fever-induced seizures, whereas phenobarbital and phetharbital elevated the threshold and prevented seizures. (Millichap JG. <u>Febrile Convulsions</u>, Macmillan, New York, 1968). See <u>Progress in Pediatric Neurology</u> II, 1994, pp16-32, and I, 1991, pp14-24, (edited by Millichap, PNB Publishers) for a compendium of more current articles on febrile seizures. -Editor. *Ped Neur Briefs* May 1995.

IBUPROFEN AND ACETAMINOPHEN ANTIPYRETIC EFFICACY

The antipyretic efficacies of ibuprofen (5 mg/kg

dose) and acetaminophen (10 mg/kg dose) were compared in 70 outpatients (mean age, 2.1 years) with a history of febrile seizures by a randomized, multiple dose, double-blind clinical study conducted at the University Hospital, Sophia Children's Hospital, and Erasmus University, Rotterdam, the Netherlands. Doses were given every 6 hours for 1 to 3 days, and rectal temperatures were recorded at 0, 2, 4, 6, 12, and 24 hours after the first dose. Ibuprofen reduced fever 0.5 degree C more than acetaminophen at 4 hours. The mean temperature was 0.26 degrees lower during ibuprofen treatment, and the highest temperature was 0.3 degrees lower. In a crossover trial and analysis, these differences in temperature were 0.66 and 0.36, respectively, in favor of ibuprofen. (Van Esch A et al. Antipyretic efficacy of ibuprofen and acetaminophen in children with febrile seizures. <u>Arch Pediatr Adolesc Med</u> June 1995;149:632-637). (Reprints: Dr Van Esch, Department of Public Health, Room Ee2091, Erasmus University, PO Box 1738, 3000 DR Rotterdam, the Netherlands).

COMMENT. The risk of recurrence of febrile seizures might be reduced by early administration of antipyretic drugs. Ibuprofen appears to be superior to acetominophen in antipyretic efficacy, but an anticonvulsant effect remains to be determined.

In laboratory studies of antipyretic agents, aspirin and acetophenetidin failed to retard the rate of temperature rise induced by radiotherm diathermy in animals, and aspirin in doses of 600 mg/kg lowered the threshold convulsive temperature and exacerbated the febrile seizure. Antipyretics in small doses may facilitate heat loss and relieve discomfort attending fever, but large doses may possibly exacerbate the tendency to febrile seizures. (Millichap JG. <u>Febrile Convulsions</u>, New York, Macmillan, 1968). -Editor. *Ped Neur Briefs* June 1995.

SERUM SODIUM AND FEBRILE SEIZURES

Serum sodium determinations were studied prospectively in 69 children with febrile convulsions followed in the Department of Paediatrics, Zuiderziekenhuis, Rotterdam, the Netherlands. Levels <135 mmol/l were found in 52%, and the mean level (134.4 mmol/l) was significantly lower compared to a group of children without fever (140.6 mmol/l) and a group with fever but no convulsions (137.6 mmol/l). Febrile seizure recurrence appeared to be correlated with a lowered serum sodium. (Hugen CAC et al. Serum sodium levels and probability of recurrent febrile convulsions. <u>Eur J Pediatr</u> May 1995;154:403-405). (Respond: Dr CAC Hugen, Department of Paediatrics, Zuiderziekenhuis, Groene Hilledijk 315. NL-3075 EA Rotterdam, the Netherlands).

COMMENT. The authors acknowledge the previous demonstration of a lowered threshold to febrile convulsions in animals with hyponatremia (Millichap JG. <u>Neurology</u> 1960;10:312-321), but overlook the previous clinical report of hyponatremia (130 mEg/l or lower) in 4 (24%) of 17 children with febrile seizures, and serum sodium of 131 - 138 mEq/l in the remaining 13 patients examined. (Millichap JG et al. Studies in febrile seizures. V. Clinical and EEG study in unselected patients. <u>Neurology</u> 1960;10:643-653; *idem.* <u>Febrile Convulsions</u>, New York, Macmillan, 1968). Serum sodium determination is important in a child with a febrile convulsion. -Editor. *Ped Neur Briefs* June 1995.

CSF GLUCOSE IN FEBRILE CONVULSIONS

The effects of convulsion and fever on the CSF and blood glucose concentrations in febrile and non-febrile children, with and without convulsions, have been studied at the Department of Paediatrics, Kuopio University Hospital and Department of Pharmacology and Toxicology, University of Kuopia, Kuopio, Finland. The concentration of glucose in the CSF was significantly higher in febrile children with and without convulsions than in non-febrile, non-convulsive children. Both fever and convulsions increased the CSF glucose levels. The body temperature plotted against the CSF glucose showed a linear correlation. Blood glucose parallelled CSF levels in all groups. Hyperglycemia and elevated CSF glucose in febrile convulsions are apparently secondary to both the fever and convulsion, not the convulsion alone. (Kiviranta T et al. The role of fever on cerebrospinal fluid glucose concentration of children with and without convulsions. <u>Acta Paediatr</u> 1995;84:1276-9). (Respond: Dr T Kiviranta, Department of Paediatrics, Kuopio University Hospital, PO Box 1777, FIN-70211, Kuopio, Finland).

COMMENT. Of 110 patients with febrile seizures examined personally, the cerebrospinal fluid was essentially normal in 86 tested. The concentration of sugar was greater than 80 mg/100 ml in 24 patients and 100 mg/100 ml or higher in 11. (Millichap JG et al. 1960). A review of the literature in the 1960s revealed 18 publications between 1934 and 1964, which included the CSF findings of 500 children with febrile convulsions. Elevations of CSF sugar were found in only three reports, in addition to my own study, the first in 1938, and these involved 37 of 68 patients tested. (Millichap JG. <u>Febrile Convulsions</u>, New York, Macmillan, 1968). The present study attempts to elucidate the mechanism of the increased CSF sugar concentration found in some children with febrile convulsions. Both fever and convulsion were found to have a role in elevating the CSF sugar levels. -Editor. *Ped Neur Briefs* Jan 1996.

FEBRILE SEIZURE DURATION AND TEMPORAL LOBE EPILEPSY

Clinical features of febrile seizures and EEG findings were compared in patients who did and did not develop later afebrile seizures among six selected families and 59 family members with febrile convulsions examined at the Department of Clinical Neurological Sciences, University of Western Ontario, London, Ontario. All six probands developed epilepsy, 5 with temporal lobe epilepsy (TLE), after onset of febrile convulsions (FC). Of 59 family members with FC, 8 (13%)

developed TLE within an average of 12 years after the first FC and 4 (7%) had other seizures. Of 213 family members without FC, only 1 had TLE. The mean duration of FC was 100+/-133 min in those with later TLE and 9+/-19 min in patients without TLE at prolonged follow-up (mean 32 years). The total number of FC, the number in one day, and age at onset did not differ significantly between groups. Of 27 patients with FC who had EEGs, 11 (41%) had epileptiform records and all but one had epilepsy. Neuropathological examination of resected temporal lobes from 5 of the patients with prolonged FC and TLE revealed mesial temporal sclerosis. (Maher J, McLachlan RS. Febrile convulsions. Is seizure duration the most important predictor of temporal lobe epilepsy? <u>Brain</u> 1995;118:1521-1528). (Respond: Dr RS McLachlan, University Hospital, 339 Windermere Road, London, Ontario, Canada N6A 5A5).

COMMENT. The duration of the febrile convulsion was the most important determinant of the later development of epilepsy and epileptiform EEGs. This finding echoes previous publications showing that prolonged febrile convulsions and seizure discharges in the EEG are the most significant criteria of a poor prognosis. (Millichap JG et al. Studies in febrile seizures. V. A clinical and electroencephalographic study in unselected patients. <u>Neurology</u> 1960;10:643-653). Millichap, JG. <u>Febrile Convulsions.</u> A monograph. New York, Macmillan, 1968). Epilepsy and recurrent afebrile seizures developed in 30% of patients with prolonged febrile seizures and in only 5% of patients with short convulsions of less than 20 min. The incidence of paroxysmal EEG tracings in children who developed epilepsy following FC was five times that observed in children with uncomplicated febrile convulsions. EEG abnormalities occurred in 36% of patients with pronged FC >20 min and in 10% of those having short FC <20 min duration.

Berg AT and Shinnar S, examining complex febrile seizures (<u>Epilepsia</u> Feb 1996;37:126-133), found a strong correlation between prolonged duration of the

FC and focal features, both in first and recurrent FC. Also, complex features tended to repeat, especially the prolonged duration, suggesting genetic or constitutional factors. The authors recommend that such children may be candidates for diazepam given at the onset of fever to abort the occurrence of a prolonged seizure. The following authors report a conflicting viewpoint, a not uncommon happening among authorities on this subject.

Knudsen FU et al, examining the long term outcome of prophylaxis for febrile convulsions (<u>Arch Dis Child</u> 1996;74:13-18), found that the prevention of new febrile convulsions by intermittent diazepam at the onset of fever offered no advantages over treatment with diazepam administered at the time of onset of a seizure. The long term prognosis in terms of subsequent epilepsy, neurological, motor, intellectual, cognitive, and scholastic ability was not influenced by the type of treatment applied in early childhood. -Editor. *Ped Neur Briefs* Feb 1996.

ELECTROLYTE ABNORMALITIES IN FEBRILE SEIZURES

The role of serum sodium in susceptibility to complicated febrile convulsions was studied in 115 children admitted with simple or complicated febrile convulsions to the Kuopio University Hospital, Finland. Sodium levels were lower in children with complex FC in comparison with those having simple convulsions. The means were 136.07 (n= 42) and 137.62 mmol l^{-1}(n=71), respectively. Sodium levels were lowest in children with repeated seizures. Levels <135 occurred in 47% of children with repeated FC and only in 8% of those with simple FC, but 50% of these simple FC cases had later complicated, repeated seizures, status epilepticus, or they developed epilepsy within 3 years. Serum potassium concentrations showed no significant changes between simple and complicated FC groups. (Kiviranta T, Airaksinen EM. Low sodium levels in serum are associated with subsequent febrile seizures.

<u>Acta Paediatr</u> Dec 1995;84:1372-4). (Respond: Dr Tuula Kiviranta, Taivallahdentie 7, FIN-70620 Kuopio, Finland).

COMMENT. Hyponatremia may increase the risk for complicated and multiple FC during the same febrile illness.

A further study by the above investigators concerns "osmolality and electrolytes in cerebrospinal fluid and serum of febrile children with and without seizures." (Kiviranta T, Tuomisto L, Airaksinen EM. <u>Eur J Pediatr</u> Feb 1996;155:120-125). CSF osmolality was lower in 60 febrile children than in 30 nonfebrile controls. The febrile groups, 36 with and 24 without seizures, did not differ, but those with repeated FC had lower CSF osmolality than the simple FC group. Differences in serum osmolality between groups were smaller than those in the CSF. Serum and CSF osmolalities showed a positive correlation. The body temperature and osmolality values were negatively correlated. Decreases in CSF sodium concentration with increasing body temperature paralleled those of CSF osmolality. Age was used as a covariant in group comparisons, since osmolality and sodium concentration in CSF correlated with age in nonfebrile children. For further reference to hyponatremia in febrile convulsions, see <u>Ped Neur Briefs</u> June 1995;9:48. -Editor. *Ped Neur Briefs* Feb 1996.

UNPROVOKED SEIZURES WITH FEBRILE SEIZURES

Unprovoked seizures occurred in 26 (6%) of 428 children followed for 2 years or more after a first febrile seizure at the Montefiore Medical Center, Bronx, NY. Risk factors for unprovoked seizures were neurodevelopmental abnormalities, complex febrile seizures, family history of epilepsy, recurrent febrile seizures, and a briefer duration of fever before the initial febrile seizure. Family history of febrile seizures, temperature and age at the initial febrile seizure were not associated risks for unprovoked seizures. (Berg AT, Shinnar S. Unprovoked seizures in children with febrile seizures: Short-term outcome.

<u>Neurology</u> Aug 1996;47:562-568). (Reprints: Dr Anne T Berg, Social Science Research Institute, Northern Illinois University, DeKalb, IL 60115). -Editor. *Ped Neur Briefs* Sept 1996.

INFANTILE SPASMS

NON-DEPOT ACTH FOR INFANTILE SPASMS

The effects and side-effects of non-depot ACTH therapy in 18 children with infantile spasms are reported from the Wilhelmina Children's Hospital, University of Utrecht, The Netherlands. In i.m. doses of 0.4 mg bid for 4 weeks, followed by gradual withdrawal over 2 weeks, non-depot ACTH resulted in complete control of spasms and normalization of the EEG in 6 (33%) patients, and a partial control in 5. Those with cryptogenic seizures responded whereas infants with congenital defects, excepting 2 with tuberous sclerosis, were refractory to treatment. Response to non-depot ACTH was comparable to that reported for depot ACTH, the incidence of side-effects was lower, and a persistent hypercortisolism was not induced. (Kusse MN et al. The effect of non-depot ACTH$_{(1-24)}$ on infantile spasms. <u>Dev Med Child Neurol</u> Dec 1993;<u>35</u>:1067-1073). (Respond: O van Nieuwenhuizen MD, PhD,Dept Child Neurology WKZ, Academisch Ziekenhuis Utecht, PO 85500, 3508 GA Utecht, The Netherlands).

COMMENT. Non-depot ACTH appears worthy of further trial in patients with West syndrome. As with depot ACTH, the dosage schedule may require controlled studies to establish optimal efficacy. Dosage based on surface area or body weight would seem more appropriate, if the mechanism of action is related to a direct effect on the brain, as suggested by these authors and by others. The relatively high frequency of serious side-effects sometimes reported with depot ACTH (eg. Riikonen R, Simell O. <u>Dev Med Child Neurol</u> 1990;<u>32</u>:203) was associated with a high dose regimen(80-140 IU daily for 6 weeks). I have favored the more conservative regimen with smaller, less toxic doses (10-20 IU daily for 2-3 weeks), a treatment schedule also followed in Japan. (see Millichap JG. <u>Progress in Pediatric Neurology</u> Chicago, PNB Publ, 1991, pp 25-26, 30-34). -Editor. *Ped Neur Briefs* Jan 1994.

ACTH EFFICACY IN SYMPTOMATIC INFANTILE SPASMS

A retrospective evaluation of 26 case records of patients with diagnoses of symptomatic infantile spasms and classic hypsarrhythmia is reported from the Division of Pediatric Neurology, University of Minnesota Medical School, Minneapolis, MN. Seventeen (65%) had complete control of spasms and 9 did not respond. Both responders and nonresponders received similar ACTH dosages (87.4 and 84.5 U/m^2, respectively). High-dose ACTH (>100 U/m^2) was not more effective than lower dose regimens. Favorable outcome was associated with late onset (>8 months of age) and prompt treatment (1 month of onset). Responders either improved or did not deteriorate in development, whereas nonresponders were more impaired neurologically. (Sher PK, Sheikh MR. Therapeutic efficacy of ACTH in symptomatic infantile spasms with hypsarrhythmia. <u>Pediatr Neurol</u> Nov/Dec 1993;<u>9</u>:451-6). (Respond: Dr Sher, Division of Pediatric Neurology, Box 486 Mayo Building, Minneapolis, MN 55455).

COMMENT. The control of seizures in responders occurred in 1.6 weeks (0.5-6), and hypsarrhythmia disappeared in all. Despite the symptomatic nature of the infantile spasms and pre-treatment neurologic abnormalities, the results of moderate and relatively short duration ACTH dosage can be satisfactory provided seizure onset is delayed until after 4 months of age and treatment is initiated promptly. High dose regimens with increased risk of serious toxicity are apparently not justified. The need for early diagnosis and treatment has been emphasized previously (Millichap JG et al. <u>JAMA</u> 1962;<u>182</u>:125). -Editor. *Ped Neur Briefs* Jan 1994.

INFANTILE SPASMS AND BIOTINIDASE DEFICIENCY

Two patients who developed infantile spasms at 1 month of age and were found to have biotinidase deficiency are reported from the Hacettepe Children's Hospital, Ankara, Turkey. The parents were consanguineous. Corticotropin had been prescribed initially with partial seizure control. When evaluated at 3 months because of seizure exacerbation, the infants were lethargic and hypotonic, one had alopecia and seborrheic dermatitis and the other's scalp hair was sparse. Metabolic and lactic acidosis developed, and biotinidase deficiency was suspected and confirmed. Both infants responded promptly to biotin, and blood pH and bicarbonate became normal within hours. At 5-11 month follow-up, seizures had not recurred, the EEG and neurologic examinations were normal, but the developmental mental scores on the Bayley Scale were severely retarded. (Kalayci O et al. Infantile spasms as the initial symptom of biotinidase deficiency. J Pediatr Jan 1994;124:103-4). (Reprints: Omer Kalayci MD, Bahcelievler 39, sokak 12/6, 06500 Ankara, Turkey).

COMMENT. Biotin responsive late onset multiple carboxylase deficiency is an autosomal recessive inherited disorder manifested by seizures, alopecia, skin rash, hypotonia, ataxia, hearing loss, and developmental retardation. Lactic acidosis and organic aciduria may be delayed. If untreated the symptoms become progressively worse and coma and death may occur. Symptoms respond rapidly to biotin 5-10 mg daily, but neurologic damage may be irreversible.(Progress in Pediatric Neurology. Chicago, PNB Publishers, 1991, pp547-550). Biotin deficiency should be considered as a possible etiology of infantile spasms.

A therapeutic trial of biotin has been recommended in all drug resistant infantile seizures, pending the results of enzyme and metabolic tests. (Ped Neur Briefs Nov 1989).

Infantile spasms or myoclonic seizures were present in 16% of 30 infants with biotinidase deficiency reported from the Medical College of Virginia, Richmond, VA. (Salbert BA, Wolf B et al. <u>Neurology</u> 1993;<u>43</u>:1351). The authors advocated neonatal mass screening for early diagnosis and avoidance of neurologic damage.(<u>Ped Neur Briefs</u> July 1993;<u>7</u>:51). -Editor. *Ped Neur Briefs* Feb 1994.

CORTICAL HYPOMETABOLISM IN WEST'S SYNDROME

The association between changes on serial PET studies and the clinical course of 12 patients with newly diagnosed West's syndrome is reported from the Departments of Pediatrics and Radiology, Nagoya University School of Medicine, Nagoya, Japan. PET with FDG revealed diffuse or focal cortical hypometabolism in 11 patients, whereas MRI showed abnormalities in only 5. In 7 patients with normal findings on a second PET, spasms ceased after treatment, whereas in 5 with persistent abnormalities on PET, spasms persisted or recurred or partial seizures developed. Patients with normal MRI and normal second PET studies had normal psychomotor development. (Maeda N, Watanabe K, Negoro T et al. Evolutional changes of cortical hypometabolism in West's syndrome. <u>Lancet</u> June 25, 1994;343:1620-23). (Dr Norihide Maeda, Dept of Pediatrics, Nagoya Univ Sch of Medicine, 65 Turuma-cho, Showa-ku, Nagoya 466, Japan).

COMMENT. PET has been found of value in the preoperative evaluation of patients with West's syndrome (Chugani HT et al. <u>Ann Neurol</u> 1990;27:406-13). It may also be used in the assessment of prognosis. See also <u>Ped Neur Briefs</u> March 1992 and <u>Progress in Pediatric Neurology II</u>, Chicago, PNB Publ, 1994, for further reference to PET and infantile spasms. -Editor. *Ped Neur Briefs* July 1994.

FOCAL SPECT AND INFANTILE SPASMS

Seven of 10 patients with infantile spasms examined by SPECT at Tokushima University School of Medicine, Japan, showed localized cerebral hypoperfusion in the temporal lobes. EEGs near time of SPECT showed corresponding focal abnormalities in 5. The MRI was less revealing, with confirmation of localized lesions in only 3. (Miyazaki M et al. Infantile spasms: localized cerebral lesions on SPECT. Epilepsia Sept/Oct 1994;35:988-992). (Reprints: Dr M Miyazaki, Department of Pediatrics, Tokushima University School of Medicine, Kuramoto-cho, Tokushima 770, Japan).

COMMENT. Infantile spasms may be associated with focal temporal lobe hypoperfusion on SPECT despite normal MRI. PET studies of infantile spasms have also shown focal abnormalities when MRI was normal. (Chugani HT et al. In: Progress in Pediatric Neurology Vol II, 1994, p35). -Editor. *Ped Neur Briefs* Dec 1994.

PET BITEMPORAL HYPOMETABOLISM IN INFANTILE SPASMS

A group of 18 infants (age range, 10 mo to 5 yr) with infantile spasms and a common metabolic pattern on positron emission tomography (PET) is reported from the Children's Hospital of Michigan, Wayne State University School of Medicine, Detroit, MI. CT and MRI scans were negative for focal abnormalities. EEGs showed bilateral or multifocal epileptogenicity. All had bilateral hypometabolism in the temporal lobes on PET. Analysis of outcome of 14 of the subjects at a mean follow-up of 4 years revealed 1) severe developmental delay; 2) absent language development; and 3) an autistic disorder in 10. The hypometabolic areas were thought to represent cortical dysplasias, but the patients were not considered candidates for cortical resection. (Chugani HT, Da Silva E, Chugani DC. Infantile spasms III. Prognostic implications of bitemporal hypometabolism on positron emission tomography. <u>Ann Neurol</u> May 1996;39:643-649). (Respond: Dr HT Chugani, Division of Pediatric Neurology and the PET Center, Children's Hospital of Michigan, 3901 Beaubien Blvd, Detroit, MI 48201).

COMMENT. Children with infantile spasms associated with bitemporal glucose hypometabolism on PET appear to comprise a homogeneous group having a poor prognosis, delayed development and severe dysphasia, and autism. They are not candidates for cortical resection. About 10% of children with infantile spasms are autistic.

PET in epilepsy is reviewed from the University Hospital Center of Liege, Belgium (Sadzot B. <u>Epilepsia</u> June 1996;37:511-514). The effect of valproate on cerebral metabolism and blood flow was investigated by deoxyglucose and ^{15}O water PET at the NIH, Bethesda, MD (Gaillard WD etal. <u>Epilepsia</u> June 1996;37:515-521). VPA reduced regional cerebral blood flow but not cerebral metabolic rate for glucose in the thalamus, an effect associated with VPA's mechanism of action in gencralized seizures. -Editor. *Ped Neur Briefs* June 1996.

INFANTILE SPASMS AND NF-1

Two patients, ages 7 and 2 years, with neurofibromatosis type 1 complicated by infantile spasms are reported from the Pediatric Institutes, Siena and Catania, Italy. ACTH and anticonvulsants were ineffective. Both children were mentally retarded and one had UBOs on MRI. The authors believe that the association of NF-1 and infantile spasms is not a coincidence and infantile spasms should be included among the clinical manifestations of NF-1. (Fois A, Tine A, Pavone L. Infantile spasms in patients with neurofibromatosis type 1. <u>Child's Nerv Syst</u> 1994;10:176-179). (Respond: Dr A Fois, Pediatric Institute, University of Siena, I-53100 Siena, Italy).

COMMENT. The authors cite 7 additional cases of infantile spasms with NF-1 in the literature, the first reference to this association originating from Japan (Kurokawa T et al. Pediatrics 1980;65:81). They include a report by Motte et al of 15 cases, all responsive to steroids and having a good mental outcome (1992, unpublished data). A reference to 2 cases reported in a population study of 135 patients with NF-1 in Wales was omitted (Huson SM et al. In: Progress in Pediatric Neurology I, 1991, Chicago, PNB Publ, p 372). Infantile spasms and hypsarrhythmia occur much less frequently with NF-1 than in tuberous sclerosis, but the association is more prevalent than expected. -Editor. *Ped Neur Briefs* Aug 1994.

EPIDEMIOLOGY OF INFANTILE SPASMS IN ICELAND

Incidence, etiology, development, EEG, response to ACTH, and follow-up of all cases of infantile spasms diagnosed in Iceland during a 10-year period are reported from the National University Hospital, Reykjavik, Iceland, and Columbia University, New York. In the period 1981 - 1990, 13 cases were identified and the cumulative incidence was 3 in 10,000 live births. Six were cryptogenic and seven were symptomatic in etiology. All had hypsarrhythmia, and all responded initially to ACTH or prednisolone. At follow-up, all in the cryptogenic group are seizure-free and of normal IQ. Those in the symptomatic group are mentally retarded, and 5 have persistent seizures. (Luovigsson P, Hauser WA et al. Epidemiologic features of infantile spasms in Iceland. Epilepsia July/Aug 1994;35:802-805). (Reprints: Dr W Allen Hauser, 630 W 168th St, New York, NY 10032).

COMMENT. The proportion of patients with a favorable outcome is relatively high compared to some studies. The dosage of ACTH was not stated, but the interval from onset of spasms to treatment was short, generally <1 - 3 weeks.

Focal variant of West syndrome. A n unusual variant of West syndrome, with focal spasms in clusters and focal delayed myelination, is reported from Nagoya University School of Medicine, Japan (Watanabe K et al. <u>Pediatr Neurol</u> 1994;11:47-49). Seizures were controlled with ACTH, and development was normal at 3 yr 5 mos.

Visual inattention and West syndrome. Of seventeen infants with visual abnormalities and occipital EEG discharges studied at Tohoku University School of Medicine, Sendai, Miyagi, Japan, two thirds developed West syndrome with hypsarrhythmia at follow-up. (Iinuma K et al. <u>Epilepsia</u> 1994;35:806-809). This study confirms previous reports of visual inattention as an early manifestation of West syndrome (see <u>Ped Neur Briefs</u> Sept 1993). -Editor. *Ped Neur Briefs* Nov 1994.

MULTIFOCAL INDEPENDENT SPIKE SYNDROME

The relationship of the syndrome of multifocal independent spikes (MIS) to hypsarrhythmia and the slow spike-wave (Lennox-Gastaut) syndrome was studied in 64 children with MIS examined during a 3-year period at the Cleveland Clinic, Ohio. Fifteen additional patients had hypsarrhythmia, 17 had generalized slow spike-wave complexes (SSWC), and 22 had MIS and SSWC in the same recording. Transitions occurred from one pattern to another in 25/40 patients with 2 or more serial EEGs at least 5 months apart. All 25 patients showed the following transition sequence: Hypsarrhthmia --> MIS --> MIS and generalized spikes --> SSWC. None of 8 patients with SSWC showed transitions, showing that SSWC is a stable pattern.

In another group of 20 patients with MIS, hypsarrhythmia, and SSWC examined prospectively over a 6 month period, sleep activated additional spike foci, increased the frequency of generalized spike discharges, and produced synchronization of bitemporal and bifrontal spike-wave discharges at 1.5-2.5 Hz, the same as SSWC. The MIS pattern lies between hypsarrhythmia and SSWC ontogenetically; it is unstable and evolves to other EEG patterns. It should be regarded as a distinct syndrome, not as a variant of the Lennox-Gastaut syndrome. (Kotagal P. Multifocal independent spike syndrome: Relationship to hypsarrhythmia and the slow spike-wave (Lennox-Gastaut) syndrome. <u>Clin Electroencephalogr</u> January 1995;26:23-29). (Reprints: Prakash Kotagal MD, Section of Pediatric Epilepsy, Desk S-51, Cleveland Clinic Foundation, 9500 Euclid Avenue, Cleveland, OH 44195).

COMMENT. The multifocal independent spikes EEG record is defined as three or more independent foci of spikes or sharp waves occurring in multiple locations in both hemispheres. The voltage of the background activity does not show the high voltage of hypsarrhythmia (ie. it is less than 200 mcV). Well developed slow spike-wave complexes are absent, but occasional generalized spike discharges occur.

The author believes that children with MIS syndrome and those with Lennox-Gastaut should not be lumped together. In the slow spike-wave syndrome (Lennox-Gastaut), generalized slow spike and slow-wave complexes at 1.5-2.5 Hz occur in a burst of three or more spike-waves in a row. The SSWC are the dominant discharges, but multifocal spikes may be seen in the same record.

The Cleveland Clinic finds the MIS syndrome to be 3-4 times as common as the Lennox Gastaut syndrome and a distinct type of symptomatic generalized epilepsy in childhood. -Editor. *Ped Neur Briefs* Jan 1995.

ASYMMETRIC HYPSARRHYTHMIA

The clinical, EEG, and radiological findings in 6 patients with the asymmetric variant of hypsarrhythmia among 26 children with infantile spasms are reported from the University of Michigan EEG Laboratory, Ann Arbor, MI. The spasms were symptomatic of cerebral dysplasia in 4, porencephaly in 1, and hypoxic-ischemic encephalopathy in 1. Focal abnormalities on neurologic exam or imaging study were found in 5 children. The abnormal EEG activity was ipsilateral to the lesion in 4 and contralateral in 1.

Of hypsarrhythmia EEGs seen in this lab, 23% were asymmetric. The EEG may show focal abnormalities that are not detected by clinical exam or imaging study. (Drury I, Beydoun A, Garofalo EA, Henry TR. Asymmetric hypsarrhythmia: Clinical electroencephalographic and radiological findings. <u>Epilepsia</u> Jan 1995;36:41-47). (Reprints: Dr I Drury, EEG Laboratory, University Hospital 1B300/0036, 1500 E Medical Center Dr, Ann Arbor, MI 48109).

COMMENT. The EEG may identify patients with infantile spasms whose lesions are amenable to surgery, even when not detected by clinical findings and imaging studies. Most cases showing asymmetric hypsarrhythmia had developmental abnormalities of the brain, primarily large cystic lesions.

Cerebral tumors and infantile spasms. Branch CE and Dyken PR report a choroid plexus papilloma and infantile spasms. (<u>Ann Neurol</u> 1979;5:302). The spasms resolved after surgery for removal of the tumor. These cases favor a primary cortical rather than brain stem origin for infantile spasms.

A generalized electrodecremental EEG resulting from a focal cortical ictal discharge and associated with partial seizures is reported in 23 patients seen at the Johns Hopkins Epilepsy Center (Arroyo S et al. <u>Epilepsia</u> 1994;35:974).

Ohtahara's syndrome and focal cortical dysplasia. The surgical treatment of an early epileptic encephalopathy with suppression-bursts (Ohtahara's syndrome) and focal cortical dysplasia is reported from Hopital Pellegrin, Bordeaux, France (Pedespan JM et al. <u>Epilepsia</u> Jan 1995;36:37-40). Infantile spasms and brief left-sided tonic unilateral seizures began at 5 days of age. The interictal EEG showed an asymmetrical suppression-burst pattern affecting the right hemisphere. MRI showed right frontotemporal cortical thickening. Seizures were resistant to AEDs and steroid therapy. The right precentral area resected showed cytoarchitectural dysplasia and ectopic neurons deep in subcortical white matter. At 1 year follow-up, the child had suffered only a "febrile seizure," and had minor developmental delay with slight left-sided weakness. Surgery may be effective in some cases of Ohtahara's syndrome.

Sarnat HB, University of Washington, Seattle, reviews "Ependymal reactions to injury" and focal dysplasias of the developing brain that may be secondary to damage to fetal ependyma. (J Neuropathol Exp Neurol January 1995;54:1-15). -Editor. *Ped Neur Briefs* Jan 1995.

ASYMMETRIC INFANTILE SPASMS

Behavioral and EEG asymmetry and asynchrony of 8,680 infantile spasms were analysed in a review of 75 consecutive video-EEG recordings performed at UCLA Medical Center, Los Angeles from 1982 to 1992. Asymmetry occurred in 25% and asynchrony in 7% of recorded spasms. The seizure EEG discharge was usually contralateral to the clinically involved side. In 12 of 60 patients (20%), more than 50% of recorded spasms were asymmetric or asynchronous. This group of patients showed the most frequent structural and functional brain abnormalities involving the contralateral central region detected by EEG, MRI, PET, and neurological examination. Partial seizures with lateralized motor behavior occurred in 50% of this group compared to only 9% of patients showing asymmetry-asynchrony in less than one third of spasms. Partial seizures were associated with clusters of infantile spasms in 35% of the children in the study. (Gaily EK et al. Asymmetric and asynchronous infantile spasms. Epilepsia Aug/Sept 1995;36:873-882). (Reprints: Dr EK Gaily, Department of Child Neurology, University of Helsinki, Children's Castle Hospital, Lastenlinnantie 2, SF-00250 Helsinki, Finland).

COMMENT. The authors suggest that this combination of asymmetric and/or asynchronous infantile spasms, partial motor seizures involving the same side of the body, and contralateral central region pathology may represent a previously undescribed and unique subset of symptomatic age-specific localization-related infantile epilepsy. The findings support the hypothesis that infantile spasms are generated by the cerebral cortex and the primary sensorimotor cortex is involved in asymmetric and asynchronous spasms. -Editor *Ped Neur Briefs* Sept 1995.

THEOPHYLLINE-INDUCED   INFANTILE SPASMS

Infantile spasms and hypsarrhythmia developed in a 6-month-old infant with asthma after 3 days treatment with theophylline at the Royal Belfast Hospital for Sick Children, Northern Ireland. Theophylline blood level was elevated to 108 mcmol/l (30 mcmol above therapeutic level). Spasms stopped and EEG became normal when nitrazepam was started and theophylline was discontinued. Nitrazepam was withdrawn at 10 months, the sleep EEG was normal at 14 months, and seizures had not recurred at 3 year follow-up. (Shields MD et al. Infantile spasms associated with theophylline toxicity. Acta Paediatr Feb 1995;84:215-217). (Respond: Dr MD Shields, Department of Child Health, Royal Belfast Hospital for Sick Children, 180 Falls Rd, Belfast BT12 6BE, Northern Ireland).

COMMENT. A direct causal relationship was considered probable because of the close temporal association of spasms and a toxic level of theophylline and the complete remission when the drug was discontinued. A dose of 6-8 mg/kg/day theophylline is usually recommended for infants <7 months of age with asthma. The toxic dose in this patient was 16 mg/kg/day.

Infantile spasms in 5 children (4 symptomatic) persisted to 5 to 14 years of age in a report from the Steele Memorial Children's Research Center, University of Arizona, Tucson (Talwar D, Griesemer DA et al. Epilepsia Feb 1995;36:151-155). -Editor. *Ped Neur Briefs* March 1995.

INFANTILE SPASM MORBIDITY vs PERINATAL MORTALITY

During a 15-year period 1968-1982, perinatal mortality in Finland declined from 19.9 to 7.4 per 1000 live births. The incidence of children with infantile spasms remained unchanged during two study periods, 1960-1977 and 1977-1991, rates of 0.41 and 0.43/1000 livebirths, respectively, with admissions to the Children's Hospital of the University of Helsinki. The proportion of low birth weight infants with infantile spasms was not different in the two periods, but the number small for gestational age decreased in the second study period. They all had severe pre-, peri-, or postnatal brain damage or other symptomatic causes for infantile spasms. In the later 77-91 compared to the earlier 60-77 period, brain malformations and tuberous sclerosis were diagnosed more frequently as causes of infantile spasms, neonatal hypoglycemia was a less frequent etiology, while idiopathic cases were of equal frequency (19%). (Riikonen R. Decreasing perinatal mortality: Unchanged infantile spasm morbidity. <u>Dev Med Child Neur</u> 1995;37:232-238).

COMMENT. Improved neuroimaging may account for the higher incidence of brain malformations detected in infants with spasms. -Editor. *Ped Neur Briefs* April 1995.

RISK FACTORS OF INFANTILE SPASMS

The role of a genetic predisposition and other risk factors for seizures was analyzed by evaluation of records of 80 children with infantile spasms admitted to 12 Danish pediatric departments during 1967-68 and 1972-73. Findings were compared with those documented in records of 474 children with other types of epilepsy and 2196 children with febrile seizures, all admitted with neurologic disorders at age 1 month to 2 years.

There was a family history of seizures in 14% of children with infantile spasms, compared to 29% in children with other epilepsies, 26% in those with febrile seizures, and 5% in children admitted for CNS infections. A family history of seizures increased the risk for infantile spasms threefold, but only in the cryptogenic cases that made up 50% of the group. Neonatal hypoxia, neonatal seizures, and CNS malformations were much stronger predictors of infantile spasms than genetic factors. The relatively low incidence of organic cases in this study was explained by the lack of available brain imaging. (Rantala H, Shields WD et al. Risk factors of infantile spasms compared with other seizures in children under 2 years of age. <u>Epilepsia</u> April 1996;37:362-366). (Reprints: Dr H Rantala, Department of Pediatrics, University of Oulu, FIN-90220 Oulu 22, Finland).

COMMENT. A family history of seizures contributes to a 3-fold risk for infantile spasms of the cryptogenic variety. Organic brain disorders and neurologic abnormalities play a much stronger role as precursors of infantile spasms. Neonatal seizures are particularly predictive of possible occurrence of infantile spasms.

Long-term outcome of West syndrome was studied in 214 children with a history of infantile spasms followed for 20-35 years or until death (31%) at the Children's Hospital, University of Helsinki, Finland. (Riikonen R. <u>Epilepsia</u> April 1996;37:367-372). Infection was the most frequent cause of death (31 of 67 patients). Eight children who died during treatment with large doses of ACTH had enlarged adrenal glands and hypertrophic cardiomyopathy. Among survivors, intelligence was normal or near normal in 24%. Factors predictive of a good prognosis included a crytogenic etiology, normal development before onset of spasms, and a good response to ACTH. Focal abnormalities in the EEG were not necessarily indicative of a poor prognosis.

Treatment with high-dose ACTH (150 U/m2/day) was superior to prednisone (2 mg/kg/day) in suppressing clinical spasms and hypsarrhythmia in the EEG in a prospective, randomized, blinded study of 29 patients (22 symptomatic and 7 cryptogenic etiologies) treated for 2 week periods at the University of Southern California, Los Angeles (Baram TZ et al. <u>Pediatrics</u> March 1996;97:375-379). Of 15 patients randomized to ACTH, 13 (87%) responded, compared to 4 (29%) of 14 given prednisone. -Editor. *Ped Neur Briefs* April 1996.

INFANTILE SPASMS IN DOWN SYNDROME

The clinical characteristics, EEG abnormalities, response to therapy, and outcome of 14 patients with infantile spasms and Down syndrome were studied at the Hopital Saint Vincent de Paul, Paris (9 cases); Universita Degli Studi de Pisa, Italy (2 cases); and Hopital de La Timone, Marseille, France (3 cases). None had antecedent cardiopathy or perinatal hypoxia. Spasms began between 4 and 18 months (mean 8 months), development was delayed before seizure onset, and visual contact deteriorated after seizure onset. Interictal EEGs showed typical hypsarrhythmia with no focal abnormality. Hydrocortisone (15 mg/kg/day for 2 weeks, and discontinuation over 2 weeks) in 10, and vigabatrin, valproate, or pyridoxine in 4 patients, controlled spasms and hypsarrhythmia within 6 months. Five with relapses within 2 months responded to further treatments. Seven remained seizure-free, and 7 developed other types of seizures resembling idiopathic generalized epilepsies, including myoclonic jerks, absences, or generalized atonic or tonic-clonic seizures, most responding readily to a combination of valproate, ethosuximide, and diazepam. None developed Lennox-Gastaut syndrome or other chronic refractory seizure disorder. Autistic features persisted in 2. (Silva ML, Cieuta C, Guerrini R, Plouin P, Livet MO, Dulac O. Early clinical and EEG features of infantile spasms in Down syndrome. <u>Epilepsia</u> Oct 1996;37:977-982). (Reprints: Dr O Dulac, Hopital Saint Vincent de Paul, 82 Ave Denfert Rochereau, 75674 Paris Cedex 14, France).

COMMENT. Infantile spasms in Down syndrome have the ictal and interictal EEG characteristics of idiopathic West syndrome, they respond relatively well to therapy, and do not generally evolve into Lennox-Gastaut or other chronic epilepsy syndrome. A delay in diagnosis may contribute to a worsening of cognitive dysfunction, and parents of Down syndrome children should be alerted to the possible development of spasms in the first year.

A case of West syndrome as the initial manifestation of congenital unilateral perisylvian cortical dysplasia is reported from University Children's Hospital, Badajoz; and Galicia General University Hospital, Santiago de Compostela, Spain (Vaquerizo-Madrid J, Eiris-Punal J, Gomez-Martin H et al. <u>Acta Neuropediatr</u> 1996;2:132-138). The child had left hemiatrophy and paresis and was developmentally delayed. Later, he had refractory epilepsy, with complex partial, atypical absence, and atonic seizures. The interictal EEG during sleep showed right sided epileptogenic activity with contralateral spread. -Editor. *Ped Neur Briefs* Oct 1996.

EPILEPTIC SYNDROMES AND ETIOLOGY

ICTUS EMETICUS INDUCED BY PHOTIC STIMULATION

Occipitotemporal seizures induced by intermittent photic stimulation in three children with brain injuries, aged 10 to 13 years, are reported from the Institute of Developmental Neuropsychiatry, University of Pisa, Italy. Infantile or early childhood seizures (infantile spasms, febrile seizures, or complex partial seizures) had been controlled and medications discontinued. All had a history of occipital spikes on the EEG. Photic stimulation induced electroclinical phenomena localized to the right occipital lobe with spread to mesial temporal limbic structures, including amygdala and hippocampus. Symptoms began with blindness, tonic eye deviation, blinking, oral automatisms, epigastric sensations, fear, reduced responsiveness, rhythmic chewing, and vomiting, appearing as a late ictal manifestation. All patients were seizure free at 1 year follow up; 2 were untreated and one had received carbamazepine. Vomiting can be a late ictal phenomenon resulting from temporal lobe spread of seizures originating in the occipital lobe. (Guerrini R et al. Occipitotemporal seizures with ictus emeticus induced by intermittent photic stimulation. Neurology Feb 1994;44:253-259). (Reprints: Dr Renzo Guerrini, Institute of Child Neuropsychiatry, University of Pisa, Via dei Giacinti 2, 56018 Calambrone, Pisa, Italy).

COMMENT. Vomiting as an ictal phenomenon is controversial and difficult to distinguish from migraine. In these patients with previous evidence of occipital epileptiform EEG discharges, visual symptoms followed by automatisms and vomiting appeared more likely to result from temporal lobe ictal involvement than a migraine secondary to an occipital seizure. The lateralization of the ictal discharge to the right hemisphere has previously been reported in 13 children with the diagnosis of ictus emeticus. (Kramer RE et al, 1988). Cyclical vomiting as a form of epilepsy in 33 children was described in 1955. (Millichap JG, Lombroso CT, Lennox WG). See Progress in Pediatric Neurology, Chicago, PNB Publishers, 1991, for further reports of ictus emeticus. -Editor. *Ped Neur Briefs* March 1994.

ICTUS EMETICUS AND NONDOMINANT TEMPORAL LOBE INVOLVEMENT

Two patients, aged 18 and 47 years, with ictal vomiting during temporal lobe seizures documented with bilateral depth electrodes are reported from the Department of Neurology, New York School of Medicine, Hospital for Joint Diseases, New York. Vomiting developed when the seizure discharge spread to the right temporal lobe of one patient. In the other patient who was left-handed and had right-hemisphere language dominance, ictal vomiting was associated with a left temporal discharge. These cases supported the localization of ictal vomiting in the nondominant temporal lobe. (Devinsky O et al. Ictus emeticus: Further evidence of nondominant temporal involvement. <u>Neurology</u> June 1995;45:1158-1160). (Reprints: Dr Orrin Devinsky, Department of Neurology, Hospital for Joint Disease, 301 East 17th St, New York, NY 10003).

COMMENT. The authors cite 16 previous reports of ictal vomiting, the first dated 1982, with right temporal foci in 14. In a 1955 report from the Children's Medical Center, Boston, 33 children with cyclic vomiting, 7 (21%) having a history of complex partial or generalized seizures and 25 (76%) with seizure discharges in the EEG, some focal with temporal localization, were thought to have a form of epilepsy. (Millichap JG, Lombroso CT, Lennox WG. <u>Pediatrics</u> 1955;15:705). Ictal vomiting is discussed in <u>Progress in Pediatric Neurology I</u>, Chicago, PNB Publ, 1991, pp46-47. -Editor. *Ped Neur Briefs* July 1995.

AUTONOMIC EPILEPSY REVIEWED

In addition to gastointestinal manifestations of epilepsy, a review of autonomic epilepsies from the Deaconess and Beth Israel Hospitals and Harvard Medical School, Boston, MA, included cardiovascular manifestations, sudden cardiac death, neurogenic pulmonary edema and other respiratory manifestations, diencephalic epilepsy, cutaneous manifestations, and urogenital manifestations. Gastrointestinal symptoms of epilepsy present as auras in adult patients with complex partial seizures, but ictal autonomic symptoms may be limited to visceral sensations, called abdominal epilepsy, especially in children. EEG abnormalities associated with ictal vomiting usually lateralize to the right or nondominant temporal lobe. (Freeman R, Schachter SC. Autonomic epilepsy. <u>Seminars in Neurology</u> June 1995;15:158-166). (Reprints: Dr Freeman, Division of Neurology, Deaconess Hospital, Suite 7H, 110 Francis Street, Boston, MA 02215).

COMMENT. "Ictus emeticus and the nondominant temporal lobe" is discussed in <u>Ped Neur Briefs</u> June 1995;9:55. Some anticonvulsants have autonomic side-effects. (Millichap JG, Ortiz WR. Nitrazepam in myoclonic epilepsies. <u>Am J Dis Child</u> 1966;112:242-248). -Editor. *Ped Neur Briefs* Aug 1995.

ANATOMY OF *DEJA VU* IN TEMPORAL LOBE EPILEPSY

Sixteen patients, ages 16 to 32 years, implanted with depth electrodes at Hopital Saint-Anne, Paris, France, had experienced a dreamy state (*deja-vu - deja vecu*, memories of complete scenes, or vague reminiscence) during sterotactic EEG (SEEG). Seizures had been present from 2 to 25 years, they began before the age of 10 years in 50% of patients, and occurred at least once a week. Etiological factors included neonatal injury (6), febrile convulsion (1), tumors (3). Most patients had dreamy states in their spontaneous seizures; the amygdala, anterior hippocampus, and temporal neocortex were all involved in recordings. They were also evoked by stimulation of the temporal neocortex (88%), anterior hippocampus (83%), or amygdala (73%). The superior temporal gyrus was more responsive than the middle temporal gyrus. (Bancaud J, Halgren E et al. Anatomical origin of *deja vu* and vivid 'memories' in human temporal lobe epilepsy. <u>Brain</u> Feb 1994;<u>117</u>:71-90). (Respond: Dr E Halgren, Clinique Neurologique, CHRU Pontchaillou, 35033 Rennes Cedex, France).

COMMENT. *Deja vu* and other dreamy states in patients with temporal lobe epilepsy may originate in and involve both medial and lateral aspects of the temporal lobe and especially the anterior hippocampus, amygdala and superior temporal gyrus. -Editor. *Ped Neur Briefs* May 1994.

FAMILIAL TEMPORAL LOBE EPILEPSY IN TWINS

A new syndrome of familial temporal lobe epilepsy is described in 38 subjects from 13 unrelated families and was first identified in 5 concordant monozygotic twin pairs at the Australian National

Health and Medical Research Council Twin Registry, University of Melbourne, Parkville, Australia. Seizure types were simple partial seizures with psychic or autonomic symptoms, infrequent complex partial seizures, and rare secondarily generalized seizures. EEGs showed focal temporal interictal epileptiform discharges in 22%. MRIs were normal. Autosomal dominant inheritance with age-dependent penetrance was likely. Some family members were affected with only mild and subtle seizure manifestations. (Berkovic SF et al. Familial temporal lobe epilepsy: A common disorder identified in twins. <u>Ann Neurol</u> Aug 1996;40:227-235). (Respond: Dr Samuel F Berkovic, Department of Neurology, Austin and Repatriation Medical Centre, Heidelberg (Melbourne), Victoria 3084, Australia).

COMMENT. Onset of familial temporal lobe epilepsy (TLE) is typically in adolescence or early adult life, whereas TLE with hippocampal sclerosis (HS) usually begins in childhood. Febrile seizures, often preceding the TLE of HS, were not increased in frequency in family members of familial TLE subjects. The mild and subtle nature of familial TLE may explain the previous infrequent reports of similar syndromes. Bray PF and Wiser WC have described the hereditary characteristics of familial temporo-central focal epilepsy, and the above authors suggest that some of their cases persisting into adulthood might represent examples of familial TLE. (<u>Pediatrics</u> 1965;36:207-211). -Editor. *Ped Neur Briefs* Sept 1996.

JUVENILE MYOCLONIC EPILEPSY

Video-polygraphic analyses of 302 myoclonic seizures (MS) in 5 patients with juvenile myoclonic epilepsy (JME) are reported from the Department of Pediatrics, Tokyo Women's Medical College, Japan. MS occurred singly or repetitively and corresponded to generalized bilaterally synchronous single or multispike-and-wave complexes at 3-5 Hz. Either distal or proximal muscles were involved, and facial jerks were infrequent. MS were asymmetrical in 4 of 5 patients and 9 to 38% of all seizures. Contraction and postmyoclonic inhibition of proximal muscles with atonia alternated with a flapping tremor during analysis of EMG in outstretched arms; myoclonic EMG potentials were suddenly disrupted when the arms dropped. Four patients fell when MS were intense. (Oguni H, Fukuyama Y et al. Video-polygraphic analysis of myoclonic seizures in juvenile myoclonic epilepsy. Epilepsia March/April 1994;35:307-316). (Reprints: Dr H Oguni, Dept Pediatrics, Tokyo Women's Medical College, 8-1 Kawada-cho, Shinjuku-ku, Tokyo 162, Japan).

COMMENT. A total of eight articles on juvenile myoclonic epilepsy were published in the March/April 1994 issue of Epilepsia. Panayiotopoulos CP et al reported a 5-year prospective study of 66 patents with JME seen at the King Khalid University Hospital, Riyadh, Saudi Arabia (Epilepsia 1994;35:285-296). Prevalence was 10.2% among 672 patients with epilepsies. Inheritance was autosomal recessive with siblings involved in 13 of 41 families.. Diagnosis had been missed before referral in 63 and even after the initial visit in one-third. Age at onset was 10 years (range 5 - 16 years). Absence seizures (in 33%) predated myoclonic jerks (in 97%) by 4 years, and generalized tonic-clonic seizures (in 79%) by 4.4 years. Myoclonic and GTC seizures occurred mainly on awakening. One-third had an essential type tremor. A combination of valproate and clonazepam was the most effective treatment. Relapse occurred in 9 of 11 patients after drug withrawal.

Clinical and EEG asymmetries were reported in 26 of 85 (31%) patients with JME seen at the Department of Neurology, Bowman Gray School of Medicine, Winston-Salem, NC. Fourteen (54%) were initially misdiagnosed as having partial seizures. (Lancman ME et al. Epilepsia 1994;35:302-306). -Editor. *Ped Neur Briefs* May 1994.

REFLEX MYOCLONIC EPILEPSY OF INFANCY

Six neurologically normal infants, aged 6-21 months, with attacks resembling benign myoclonic epilepsy of infancy but occurring as reflex responses to auditory and tactile stimuli are reported from Bambino Gesu Children's Hospital, Rome, Italy. An excessive startle response caused symmetric jumping of limbs, arms more than legs. Spontaneous attacks developed in 4, particularly in sleep. A family history of epilepsy or febrile convulsions was elicited in 5. Remissions occurred in 4-14 months, spontaneously or in response to valproate. EEGs showed short generalized spike- or polyspike-and-wave discharges. (Ricci S et al. Reflex myoclonic epilepsy in infancy: A new age-dependent idiopathic epileptic syndrome related to startle reaction. <u>Epilepsia</u> April 1995;36:342-348). (Reprints: Dr S Ricci, Section of Neurophysiology, Bambino Gesu Children's Hospital, IRCCS, Piazza S Onofrio 4, 00165 Rome, Italy).

COMMENT. In addition to the reflex nature of these attacks, the abnormal EEG appears to distinguish this syndrome from benign myoclonic epilepsy in infancy. Therapy with anticonvulsants seemed justified when attacks occurred spontaneously and frequently, from 5 to 20 times daily. -Editor. *Ped Neur Briefs* May 1995.

EPILEPSY WITH MYOCLONIC ABSENCES

Resistance to therapy and learning disabilities are stressed as frequent complications of the syndrome of "epilepsy with myoclonic absences" reported in 8 children , ages 6 to 16 years, seen at the University Hospital of Wales in a 10 year period. The mean age at onset was 4.9 years. Febrile seizures had occurred in siblings of 3 patients. Myoclonic absences were brief, and they could be precipitated by hyperventilation. Loss of awareness was associated with bilateral jerking of the head and upper limbs, and the EEG showed rhythmic 3 c/s spike-wave discharges. The majority had generalized tonic-clonic or astatic seizures and cerebellar ataxia in addition. All became learning disabled and 7 had behavioral problems, including restlessness and impulsiveness. Treatment with lamotrigine and valproate was partially effective. (Manonmani V, Wallace SJ. Epilepsy with myoclonic absences. <u>Arch Dis Child</u> April 1994;70:288-290). (Respond: Dr Wallace, Dept Paediatric Neurology, University Hospital of Wales, Heath Park, Cardiff CF4 4XW, Wales, UK).

COMMENT. The response to lamotrigine (LTG) reported by Wallace in this and a previous report is in contrast to the experience of Schlumberger E et al at the Hopital Saint Vincent de Paul, Paris, France. (<u>Epilepsia</u> March/April 1994;35:359-367). Of 9 patients with myoclonic absence epilepsy treated with LTG, none was seizure-free at 3 months, 4 improved and 5 were unchanged. Side effects included skin rash, especially when LTG was added to VPA therapy, ataxia, drowsiness, and vomiting. The differentiation of this syndrome from typical absence epilepsy is important because of the poor response to treatment and the unfavorable long term outcome. -Editor. *Ped Neur Briefs* June 1994.

GENETICS OF EARLY CHILDHOOD ABSENCE EPILEPSY

The clinical and EEG family data of 140 cases of early childhood epilepsy with absences selected from the epilepsy family archive are reported from the Neuropaediatric Department of the University of Kiel, Germany. Patients with absences manifesting between the 1st and 5th year of age were selected for study. Two groups were formed: 1) GTCS, those presenting with generalized tonic-clonic seizures (90 cases); and 2) non-GTCS, presenting with absences (50 cases). GTCS at onset were afebrile or febrile. In 43% of probands absence were combined with myoclonic and/or myoclonic astatic seizures. Parents and their sibs of group 1 had seizures twice as often as parents and sibs in group 2. The EEG of relatives showed elevated incidences of spike and wave and photosensitivity in both groups. However, in parents of the non-GTCS group, EEG abnormality was more frequent than in parents of the GTCS group. Mothers' EEG was the best predictor of seizure risk in probands' siblings. Early childhood epilepsy with absences overlaps with early onset GTCS and myoclonic astatic epilepsy on one hand and with childhood absence epilepsy on the other. This syndrome could not be regarded as a specific entity. The analysis supports the assumption of heterogeneity within early childhood absence epilepsy. (Doose H. Absence epilepsy of early chidhood - genetic aspects. <u>Eur J Pediatr</u> May 1994;153:372-377). (Respond: Dr H Doose, Norddeutsches Epilepsie-Zentrum, D-24223 Raisdorf, Germany).

COMMENT. Three type of absence epilepsy are distinguished by the International Classification: 1) childhood absence with absence as presenting symptom, 2) juvenile absence with or without GTCS, and 3) epilepsy with myoclonic absences. Absence epilepsy of early childhood has not been distinguished as a specific entity, although Doose has demonstrated some characteristics which might allow differentiation from childhood absence. These include: onset before 5 years of age with absences or GTCS, male preponderance, associated myoclonic and/or myoclonic astatic seizures, poor response to AEDs, and unfavorable psychologic and social development in children with GTCS. The clinical and family data reported here are considered to support genetic heterogeneity within the disorder. Both non-GTCS and GTCS forms of the syndrome appear to be part of the larger spectrum of idiopathic generalized epilepsies of childhood. -Editor. *Ped Neur Briefs* June 1994.

MECHANISMS OF ABSENCE SEIZURES

A unifying hypothesis for the pathogenesis of absence seizures, involving the thalamocortical circuitry, is proposed in a neurological progress report from the University of Southern California School of Medicine, Childrens Hospital Los Angeles. Abnormal oscillatory rhythms generated in the circuit involve g-aminobutyric acid (GABA)B-mediated inhibition alternating with glutamate-mediated excitation which triggers a low-threshold calcium current in neurons of the nucleus reticularis thalami. The process is modulated by pathways utilizing various neurotransmitters and projected onto the thalamus and cortex, generating bilaterally synchronous spike wave discharges and absence seizures. Ethosuximide and trimethadione block absence seizures by reducing the low-threshold calcium current via a direct action at the T-type calcium channel. Other anti-absence seizure medications have indirect effects on this calcium current within the thalamus. (Snead OC III. Basic mechanisms of generalized absence seizures. <u>Ann Neurol</u> Feb 1995;37:146-157). (Respond: Dr Snead, Box 82, 4650 Sunset boulevard, Los Angeles, CA 90027).

COMMENT. A knowledge of the mechanisms of absence seizures should facilitate the development of more specific antiepileptic medications and the avoidance of drugs (eg. phenytoin and carbamazepine) that exacerbate absence attacks. For an excellent review of mechanisms of antiepileptic drug action see Talwar D, 1990, and commentary, <u>Progress in Pediatric Neurology</u> I, 1991, pp94-5. -Editor. *Ped Neur Briefs* March 1995.

OUTCOME OF ABSENCE EPILEPSY

A meta-analysis of 2303 patients with a diagnosis of absence epilepsy (AE), derived from 26 publications on 23 study cohorts, was conducted at Leiden University Hospital, The Netherlands. Age at onset of AE, stated for 60%, was as follows: 73% before puberty, 18% between 12 and 17 years, and 8% in adulthood, not conforming to strict AE criteria. Despite application of the 1989 diagnostic classification criteria of the International League against Epilepsy, the outcome definitions differed substantially due to heterogeneity in inclusion criteria and length of follow-up. Remission rates varied from 0.21 to 0.89, the poorest outcomes occurring in patients who developed generalized tonic-clonic seizures (GTCS) and in studies with longer follow-up periods. In the 50 percent with AE and GTCS, the proportion seizure free at follow-up was only 0.35, whereas in the 50 percent with absence seizures alone, 0.78 were seizure free. The prognosis for AE suggested by this meta-analysis was worse than previously stated, and the results would not permit an early prediction of outcome in individual patients presenting with absence seizures. (Bouma PAD, Westendorp RGJ, van Dijk JG, Peters ACB, Brouwer OF. The outcome of absence epilepsy: a meta-analysis. <u>Neurology</u> Sept 1996;47:802-808). (Reprints: PAD Bouma MD, Department of Neurology, Leiden University Hospital, PO Box 9600, 2300 RC Leiden, The Netherlands).

COMMENT. The main purpose of this study was to determine if the outcome of absence epilepsy could be predicted with certainty at the time of diagnosis in the individual patient. The authors conclude that early prognostication is not feasible because of the extensive heterogeneity of calculated remission rates. Generally, the outcome should be more pessimistic than that currently accepted. If the AE is "pure" and uncomplicated by tonic clonic seizures (GTCS), the outcome may be good and remission rates favorable. In long-term follow-up, however, a 50% chance of developing GTCS is accompanied by a poorer outcome and lower remission rates.

In a previous study of childhood epilepsies which showed an overall remission rate of 0.71 after AED withdrawal, predictors of relapse were adolescent age at onset, symptomatic epilepsies, and an abnormal interictal EEG (Berg AT, Shinnar S. Relapse following discontinuation of antiepileptic drugs: a meta-analysis. <u>Neurology</u> 1994;44:601-608). An identical remission rate was reported by Camfield and colleagues in a study in which patients with absence and minor motor seizures were excluded and seizure type was not of predictive value.(see <u>Progress in Pediatric Neurology II</u>, PNB Publ, 1994, for further discussion of outcome studies in childhood epilepsies). Greater attention to EEG characteristics, especially form of spike-wave complexes and duration of paroxysms, at the time of diagnosis and later at AED withdrawal could be more revealing in future outcome studies.

Accidental injuries, especially bicycle accidents, pose a 27% risk during absence seizures in children, according to a study of 59 patients at the IWK-Grace Health Centre and Dalhousie University, Halifax, Nova Scotia (Wirrell EC, Camfield PR, Camfield CS, Dooley JM, Gordon KE. Accidental injury is a serious risk in children with typical absence epilepsy. <u>Arch Neurol</u> 1996;53:929-932). -Editor. *Ped Neur Briefs* Oct 1996.

PROPOFOL ANESTHESIA-INDUCED SEIZURES

A case of a healthy young man who developed seizures and generalized paroxysmal fast activity in the EEG following use of propofol for anesthesia in minor surgery is reported from the Department of Neurology, University of South Alabama, Mobile, AL. Myoclonic jerking and obtundation developed shortly after anesthesia and a generalized seizure associated with EEG paroxysmal fast activity and controlled with divalproex occurred the following day. (Nowack WJ, Jordan R. Propofol, seizures and generalized paroxysmal fast activity in the EEG. <u>Clin Electroencephalogr</u> July 1994;25:110-114). (Reprints: William J Nowack MD, Dept of Neurology, Univ of South Alabama, Mobile, AL 36617).

COMMENT. Propofol anesthesia has been associated with seizures, myoclonic jerking and opisthotonic posturing. Spikes, polyspikes and spike wave complexes in the EEG have also been reported. The fast activity in the EEG in the above case was considered to be epileptiform, resolving after short-term anticonvulsant therapy. -Editor. *Ped Neur Briefs* July 1994.

PROLONGED QT SYNDROME PRESENTING AS EPILEPSY

Two patients, ages 19 and 12 years, and a review of 8 previous cases of prolonged QT syndrome presenting as epilepsy are reported from the Department of Neurology and Hospital for Joint Diseases

Epilepsy Center, New York University, New York. The 19 year old woman presented with "blackout spells" at 13 years. Some were a transient light-headedness and weakness, while other attacks progressed to tonic-clonic seizures with loss of consciousness. CT, EEG, ECG, and Holter monitor were normal. Echocardiogram showed mitral valve prolapse. Carbamazepine was ineffective, and within 2 months she was found dead at home. Review of ECGs revealed a prolonged QT interval, previously unrecognized. The 12 year old boy was referred with intractable seizures since 4 years of age. He also had "panic attacks" with tachycardia, dyspnea, palm sweating, and limpness. Numerous AEDs were without benefit. EEG and ECG were normal. A Holter monitor revealed ventricular tachycardia and prolonged QT syndrome. Of a total of 10 patients, 5 had family histories consistent with congenital prolonged QT syndrome (ie. sudden death or deafness). The first convulsion occurred at an average age of 4 years. Time to diagnosis ranged from 1 to 28 years. Presyncope and "lifelessness" prior to seizures were common complaints. The beta blocker, propranolol, the mainstay of therapy, is successful in most patients. Some require a pacemaker or implantable cardiac defibrillator. (Pacia SV et al. The prolonged QT syndrome presenting as epilepsy: A report of two cases and literature review. <u>Neurology</u> Aug 1994;44:1408-1410). (Reprints: Dr Steven Pacia, Dept of Neurology, Hospital for Joint Diseases, 301 East 17th St, New York, NY 10003).

COMMENT. Diagnosis of this life-threatening condition may be difficult, but several factors should alert the neurologist to the cardiac origin of the seizures: 1) history of tachycardia, and presyncopal or lifeless feelings prior to onset of convulsive attacks; 2) normal neurologic exam and EEG: 3) family history of deafness, cardiac arrhythmia, or unexpected sudden death; and 4) lack of response to antiepileptic drugs. Familial, autosomal recessive or dominant, and acquired types of prolonged QT interval are recognized. The mortality may be as high as 70% if unrecognized and untreated. -Editor. *Ped Neur Briefs* Sept 1994.

VIDEO GAME-INDUCED SEIZURES

Fifteen patients, ages 9 to 15 years, who experienced epileptic seizures while playing video games are reported from St Thomas's Hospital, London, UK. An additional 20 patients in 12 reports in the literature are reviewed, and 3 further patients are described in an addendum. The majority had the first seizure as a result of the video game. Seizure patterns were generalized tonic clonic in two thirds; some had absence and 30% had juvenile myoclonic epilepsy. Photosensitivity occurred in 70%, while excitement, fatigue, sleep deprivation, and cognitive processing were important precipitants in others. Partial, mainly occipital, seizures occurred in 29%. Management was individualized, and AEDs were not always necessary. (Ferrie CD et al. Video game induced seizures. <u>J Neurol Neurosurg Psychiatry</u> Aug 1994;57:925-931). (Respond: Dr CD Ferrie, Dept Clinical Neurophysiology and Epilepsy, St Thomas's Hospital, London SE1 7EH, UK).

COMMENT. Video game seizures are reflex epilepsies, generalized or partial, and a feature of various idiopathic epileptic syndromes. Both photic and non-photic precipitants are involved. The avoidance of the precipitant may prevent the progression of minor absences, jerks, or visual phenomena to a generalized tonic clonic epilepsy.

See <u>Ped Neur Briefs</u> April 1994, p 28, for a previous report of 10 patients seen at the University of Washington, Seattle, and a review of 20 cases cited in the literature. The comment that video game related seizures are more common than previously recognized appears to be confirmed. -Editor. *Ped Neur Briefs* Sept 1994.

VISUALLY INDUCED SEIZURES

Photosensitivity and pattern sensitivity were evaluated in 67 reactive epileptic children, aged 4 - 19 years, at Universita "La Sapienza," Rome, Italy. Fifty-one percent showed sensitivity to both light and pattern, 33% showed photosensitivity, and 16% were pattern sensitive. Pattern sensitive patients without photosensitivity had a higher incidence of focal symptomatic epilepsies, neurologic abnormalities, and focal EEGs. The EEG in pattern sensitive children showed focal polyspikes, spikes, slow or sharp waves in occipital regions, whereas photosensitive patients had more frequent generalized polyspike-wave and spike-wave complexes in the EEG. (Brinciotti M et al. Pattern sensitivity and photosensitivity in epileptic children with visually induced seizures. <u>Epilepsia</u> July/August 1994;35:842-849). (Reprints: Dr M Brinciotti, Instituto di Neuropsichiatria Infantile, Universita "La Sapienza," Via dei Sabelli 108, 00185 Rome, Italy).

COMMENT. Patients with pattern sensitivity are at risk of focal, symptomatic seizures and neurologic abnormalities, whereas those with photosensitivity have generalized seizure patterns.

Video-game epilepsy. Kasteleijn-Nolst Trenite DGA, of the Instituut voor Epilepsiebestrijding, Heemstede, the Netherlands, comments on video-game epilepsy (<u>Lancet</u> Oct 22, 1994;344:1102-3). 50 cases have been published world wide. Mean age is 13 years, and 75% are male. One-third had a prior spontaneous or visually induced non-video-game seizure, and 50% showed epileptiform EEG discharges with photic stimulation. Only 5% of epileptic patients in general are sensitive to photic stimulation.

The video game is a specific provocative factor in predisposed "photosensitive" epileptic patients. These patients are also sensitive to television (40%), flickering sunlight (35%), disco lights (25%), and striped patterns such as venetian blinds and escalators (10%). In video game epilepsy, precipitating factors might include color, flashing lights or patterns, the cognitive content, and lack of sleep.

Studies in the Netherlands show that viewing a "flashing" program on a 50 Hz television in close proximity to the set is the most provocative stimulus. A video game is more provocative than a picture with less color and movement. Children should be kept at a distance of at least 2 m from a television screen. (see <u>Ped Neur Briefs</u> Sept 1994). -Editor. *Ped Neur Briefs* Nov 1994.

SELF-INDUCED PHOTOGENIC SEIZURES

The characteristics of photogenic self-induced seizures and their treatment by optical filters in a 2-year-old boy with severe myoclonic epilepsy in infancy are reported from the National Epilepsy Center, Shizuoka Higashi Hospital, Japan. Between 17 and 20 months of age the boy began to induce absences and/or myoclonic jerks by flickering hand movements (FHM) and forced eye closure (FEC). Continuous wearing of a filter decreased the average daily frequency of FHM and, after 10 days, FHM disappeared even without a filter. FHM could also be inhibited by a blank goggle frame, but this placebo effect gradually subsided, while the filter effects were maintained. Optical studies showed that a degree of absorption from 600-700 nm accounted for the filter effect. Blue-tinted contact lenses were tolerated better than goggles and could not be removed. Photosensitivity was gradually reduced and FHMs were not resumed after a period of 6 months, even after removal of the lenses. (Takahashi Y, Seino M et al. Self-induced photogenic seizures in a child with severe myoclonic epilepsy in infancy: Optical investigations and treatments. <u>Epilepsia</u> July 1995;36:728-732). (Reprints: Dr Y Takahashi, Department of Pediatrics, Gifu University School of Medicine, 40 Tsukasa, Gifu 500, Japan).

COMMENT. Tinted contact lenses were effective in reduction of photosensitivity in a 2-year-old child. The authors recommend continuous use of tinted contacts during daytime from morning to evening in young patients with photogenic seizures. -Editor. *Ped Neur Briefs* July 1995.

ELECTRONIC SCREENS AND FIRST SEIZURE

The incidence of a first seizure triggered by electronic screen games in subjects without a history of epilepsy was determined by reviewing reports from 118 EEG departments in Great Britain during two 3-month periods, and analysing the data at the National Society for Epilepsy, and Department of Clinical Neurophysiology and Institute of Neurology, National Hospital, London, UK. The EEG showed a photoparoxysmal response, or there was clinical evidence of photosensitivity, repeat seizures on further exposure to the games, and/or occipital spikes in the resting EEG. The age range of 103 patients was 7 to 19 years. Within this age group, the annual incidence of first seizures triggered by playing electronic screen games was estimated at 1.5/100,000. (Quirk JA, Fish DR et al. First seizure associated with playing electronic screen games: a community-based study in Great Britain. <u>Ann Neurol</u> June 1995;37:733-737). (Respond: Dr Fish, The National Society for Epilepsy, Chalfont St Peter, Gerrards Cross Bucks SL9 0RJ, UK).

COMMENT. TV-induced seizures are likely to be less common in America than in Great Britain because of differences in flicker rate patterns (60 Hz vs 50 Hz). Computers vary in flicker rate, and their tendency to induce seizures is independent of the main frequency. Sleep deprivation was a contributing factor in patients in this study. The length of play sessions was not a hazard. -Editor. *Ped Neur Briefs* July 1995.

READING EPILEPSY

The electroclinical manifestations and natural history of reading epilepsy (RE) in 20 patients diagnosed between 1949 and 1989 are reported from the Mayo Clinic, Rochester, Minnesota. Age at onset ranged from 10 to 46 years (median 17 years). Juvenile myoclonic epilepsy occurred in 4, and a positive family history for epilepsy in 4, with RE in 1. Seizures were myoclonic, involving orofacial and jaw muscles, and the upper limbs also in 5. Generalized tonic-clonic seizures occurred at least once in 16. The EEG showed generalized spike or spike-and wave discharges in 15 cases and left hemisphere discharges in 5. RE was persistent into late adult life but not progressive; it responded to valproic acid. Higher cognitive processes acting as trigger mechanisms other than reading included calculation in 6, speaking under stress in 5, writing in 2, and playing chess in 1. (Radhakrishnan K, Silbert PL, Klass DW. Reading epilepsy. An appraisal of 20 patients diagnosed at the Mayo Clinic, Rochester, Minnesota, between 1949 and 1989, and delineation of the epileptic syndrome. <u>Brain</u> Feb 1995;118:75-89). (Respond: Donald W Klass MD, Section of Electroencephalography, Mayo Clinic, 200 First Street SW, Rochester, MN 55905).

COMMENT. The authors dedicate their article to Dr Reginald G Bickford on his 81st birthday and we add our congratulations! Bickford (1954) and Bickford, Klass et al (1956) first described the syndrome of reading epilepsy and stressed the importance of precipitating factors in the mechanism of seizures and EEG epileptiform discharges in general.

Christie S (1988) found a combination of factors involved in the precipitation of reading epilepsy: saccadic eye movements, articulation, and difficulty of linguistic content. Bickford had alluded to the degree of difficulty of reading matter in his original article. (See <u>Progress in Pediatric Neurology</u> I, 1991, p45). -Editor. *Ped Neur Briefs* May 1995.

READING-INDUCED ABSENCE SEIZURES

A 12-year-old girl with a 2-year history of absence seizures induced by reading and diagnosed by video EEG is reported from The University of Texas Southwestern Medical Center, Dallas, and Riyadh Armed Forces Hospital, Saudi Arabia. The reading of complex material especially, either silently or aloud, produced staring episodes lasting several seconds and occasionally followed by headaches. Attacks were one to two a day at first and later increased to five to six daily.

Two siblings had a history of febrile seizures. Routine EEG, including hyperventilation and photic stimulation, was normal. Video-EEG showed no spontaneous seizures in a 6-hour baseline period, but hyperventilation induced generalized 3-Hz spike-and-wave discharges and a clinical absence seizure. Reading in Arabic from the Koran for 30 seconds induced an absence seizure lasting 30 seconds. The reading challenge repeated several times at 10-minute intervals induced absences within 30 seconds. Valproate therapy given for 2 years controlled seizures, and she has been seizure-free for 9 months since stopping treatment. The EEG is normal, both during prolonged reading and hyperventilation. (Singh B et al. Reading-induced absence seizures. Neurology August 1995;45:1623-1624). (Reprints: Dr Balbir Singh, Department of Pediatric Neurology, University of Texas Southwestern Medical Center, 5323 Harry Hines Blvd, Dallas, TX 75235).

COMMENT. The electroclinical manifestations and natural history of reading epilepsy in 20 patients was recently reported from the Mayo Clinic (see Ped Neur Briefs May 1995). Seizures were myoclonic, involving orofacial and jaw muscles, and generalized tonic-clonic seizures occurred in 16. The reading epilepsy persisted into late adult life. It resonded to valproic acid. The reading-induced absence seizures in the present report appear to be unique and previously unreported. The precipitating stimuli for reading epilepsy are reviewed in Progress in Pediatric Neurology I, PNB Publ, 1991, pp 45-46. -Editor. *Ped Neur Briefs* Sept 1995.

ADHD AND EPILEPSY

The safety of methylphenidate (MPH), 0.3 mg/kg, in 9 boys and 8 girls, ages 6 to 16 years, with ADHD and epilepsy, studied in Jerusalem, Israel, was reported at the Annual Meeting of the Child Neurology Society, Oct 2-8, 1994, in San Francisco, CA. Of 17 patients treated with MPH for 1-month, following a placebo period of 1-month, 15 children who were seizure-free had no recurrence of seizures, while 2 with 1 to 2 seizures weekly before MPH had a moderate exacerbation of epilepsy. The EEGs showed no "major" changes. AED levels (CBZ and VA) were therapeutic during placebo and MPH periods. ADHD symptoms were benefited by MPH in 12 patients. (Gross-Tsur V et al. Methylphenidate for children with epilepsy and attention deficit hyperactivity disorder. <u>Ann Neurol</u> Sept 1994;36:501 [abstr]).

COMMENT. The authors recommend caution in the use of methylphenidate in ADHD children with an active seizure disorder. The PDR states that: "In the presence of seizures, the drug (MPH) should be discontinued." Based on the present and previous reports there appears to be some justification for trials of MPH in selected patients with ADHD and epilepsy whose seizures are controlled with antiepileptic drugs. Pemoline (Cylert) is generally considered to have less tendency to lower seizure threshold than MPH.

EEG and ADHD. The indications for an electroencephalogram in ADHD patients considered for stimulant medications include the following: 1) a history of seizures; 2) the occurrence of "daydreaming' or other complaints suggestive of absence attacks; 3) family history of epilepsy; 4) abnormal neurologic signs. Methylphenidate treated ADHD patients showing epileptiform discharges in the EEG should receive concomitant AED therapy. Children with ADHD have a 7% incidence of epileptiform EEGs. (<u>Ped Neur Briefs</u> Oct 1989; <u>Progress in Pediatric Neurology I</u>, 1991, p 190). -Editor. *Ped Neur Briefs* Oct 1994.

EPILEPSY AND HYPERKINETIC BEHAVIOR

A 4-year-old boy with benign partial epilepsy and hyperkinetic behavior between seizures is reported from Sapporo Medical University, Japan. Hyperactivity was noted at age 3, and seizures began at 4 years 6 months. Attacks consisted of a terrified expression, crouching, and rubbing his forehead on the floor. They occurred in sleep and awake. An ictal EEG in sleep showed theta rhythm, predominant over the left hemisphere, followed by voltage depression, but no spike and wave complexes. Both seizures and hyperkinetic behavior responded to carbamazepine. The epilepsy was characterized as benign partial epilepsy with affective symptoms. (Wakai S et al. Benign partial epilepsy with affective symptoms: Hyperkinetic behavior during interictal periods. Epilepsia July/Aug 1994;35:810-812). (Reprints: Dr S Wakai, Dept Pediatrics, Sapporo Medical University, School of Medicine, South 1 West 16, Chuo-ku, Sapporo, 060, Japan).

COMMENT. Behavioral and emotional disorder as a form of epilepsy is a controversial topic, and the response to antiepileptic drugs in treatment is not proof of epilepsy. This patient tends to support the concept of a specific epileptic syndrome, BPEAS, but the EEG evidence could be more convincing.

A multicenter Japanese study provided evidence against the concept of a so-called "masked epilepsy" in some hyperkinetic children. A comparison of the emotional and behavioral problems of 53 children having epileptiform EEG discharges and those of children without this EEG abnormality showed no significant differences. The authors concluded that the emotional and behavioral problems were coincidental and not directly related to the epileptiform discharges. (Okubo Y et al. Epileptiform EEG discharges in healthy children: Prevalence, emotional and behavioral correlates, and genetic influences. Epilepsia July/Aug 1994;35:832-841). -Editor. *Ped Neur Briefs* Nov 1994.

PSYCHOSES AND EPILEPSY: PARADOXICAL NORMALIZATION

Five children aged 2.5 to 9 years who developed paradoxical, or forced normalization (acute psychiatric symptoms with abrupt cessation of seizures and normalized EEG) are reported from the Shaare Zedek Medical Center, Jerusalem. Three had Lennox-Gastaut syndrome, and 2 had simple motor and complex partial seizures. They had been treated with ACTH, valproic acid, carbamazepine, or vigabatrin. One patient at age 9 years was having multiple daily seizures despite phenobarbital, phenytoin, and carbamazepine. Within 7 days of initiating a second trial of ACTH gel (80 U/day) for Lennox-Gastaut syndrome, seizures ceased and EEG epileptic activity disappeared. Concomitantly, his behavior changed; he became disoriented, aggressive, hyperactive, dyspraxic, and dysphasic. ACTH was discontinued, he remained seizure-free, but his behavior necessitated psychiatric hospitalization. He gradually improved over 5 years, but as an adult he is retarded (IQ 55). He has no seizures, no antiepileptic therapy, and his EEG is normal. The behavioral manifestations in this patient were classified as organic mental syndrome; in the remaining patients they were a schizophrenia-like psychosis in 1, and autistic withdrawal in 3. (Amir N, Gross-Tsur V. Paradoxical normalization in childhood epilepsy. Epilepsia Sept/Oct 1994;35:1060-1064). (Reprints: Dr N Amir, Neuropediatric Unit, Shaare Zedek Medical Center, Jerusalem, Israel 91031).

COMMENT. Psychiatric complications have been reported in adolescents and adults with absence epilepsy. Paroxysmal normalization (PN) was triggered by ethosuximide and methsuximide. The authors found no previous case of PN reported in childhood epilepsy. In 2 of their patients with a typical history of PN, the discontinuance of treatments (ACTH and vigabatrin) resulted in seizure recurrence and a concomitant psychiatric remission. In patient 1, described above, withdrawal of ACTH caused neither seizure recurrence nor change in behavior. Usually, discontinuation of the offending antiepileptic drug is sufficient to reverse the psychiatric symptoms.

This syndrome was particularly common during trials of phenacemide (Phenurone) in the early 1950s, and some drugs appear to have a greater propensity than others to cause personality changes. ACTH is more likely to cause psychiatric side-effects in older children and adults than in infants and young children. As the authors suggest, the association between epilepsy and psychosis is age-dependent.

-Editor. *Ped Neur Briefs* Dec 1994.

PRENATAL EVENTS AND CNS MIGRATION DISORDERS

The role of pre-, peri-, and postnatal environmental factors and genetic predisposition in the genesis of neuronal migration disorders (NMD) in 40 patients with epilepsy was determined by standardized questionnaires at the Montreal Neurological Institute and Hospital, Canada. Potentially harmful prenatal events (maternal trauma, medications, roentgenograms, infections) were reported in pregnancy histories of 58% of patients with NMD compared to 15% of 40 epileptic controls without NMD. In contrast, peri- and postnatal factors were present in only 22% of NMD patients compared to 50% of controls. Genetic factors (family history of epilepsy, mental retardation, or CNS malformation) occurred in 13 and 20% of families, respectively. Stillbirths occurred in 3% of NMD sibling pregnancies, but none in controls. Prenatal environmental factors are important in the cause of NMD. (Palmini A, Andermann E, Andermann F. Prenatal events and genetic factors in epileptic patients and neuronal migration disorders. Epilepsia Sept/Oct 1994;35:965-973). (Reprints: Dr E Andermann, Montreal Neurological Institute, 3801 University St, Montreal, Quebec H3A 2B4, Canada).

COMMENT. Maternal physical trauma in the first trimester was the most significant factor associated with NMD. Genetic factors are important in lissencephaly.

Dr Harvey B Sarnat comments on advances in neuroblast migratory disorders in Progress in Pediatric Neurology II, PNB Publishers, 1994, pp279-280. Morphological and metabolic abnormalities of the ependyma, and congenital cytomegalovirus were documented as causes, as well as new experimental data on neuroblast migration mediated by radial glial cells. -Editor. *Ped Neur Briefs* Dec 1994.

CEREBRAL CORTICAL DYSGENESIS AND EPILEPSY IN ADULTS

The clinical, EEG and neuroimaging features in 100 adult patients with cerebral cortical dysgenesis (CD) were reviewed at the National Hospital for Neurology and Neurosurgery, St Mary's Hospital, London, and the National Society for Epilepsy, Chalfont St Peter, Gerrards Cross, UK. Patients had medically refractory epilepsy with onset at a median age of 10 years. Only 15% had a history of status epilepticus. Diagnosis was by neuroimaging in 70. EEGs were abnormal in 95%. Of 35 patients treated by surgery, 15 were completely seizure-free. Demonstration of subtle forms of CD by MRI lessen the incidence of cryptogenic epilepsy in adult patients. (Raymond AA et al. Abnormalities of gyration, heterotopias, tuberous sclerosis, focal cortical dysplasia, microdysgenesis, dysembryoplastic neuroepithelial tumour and dysgenesis of the archicortex in epilepsy. Clinical, EEG and neuroimaging features in 100 adult patients. <u>Brain</u> June 1995;118:629-660). (Respond: Dr DR Fish, Department of Clinical Neurophysiology, National Hospital for Neurology and Neurosurgery, Queen Square, London WC1N 3BG, UK).

COMMENT. The heterogeneity of abnormalities associated with CD in adults with epilepsy, as listed in the title of this article, was associated with varied clinical, EEG and MRI features. Compared to children with epilepsy and CD, these adult patients had a relatively low frequency of delayed milestones (12%), mental retardation (11%) and neurologic deficits (17%). -Editor. *Ped Neur Briefs* Aug 1995.

MENINGOMYELOCELE AND EPILEPSY

The prevalence of seizures and epilepsy and the occurrence of other brain malformations or structural abnormalities were examined in 81 children with meningomyelocele followed at the multidisciplinary Children's Clinics for Rehabilitative Services, University of Arizona Health Sciences Center, Tucson,

AZ. Seventeen (21%) had seizures during follow-up ranging from 1.3 to 16 years. Fourteen (17%) had epilepsy and 5 had seizures controlled by anticonvulsant drugs. CNS pathology in addition to the shunted hydrocephalus included encephalomalacia in 7, cerebral malformations in 2, and calcifications in 1. (Talwar D et al. Epilepsy in children with meningomyelocele. <u>Pediatr Neurol</u> July/August 1995;13:29-32). (Respond: Dr Talwar, Department of Pediatrics, University of Arizona Health Sciences Center, 1501 North Campbell Avenue, Tucson AZ 85724).

COMMENT. Although epilepsy in children with meningomyelocele occurs mainly in those with shunted hydrocephalus, structural cerebral abnormalities other than the shunt may be important causes. -Editor. *Ped Neur Briefs* Aug 1995.

EARLY SEIZURES AND HIPPOCAMPAL PATHOLOGY

The relation of childhood seizures to hippocampal neuron loss, mossy fiber synaptic reorganization, and eventual hippocampal sclerosis was investigated at the Brain Research Institute, University of California, Los Angeles, and the Cleveland Clinic Foundation, OH. Surgical epilepsy cases had generalized seizures and extra-hippocampal prenatal cortical dysplasia or postnatal ischemic and encephalitic lesions, or complex partial hippocampal epilepsy. Extra-hippocampal childhood seizures of prenatal or postnatal etiology were associated with moderate fascia dentata and minimal Ammon's horn neuron losses and signs of aberrant mossy fiber sprouting. Children with mesial temporal epilepsy showed patterns of neuron loss and mossy fiber sprouting, typical of adult form hippocampal sclerosis, whereas repeated extra-hippocampal generalized seizures were not associated with progressive hippocampal damage and sclerosis. (Mathern GW, Babb TL, Mischel PS et al. Childhood generalized and mesial temporal epilepsies demonstrate different amounts and patterns of hippocampal neuron loss and mossy fibre synaptic reorganization. <u>Brain</u> June 1996;119:965-987). (Respond: Gary W Mathern MD, Division of Neurosurgery, Reed Neurological Research Center, UCLA Medical Center, Los Angeles, CA 90095).

COMMENT. The authors conclude that childhood seizures can damage postnatal development of hippocampal granule cells, contributing to chronic hippocampal complex partial epilepsy. Generalized seizures are not a cause of hippocampal sclerosis. -Editor. *Ped Neur Briefs* Aug 1996.

EPISODIC HYPERSOMNOLENCE EPILEPSY

A 4 year old child who had complex partial seizures alternating with sleep that presented as episodic hypersomnolence is reported from the Mayo Clinic, Rochester, MN. The hypersomnolence lasting 24-72 hrs was preceded by irritability and hyperkinesia for 48-96 hrs. The intervals between episodes ranged from 10-60 days. The EEG showed left occipital spikes in sleep. Prolonged recording during hypersomnolence showed right temporal seizure discharges. Phenytoin controlled the episodic hypersomnolence, with no recurrence at 19 yr follow-up. Complex partial seizures followed by postictal somnolence occurred occasionally between 5 and 11 yrs of age. CT was normal. Behavioral problems required special education and methylphenidate. He graduated from high school and has a manual labor job. (Wszolek ZK, Groover RV, Klass DW. Seizures presenting as episodic hypersomnolence. <u>Epilepsia</u> Jan 1995;36:108-110). (Reprints: Dr DW Klass, Section of Electroencephalography, Mayo Clinic, 200 First St SW, Rochester, MN 55905).

COMMENT. The EEG recording showing right temporal seizure discharges during the period of hypersomnolence. and the excellent response to phenytoin suggest that the episodic sleep disorder may be regarded as a seizure phenomenon. Lennox WG refers to "sleeplike episodes" and somnambulism as forms of epilepsy, but does not describe a case similar to the above report. (<u>Epilepsy and Related Disorders</u>. Boston, Little, Brown, 1960).

A young man presented with episodes of unexplained hypersomnolence lasting 24-48 hrs in my own practice. An EEG between episodes showed occasional temporal sharp waves. CT and metabolic studies were normal. An EEG recording during an attack could not be obtained. A trial of phenytoin was successful in this case, and attacks recurred when treatment was discontinued. A seizure disorder was suspected but not proven.

Sleep disorders with central hypoventilation syndrome and seizures is reviewed in <u>Progress in Pediatric Neurology II</u>, Chicago, PNB Publ, 1994, pp 192-4. -Editor. *Ped Neur Briefs* Jan 1995.

MECHANISM OF OPSOCLONUS-MYOCLONUS SYNDROME

Cerebrospinal fluid measurements of the serotonin metabolite 5-hydroxyindoleacetic acid (5-HIAA) and the dopamine metabolite homovanillic acid (HVA) in samples from 27 children with opsoclonus-myoclonus syndrome and 47 controls are reported from the National Pediatric Myoclonus Center, Children's Research Institute, Washington, DC, and other centers. The mean age at onset was 1.5 years, and patients were symptomatic for 3 years before evaluation. Treatment with ACTH in 65% of patients had been discontinued for a mean of 27 months before collection of CSF. The etiology was paraneoplastic (46%) or infectious. EEGs were not epileptiform. Concentrations of 5-HIAA and HVA were 30-40% lower in patients compared to controls. Biochemical heterogeneity was evident since low CSF levels of 5-HIAA were not found in all patients with opsoclonus. Lowest values were present in younger patients < 4 years of age, when control values were at their highest, suggesting an impairment of ontogenesis of central serotonergic systems. (Pranzatelli MR et al. Cerebrospinal fluid 5-hydroxyindoleacetic acid and homovanillic acid in the pediatric opsoclonus-myoclonus syndrome. <u>Ann Neurol</u>

Feb 1995;37:189-197). (Respond: Dr Pranzatelli, National Pediatric Myoclonus Center, Children's Research Institute, 111 Michigan Avenue, NW, Washington, DC 20010).

COMMENT. Opsoclonus and myoclonus have been induced by various neurotransmitters and chemicals that alter serotonergic or noradrenergic mechanisms, eg. tricyclic antidepressants, and the chlorinated insecticides, chlordecone and DDT. Low CSF 5-HIAA levels have also been reported in patients with progressive myoclonus epilepsy of the Unverricht-Lundborg type, and other myoclonic disorders. -Editor. *Ped Neur Briefs* March 1995.

SUPPLEMENTARY SENSORIMOTOR SEIZURES

The diagnosis, clinical features, video EEG and MRI findings, medical and surgical treatment, pathology, and prognosis in eleven children and adolescents with supplementary sensorimotor area seizures (SSMA) are reported from the Departments of Neurology, Neurosurgery, and Radiology, Cleveland Clinic Foundation, Cleveland, Ohio. Mean age at onset was 5.8 years, and the diagnosis was made by vertex sharp waves on prolonged video EEG (3 to 7 days) at a mean age of 12 years. Neurologic exam was normal, except for 2 patients with a focal decrease in hand coordination, and routine EEGs were frequently normal. Seizures were usually bilateral and tonic, affecting proximal limb muscles, frequent, occurring daily, refractory to medication, without loss of cosciousness, and mainly during sleep. MRI revealed a low-grade tumor or focal cortical dysplasia in 5 patients. Six had cortical resection after confirmation of SSMA by subdural EEG, and 5 were benefited. (Bass N, Wyllie E et al. Supplementary sensorimotor area seizures in children and adolescents. J Pediatr April 1995;126:537-544). (Reprints: Elaine Wyllie MD, Head, Pediatric Epilepsy Program, Cleveland Clinic Foundation, Desk S51, 9500 Euclid Ave, Cleveland, OH 44195).

COMMENT. SSMA seizures differ from generalized

TC seizures in preservation of consciousness, and from perirolandic benign focal epilepsy of childhood in bilaterality and proximal gross flailing movements. Preserved consciousness and gross bilateral, proximal limb movements are the principal distinguishing features of SSMA. Brevity and nocturnal predominance are other characteristic features. Prolonged video EEG and MRI are important in diagnosis, and surgery should be considered in refractory patients. The neuropsychological and behavioral abnormalities often found in adolescents with frontal lobe seizures or damage (see <u>Progress in Pediatric Neurology</u> I, 1991, p71, and Vol II, 1994, p180-3) were not evident in these patients with lesions in the supplementary SM area.

Auras and sensory manifestations may be more difficult to elicit in children than in adults. Auras in 5 of the above patients included crawling, tingling or heavy sensations of the limbs and one complained of epigastric discomfort. Similar sensations were described in case reports of Penfield W, and Jasper H. <u>Epilepsy and the Functional Anatomy of the Human Brain.</u> Little, Brown, Boston, 1954, p398. -Editor. *Ped Neur Briefs* May 1995.

SUPPLEMENTARY SENSORIMOTOR SEIZURES

The electroclinical and neuroimaging features, and response to antiepileptic drugs in 12 children with seizures involving the supplementary sensory motor area (SSMA) are reported from the British Columbia's Children's Hospital, Vancouver, BC, Canada. SSMA seizures were characterized by bilateral tonic posturing of upper or lower extremities, preserved consciousness, and no postictal confusion. Sensory auras, speech arrest, and abnormal vocalization were frequent symptoms. Ictal EEGs showed abrupt generalized attenuation of background activity and diffuse beta activity, followed by theta or delta frontal activity or generalized rhythmic midline slowing. Interictal recordings were normal in 50%. Delayed cognitive development occurred in 3 patients. One patient had tuberous sclerosis and one had a hypothalamic hamartoma. Brain imaging was normal in the remaining 10 patients. Seizures were responsive to AEDs in 50% of cases. (Connolly MB et al. Seizures involving the supplementary sensorimotor area in children: A video-EEG analysis. <u>Epilepsia</u> October 1995;36:1025-1032). (Reprints: Dr K Farrell, Division of Neurology, Department of Pediatrics, University of British Columbia, British Columbia's Children's Hospital, 4480 Oak St, Vancouver, BC, Canada V6H 3V4).

COMMENT. Supplementary SM seizures in adults with surgical lesions are described by Penfield W and Jasper H in their classic "Epilepsy and the Functional Anatomy of the Human Brain," Boston, Little Brown, 1954. In one patient with a scar in the right posterior frontal region adjacent to the longitudinal sinus, attacks were ushered in by a sensation in the left foot. This was followed by turning of the head and eyes to the left, raising of the left hand and tonic posturing of both legs. Clonic movements followed. There was no loss of consciousness unless a generalized seizure occurred. Attacks in children are similar to those described in adults. Diagnosis is often difficult because of frequent normal interictal EEG and subtle ictal EEG abnormalities. Repeated video/EEG recordings may be required to establish a clear electroclinical pattern. -Editor. *Ped Neur Briefs* Oct 1995.

ACUTE LYMPHOBLASTIC LEUKEMIA AND SEIZURES

The incidence, timing, etiologies, and recurrence rate of seizures among 127 pediatric patients with acute lymphoblastic leukemia (ALL) were determined at the Schneider Children's Hospital, and the Long Island Jewish Medical Center, New York. Of 17 patients (13%) who developed one or more seizures, 16 had seizures during antileukemic treatment, almost always related to intrathecal methotrexate or subcutaneous L-asparaginase. The long-term recurrence risk of seizures was low, occurring only in 2 patients (12%) who had static encephalopathy and neurologic deficits.

Chronic antiepileptic drug therapy was restricted to patients with recurrent seizures and structural cerebral lesions. (Maytal J et al. Prognosis and treatment of seizures in children with acute lymphoblastic leukemia. <u>Epilepsia</u> August 1995;36:831-836). (Reprints: Dr J Maytal, Division of Pediatric Neurology, Schneider Children's Hospital, New Hyde Park, NY 11042).

COMMENT. Seizures occurring in children with ALL in this study were related to side-effects of chemotherapy. None had seizures secondary to CNS leukemic relapse. Phenytoin was the drug of choice for the control of the acute seizures because of its relative lack of behavioral and sedative adverse effects. Carbamazepine and valproate were avoided because of potential bone marrow suppression and the lack of intravenous preparations. -Editor. *Ped Neur Briefs Aug 1995.*

HEMIFACIAL SEIZURES AND CEREBELLAR GANGLIOGLIOMA

A female infant with cerebellar ganglioglioma who developed hemifacial seizures from the first day of life is reported from the Miami Children's Hospital, FL. When investigated at 6 months of age there were daily episodes of left hemifacial contraction, resistant to medication, head and eye deviation to the right, nystagmoid jerks to the right, autonomic dysfunction, while consciousness was retained. MRI at 2 months showed a mass in the left cerebellar hemisphere. The scalp EEG recordings were normal, while interictal and ictal intracranial EEGs revealed focal spikes, confirming seizures arising in the region of the left cerebellar mass. Partial resection of a ganglioglioma at 3 months was accompanied by remission of seizures. Six previous reports of infants with hemifacial spasms and cerebellar mass lesions are cited in the literature and reviewed, 3 having gangliogliomas. (Harvey AS, Jayakar P, Duchowny M, Resnick T, Renfroe JB et al. Hemifacial seizures and cerebellar ganglioglioma: an epilepsy syndrome of infancy with seizures of cerebellar origin. <u>Ann Neurol</u> July 1996;40:91-98). (Respond: Dr Jayakar, Neuroscience Center, Miami Children's Hospital, 3100 SW 62nd Ave, Miami, FL 33155).

COMMENT. The authors describe a syndrome of infantile focal facial seizures associated with cerebellar ganglioglioma. Seizures associated with cerebellar tumors in infants and children have been described previously. The term "ictus infratentorialis" was coined by Penfield and Jasper for attacks of opisthotonus, syncope, vertigo, and focal clonic movements occurring in patients with infratentorial tumors. In a study at the Mayo Clinic of 291 children with intracranial tumors, seizures occurred in 17% of the total group, in 25% of those with supratentorial and in 12% of infratentorial tumors. None had gangliogliomas. (Backus RE, Millichap JG. The seizure as a manifestation of intracranial tumor in childhood. <u>Pediatrics</u> June 1962;29:978-984). -Editor. *Ped Neur Briefs* Aug 1996.

PREVALENCE OF EPILEPSY IN 10-YEAR-OLDS

The prevalence of epilepsy and seizure types among 10-year-old children in metropolitan Atlanta were ascertained from EEG laboratories and other sources and reported from the Centers for Public Health Research, Battelle; Division of Birth Defects, Center for Disease Control and Prevention; and Children's Epilepsy Center, Scottish Rite Children's Medical Center, Atlanta, GA. For the 538 patients identified, the lifetime prevalence of childhood epilepsy was 6 per 1000 10-year-old children. Boys outnumbered girls, especially among black children. Partial and secondarily generalized seizures accounted for 58% and generalized seizures for 35%. Coexisting developmental disabilities affected 35%. Mental retardation occurred in 30% of whom two thirds were severely retarded, cerebral palsy in 18%, visual impairment in 5%, and hearing impairment in 2%. Forty percent had a first seizure before 2 years of age and 55% before 4 years. (Murphy CC et al. Prevalence of epilepsy and epileptic seizures in

10-year-old children: Results from the Metropolitan Atlanta developmental disabilities study. <u>Epilepsia</u> Aug/Sept 1995;36:866-872). (Reprints: Dr CC Murphy, Centers for Disease Control and Prevention, Division of Birth Defects and Developmental Disabilities, 4770 Buford Highway, Mailstop F-15, Atlanta, GA 30341).

COMMENT. A higher rate for epilepsy of 9.8 per 1000 children <15 years found by Hauser WA, (1994) in Rochester, MN was thought to reflect a more complete case ascertainment in a well-defined stable population. Children with milder forms of epilepsy and those no longer under medical care may have been missed in the Atlanta study. Prevalence rates for active epilepsy may be lower than rates for lifetime prevalence. -Editor. *Ped Neur Briefs* Sept 1995.

IDIOPATHIC GENERALIZED EPILEPSY SYNDROMES

The clinical features of 101 patients with idiopathic generalized epilepsy beginning in adolescence were studied by standardized interview at the Department of Neurology, Austin Hospital, and the Department of Medicine, The University of Melbourne, Australia. Nonconvulsive seizures (myoclonic or absence) occurred in 84 patients, of whom 75 also had generalized tonic clonic seizures (GTCS). GTCS occurred alone in 17 patients. A group with myoclonic but not absence seizures (21 patients) corresponded to the ILAE syndrome of juvenile myoclonic epilepsy. A group with absence but not myoclonic seizures (37) resembled juvenile absence epilepsy. A group of 26 patients shared the features of juvenile myoclonic and juvenile absence epilepsies. Epilepsy with GTCS on awakening was not a specific entity. Seven patients with only GTCS, occurring neither on awakening nor in the evening period of relaxation, were not included in the current ILAE syndrome classification. (Reutens DC, Berkovic SF. Idiopathic generalized epilepsy of adolescence: Are the syndromes clinically distinct? <u>Neurology</u> August 1995;45:1469-1476). (Reprints: Dr Samuel F Berkovic,

Department of Neurology, Austin Hospital, Heidelberg (Melbourne), Victoria 3084, Australia).

COMMENT. The authors conclude that some patients with idiopathic generalized epilepsy of adolescence are not included in the current ILAE syndromic classification and those that correspond to classified syndromes show overlap, suggesting genetic relationships. A substantial group of patients shared features of both juvenile myoclonic and juvenile absence epilepsies. -Editor. *Ped Neur Briefs* Sept 1995.

HEREDITARY ROLANDIC EPILEPSY AND SPEECH DYSPRAXIA

A syndrome of nocturnal oro-facio-brachial partial seizures, secondarily generalized partial seizures, centro-temporal epileptiform discharges, associated with oral and speech dyspraxia and cognitive impairment, is described in a family of 9 affected members in three generations reported from Austin Hospital, Heidelberg (Melbourne), the University of Melbourne, and the Royal Children's Hospital, Melbourne, Australia. All affected individuals had nocturnal rolandic seizures limited to midchildhood. Inheritance of epilepsy and speech dyspraxia was autosomal dominant, with 100% penetrance for speech dyspraxia. Clinical anticipation was noted across the three generations of affected individuals, with increasingly severe speech dyspraxia, epilepsy as well as cognitive impairment. The syndrome has features resembling benign rolandic epilepsy (BRE) and may help in identifying the gene for BRE which is unassociated with clinical anticipation. It differs from the syndromes of Landau-Kleffner and epilepsy with continuous spike and wave during slow-wave sleep. (Scheffer IE et al. Autosomal dominant rolandic epilepsy and speech dyspraxia: a new syndrome with anticipation. <u>Ann Neurol</u> October 1995;38:633-642).

(Respond: Dr Scheffer, Department of Neurology, Austin Hospital, Heidelberg (Melbourne), Victoria, Australia).

COMMENT. The authors suggest that this new syndrome, with its known genetic basis, may help to clarify the relationship between benign rolandic epilepsy, a benign syndrome, and Landau-Kleffner and CSWSS, more severe syndromes.

Symptoms and findings in the Landau-Kleffner (LKS) and continuous spike-and-wave during slow sleep (CSWSS) syndromes are compared in a report from the Department of Child Neurology, University of Helsinki, Children's Castle Hospital, Helsinki, Finland. (Granstrom M-L et al. <u>Epilepsia</u> 1995;36(suppl 4):123). Bilateral epileptiform activity was found in sleep EEGs in 5 of 6 LKS children and in all 11 children with CSWSS.

All LKS children had auditory agnosia and deterioration of expressive language, 4 had attention deficit disorders, and 2 became clumsy or ataxic. Six children with CSWSS had deterioration of expressive language, motor skills and general intelligence, and 4 had hyperkinesia and delayed development. Epileptic seizures occurred in all LKS and in 8 CSWSS children.

Mean age at diagnosis was 5 years for LKS and 6 and 1/2 years for CSWSS. MRI/CT was abnormal in 1 LKS and 5 CSWSS patients. LKS usually affects previously normal children whereas CSWSS occurs in children with pre- or perinatal pathology and previously abnormal development. An overnight EEG is recommended in children with developmental arrest, loss of speech, and/or major behavioral problems. Four additional abstracts of papers on Landau-Kleffner syndrome were included in the program at the Annual Meeting of the American Epilepsy Society, Baltimore, Dec 1-6, 1995. -Editor. *Ped Neur Briefs* Nov 1995.

SPECT AND EEG IN LANDAU-KLEFFNER SYNDROME

Five right-handed children with Landau-Kleffner syndrome (LKS) were studied with EEG and single-photon emission computed tomography (SPECT) before and after 6 months of corticosteroid therapy at the Universities of Estadual de Campinas and Sao Paulo,

Brasil. EEGs showed both focal and generalized spikes, and spike-wave bitemporal discharges. MRI was normal. Brain SPECT showed abnormal perfusion in the left temporal lobe. Steroids and AEDs had no significant beneficial effects on either aphasia or behavior. (Guerreiro MM et al. Brain single photon emission computed tomography imaging in Landau-Kleffner syndrome. <u>Epilepsia</u> Feb 1996;37:60-67). (Reprints: Dr MM Guerreiro, Rua Camargo Paes 637, 13073-350 Campinas, Sao Paulo, Brazil).

COMMENT. Landau-Kleffner syndrome is an acquired epileptic aphasia or verbal auditory agnosia affecting children between 2 and 5 years of age and characterized by profound language dysfunction, seizures, and/or a paroxysmal EEG abnormality, and associated with a generally poor prognosis. The EEG abnormality is frequently bilateral and localization of a focal temporal lesion is often difficult. Brain SPECT in the above study, and previously reported by Morrell et al, may show hypoperfusion of the left temporal cortex.

Subpial intracortical transection in LKS. Morrell and colleagues at Rush-Presbyterian-St Luke's Medical Center and Epilepsy Center, Chicago, describe a methohexital suppression test which permits epileptiform potentials to stand out in an otherwise flat EEG. Using this technique to define a unilateral origin for the bilateral epileptiform discharge, 14 children with LKS were treated surgically by subpial intracortical transection. Eleven (79%) are now speaking, and 7 of these no longer require speech therapy. This method of treatment in selected cases appears superior to corticosteroids which have at best a temporary beneficial effect. (Morrell F et al. Landau-Kleffner syndrome. Treatment with subpial intracortical transection. <u>Brain</u> 1995;118:1529-1546). -Editor. *Ped Neur Briefs* Feb 1996.

PAINFUL HAND SEIZURES

A 14-year-old boy with habitual painful seizures of the backs of both hands since age 4 is reported from the Department of Pediatric Neurology, Osaka Medical Center, Japan. He had three febrile convulsions from one to three years of age. Painful hand seizures occurred 5 - 15 times daily, lasting 15 - 60 seconds, and occasionally followed by loss of consciousness and postictal confusion but no secondarily generalized seizures. Seizures were resistant to conventional medications until 13 years of age, when they showed some response to polytherapy with carbamazepine, valproate, and clorazepate. Interictal EEG showed frequent spikes and spike-waves over the right frontopolar area with spread to the left frontal region. Ictal EEG showed right temporal 4-6Hz rhythmic activity after a pain sensation. CT and MRI were normal. SPECT showed right temporal hypoperfusion. These secondary sensory seizures were thought to originate from the S2A area. (Otani K et al. Bilateral painful epileptic seizures of the hands. <u>Dev Med Child Neurol</u> Oct 1995;37:933-936). (Respond: Dr K Otani, Department of Pediatric Neurology, Osaka Medical Center, 840 Murodo-cho, Izumi, Osaka 590-02, Japan).

COMMENT. The authors cite 4 reports including eight previous patients with secondary sensory seizures published in the last 40 years, the first involving 2 patients of Penfield and Jasper (1954). One study was entitled 'Sensory seizures mimicking a psychogenic seizure.' (Lessor RP et al. <u>Neurology</u> 1983;33:800). It is certainly conceivable that the diagnosis is sometimes overlooked and the symptoms misinterpreted as psychogenic. -Editor. *Ped Neur Briefs* Jan 1996.

NOCTURNAL FRONTAL LOBE EPILEPSY

The electroclinical pattern of 33 patients with familial, autosomal dominant, nocturnal frontal lobe epilepsy was studied, including video-polysomnographic monitoring in 12, at the University of Milano, School of Medicine, Italy. The syndrome is characterized by clusters of brief nocturnal motor seizures during sleep, beginning in childhood and persisting throughout adult life. The motor seizures during sleep varied from thrashing hyperkinetic activity to tonic extension with clonic movements. The most frequently repeated patterns included pelvic thrusting, facial grimacing and moaning, and dystonic posturing. Some had sudden elevation of the head and an expression of fear. Misdiagnoses included benign nocturnal parasomnias, including nightmares, night terrors, and somnambulism. Diurnal episodes in 58% included generalized shivering followed by loss of consciousness, and complaints of tingling and daytime sleepiness. Interictal and ictal EEGs showed nonspecific patterns (atypical K-complexes), or epileptiform abnormalities (in 58% of patients), consisting of bilateral or right frontal spikes, during stage 2 non-REM sleep. Normal EEGs were recorded during wakefulness. Both nocturnal and diurnal attacks were controlled by carbamazepine or clonazepam. (Oldani A, Zucconi M, Ferini-Strambi L, Bizzozero D, Smirne S. Autosomal dominant nocturnal frontal lobe epilepsy: electroclinical picture. Epilepsia October 1996;37:964-976). (Reprints: Dr A Oldani, Sleep Disorders Center, IRCCS H San Raffaele, via Prinetti 29, 20127 Milano, Italy).

COMMENT. Nocturnal frontal lobe epilepsy is often misdiagnosed as nightmares, night terrors, or somnambulism. Nocturnal paroxysmal dystonia is also considered in the differential diagnosis. EEGs are frequently nonspecific, and video-polysomnographic monitoring is often essential. If the diagnosis is suspected but unconfirmed by EEG, a trial of antiepileptic drugs may still be warranted. -Editor. *Ped Neur Briefs* Oct 1996.

RISK OF SEIZURE RECURRENCE AFTER FIRST SEIZURE

The long-term recurrence risk after a first unprovoked seizure was determined in a prospective study of 407 children, followed for a mean of 6.3 years, at the Montefiore Medical Center, Albert Einstein College of Medicine, Bronx, New York. Seizures recurred in 42%; the cumulative risk of seizure recurrence at 1, 2, 5, and 8 year follow-up was 29%, 37%, 42%, and 44%, respectively. One-half recurrences had occurred within 6 months, and almost 90% within 2 years. Risk factors for seizure recurrences included a remote symptomatic etiology, abnormal EEG, nocturnal seizures, prior febrile seizures, and Todd's paresis. Children with the most favorable prognosis (21% recurrence risk after 5 years) had a cryptogenic first seizure while awake and a normal EEG. (Shinnar S, Berg AT, Moshe SL et al. The risk of seizure recurrence after a first unprovoked afebrile seizure in childhood: an extended follow-up. <u>Pediatrics</u> Aug 1996;98:216-225). (Reprints: Shlomo Shinnar MD, Epilepsy Management Center, Montefiore Medical Center, 111 E 210th St, Bronx, NY 10467).

COMMENT. This study is important because of the large number of patients included and the long duration of follow-up. In addition to acquired symptomatic etiology and EEG dysrhythmia, factors frequently associated with an increased risk of seizure recurrence in other studies, sleep related seizures, prior febrile seizures, and Todd's paresis were demonstrated as risk factors. Cryptogenic seizures while awake and a normal EEG were predictive of a good prognosis and a low rate of recurrence.

In a further report, these authors correctly point out that the control of seizures by AEDs and a favorable long-term remission is only part of the goal of therapy. Heightened self-esteem, improved school achievement, and social acceptance by peers are other important considerations. Although the prognosis of epilepsy is determined largely by the underlying cause and associated neurologic abnormalities, the control of seizures by AEDs improves the quality of life and is justification for rational therapy. (Shinnar S, Berg AT. Does antiepileptic drug therapy prevent the development of "chronic" epilepsy? <u>Epilepsia</u> Aug 1996;37:701-708). -Editor. *Ped Neur Briefs* Oct 1996.

ETIOLOGY AND MORTALITY OF EPILEPSY

Standard mortality ratios (SMRs) of patients with newly diagnosed epilepsy were determined in a prospective national population-based study at the Epilepsy Research Group, National Hospital, London; Chalfont Centre for Epilepsy; and the Institute of Public Health, Cambridge, UK. Of 1091 patients attending one of 275 UK general practices from 1984-1987, 564 were classified as definite epilepsy, 228 as possible epilepsy, 220 as febrile seizures, and 79 as not epilepsy after 6 months follow-up. Over a median follow-up of 6.9 years, the SMR for patients with definite epilepsy was 3.0. It was highest during the first year after diagnosis (5.1), and declined to 2.5 at 3 years and 1.3 at 5 years. The SMR was highest in cases of remote symptomatic epilepsy (4.3), it was 2.9 with acute symptomatic epilepsy, 1.6 with idiopathic epilepsy, and 0 for febrile seizures. The commonest causes of death were pneumonia, cancer, and stroke. (Cockerell OC et al. Mortality from epilepsy: results from a prospective population-based study. <u>Lancet</u> Oct 1, 1994;344:918-921). (Respond: Dr OC Cockerell, Chalfont Centre for Epilepsy, Chalfont St Peter, Bucks SL9 0RJ, UK).

COMMENT. The high mortality in patients with epilepsy was due mainly to the underlying cause, although idiopathic epilepsy itself carries an increased risk. The death rate was highest in the first year after diagnosis, the result of associated diseases such as stroke and tumor, and then decreased progressively. Heart disease was not a factor. An increased incidence of suicide previously reported in patients with epilepsy was not confirmed in this study.

Heautoscopy, epilepsy, and suicide. A 21 year-old man with complex partial seizures who tried to commit suicide during the experience of heautoscopy is reported from the University Hospital, Zurich, Switzerland. As the classic *doppelganger* experience, heautoscopy, the reduplicative hallucination of one's own person, combines features of autoscopy (a mirror reflection of one's body) and an out of body experience (illusion of physical separation from one's own body). Seizures associated with heautoscopy usually originate in parietal or deep temporal foci. (Brugger P et al. J Neurol Neurosurg Psychiatry July 1994;57:838). -Editor. *Ped Neur Briefs* Nov 1994.

SUDDEN UNEXPLAINED DEATH AND EPILEPSY

The incidence of sudden unexplained death (SUD) among patients less than 50 years old with refractory epilepsy was determined at Boston University Medical Center, Lexington, MA, and Department of Epidemiology, Glaxo Wellcome, Research Triangle Park, NC. Subjects receiving two or more anticonvulsants concurrently were identified from the General Practice Research Database in the UK and their clinical records were reviewed. Of 4150 patients with refractory epilepsy, 612 (15%) were under 20 years of age. For all subjects, including both idiopathic and acquired epilepsies, the incidence rate of highly probable SUD was 1.5/1000 person-years; for highly probable and possible categories combined, the incidence rate was 2.2/1000 person-years. The respective rates for idiopathic and acquired epilepsy separately were 2.4 and 1.0/1000 person-years. Of a total of 15 subjects with SUD and epilepsy, 8 male and 7 female, 2 (13%) were younger than 20 years. (Derby LE, Tennis P, Jick H. Sudden unexplained death among subjects with refractory epilepsy. Epilepsia Oct 1996;37:931-935). (Reprints: Dr LE Derby, Boston Collaborative Drug Surveillance Program, 11 Muzzey Street, Lexington, MA 02173).

COMMENT. Idiopathic refractory epilepsy was associated with an estimated risk of sudden unexplained death of 2.4/1000 person-years, whereas the risk with acquired refractory epilepsy was 1.0/1000. A previous study has estimated a higher risk of SUD in patients with acquired epilepsy. The authors concede that relevant information on the cause of epilepsy may have been omitted in some records, leading to an overascertainment of idiopathic cases.

Male sex, the need for multiple AEDs, and use of psychotropic drugs were risk factors for SUD in a Canadian study which showed an overall rate of 1.35/1000 person-years. (see <u>Ped Neur Briefs</u> Jan 1995;9:1 for review and commentary). Cardiac causes for idiopathic seizures and a normal EEG, a possible explanation for some cases of SUD, especially in adolescent males, should always be considered when AEDs are ineffective. -Editor. *Ped Neur Briefs* Oct 1996.

SUDDEN UNEXPLAINED DEATH IN TREATED EPILEPSY

The overall incidence of sudden unexplained death in persons with epilepsy (SUDEP) was measured, and subgroups with a high risk of SUDEP were identified among a cohort of 6,044 persons aged 15-49 years listed in the Saskatchewan Health prescription drug file. The file contained all outpatient drug prescriptions since 1976. Anyone who had filled four or more prescriptions for antiepileptic drugs (AEDs) between 1976 and 1987 was included in the cohort analysed. Subjects with cancer or heart problems and those without epilepsy were excluded. For 153 of 163 deaths occurring in the final cohort of 3,688 subjects, copies of death certificates and autopsy reports of potential SUDEP cases were examined. There were 18 definite/probable SUDs and 21 possible SUDEPs, with an incidence of 0.54 to 1.35 SUDEP per 1,000 person-years. SUDEP incidence was highest in males with a history of treatment with three or more AEDs and four or more psychotropic drug prescriptions. A 1.7-fold increase in risk of SUDEP occurred for each increment in maximum number of AEDs. (Tennis P, Cole TB, Annegers JF, Leestma JE, McNutt M, Rajput A. Cohort study of incidence of sudden unexplained death in persons with seizure disorder treated with antiepileptic drugs in Saskatchewan, Canada. <u>Epilepsia</u> January 1995;36:29-36). (Reprints: Dr P Tennis, ESP Division, Burroughs Wellcome Co, 3030 Cornwallis Rd, Research Triangle Park, NC 27709).

COMMENT. Male sex, multiple AEDs, and use of

psychotropic drugs are risk factors for SUD in persons with epilepsy. Severity and persistence of seizures are major risk factors. Some patients with potential cardiac causes, which can be important in the adolescent age group, were excluded from this study. Among the causes of death listed on the death certificates, cardiac related episodes accounted for six (12%), drowning occurred in 5, and aspiration in 7. A careful cardiac evaluation is recommended in young males with seizures of undetermined origin and a normal EEG, especially when a response to antiepileptic drugs is lacking. -Editor. *Ped Neur Briefs* Jan 1995.

METABOLIC DISORDERS AND SEIZURES

GABA SYNTHESIS AND PYRIDOXINE SEIZURES

A reduction in pyridoxal-5-phosphate (PLP) dependent enzyme, glutamic acid decarboxylase (GAD),which synthesizes GABA, is reported in a 3 month-old infant with seizures responsive to pyridoxine treated at University of California, Davis. The infant had asynchronous jerking of arms and legs and lip smacking at birth which responded to phenobarbital and phenytoin. MRI showed enlarged ventricles, and the EEG demonstrated bitemporal and left frontal epileptiform activity. Seizures recurred at 7 weeks and were not responsive to phenobarbital and carbamazepine. When admitted at 3 months, 100 mg pyridoxine IV stopped a seizure within 5 minutes. Anticonvulsants were discontinued and electrographic and clinical seizure activity was controlled with oral pyridoxine 25 mg daily. PLP independent GAD activities measured in skin fibroblasts of the patient and 5 controls were similar, whereas the patient's PLP dependent GAD activity was reduced. (Gospe SM Jr, et al. Reduced GABA synthesis in pyridoxine-dependent seizures. <u>Lancet</u> May 7 1994;343:1133-34). (Respond: Dr Sidney M Gospe Jr, Division of Child Neurology, University of California, Davis Medical Center, 2315 Stockton Boulevard,

Sacramento, CA 95817, USA).

COMMENT. An alteration in the function of pyridoxal phosphate dependent, glutamic acid decarboxylase appears to be responsible for the autosomal recessive syndrome of pyridoxine dependent epilepsy. -Editor. *Ped Neur Briefs* June 1994.

GLUTAMATE IN PYRIDOXINE-DEPENDENT EPILEPSY

Cerebrospinal fluid levels of glutamate, g-aminobutyric acid, and pyridoxal-5-phosphate examined in a patient with pyridoxine dependency while on and off vitamin B6 treatment are reported from Universitat Munchen, and Universitats-Nervenklinik, Wurzburg, Germany. Seizures began at age 3 weeks. Despite phenobarbital, status epilepticus occurred at 3 months and was followed by infantile spasms and hypsarrhythmia. The addition of ACTH and vitamin B6 controlled the seizures and the EEG became normal. Seizures recurred on each of several occasions when vitamin B6 was withdrawn. CSF glutamate was elevated 200-fold, whereas GABA and PLP were normal. After vitamin B6 (5 mg/kg BW/day) was reintroduced, seizures stopped and the EEG was normal, but CSF glutamate was still elevated 10 fold. A dose of 10 mg/kg BW/day vitamin B6 lowered the CSF glutamate to normal levels and controlled seizures, without apparent side-effects. At age 45 months, development was normal; the head circumference having dropped from the 25th at birth to the 3rd percentile at 3 months was further reduced during ACTH treatment but rebounded and grew to a 50th percentile after vitamin B6.(Baumeister FAM, Egger J et al. Glutamate in pyridoxine-dependent epilepsy: Neurotoxic glutamate concentration in the cerebrospinal fluid and its normalization by pyridoxine. Pediatrics Sept 1994;94:318-321).

COMMENT. The authors emphasize that control of seizures alone may not suffice in treating pyridoxine dependency. In order to prevent mental retardation, it is important to adjust the dose of vitamin B6 to normalize CSF glutamate levels, but using the minimum effective dosage to avoid neuropathic side effects.

Glutamate is an excitatory neurotransmitter and neurotoxin, and elevated brain concentrations in infants with pyridoxine dependency may explain frequent occurrence of psychomotor retardation despite remission of seizures with vitamin B6. -Editor. *Ped Neur Briefs* Sept 1994.

ACUTE ISONIAZID NEUROTOXICITY

An increased incidence of acute isoniazid (INH) neurotoxicity correlating with a resurgence of tuberculosis (TB) in New York City is reported from the Children's Medical Center of Brooklyn and the Department of Emergency Medicine, State University of New York, Health Science Center at Brooklyn. Nine patients receiving INH prophylaxis for TB between 1991 and 1994 developed refractory seizures, metabolic acidosis, vomiting, and/or coma after accidental or suicidal ingestion of toxic doses of INH (14 - 99 mg/kg). Eight patients were adolescents and one was a 5-day-old infant. Symptoms began within 45 - 150 min (aver, 90 min). IV pyridoxine controlled seizures. (Shah BR et al. Acute isoniazid neurotoxicity in an urban hospital. Pediatrics May 1995;95:700-704). (Reprints: Binita R Shah MD, Box 49, Department of Pediatrics, Children's Medical Center of Brooklyn, State University of New York, Health Science Center at Brooklyn, 450 Clarkson Ave, Brooklyn, NY 11203).

COMMENT. In children receiving prophylactic treatment for tuberculosis who present with an acute onset of seizures refractory to anticonvulsants, isoniazid toxicity should be suspected and pyridoxine administered intravenously.

Pyridoxine reverses the depletion of GABA caused by INH and restores the balance of inhibitory and excitatory neurotransmitters in the brain. If the amount of INH ingested is known, the dose of pyridoxine is limited to a gram-for-gram replacement, and is given in 15 to 30 minutes. Multiple excessive doses of pyridoxine may result in sensory loss and should be avoided. INH inhibits phenytoin metabolism and may lead to phenytoin toxicity. Diazepam can be used to supplement the specific anticonvulsant effect of the pyridoxine in INH induced seizures that are severe or prolonged. -Editor. *Ped Neur Briefs* June 1995.

PYRIDOXINE-DEPENDENT SEIZURES AND MRI ABNORMALITY

An infant with pyridoxine-dependent seizures and MRI, PET, and EEG evidence of diffuse structural or functional brain disease is reported from the University of New Mexico Health Sciences Center, Albuquerque, NM, and the UCLA School of Medicine, Los Angeles, CA. Seizures began at 10 weeks, and status epilepticus occurred four times between 3 and 7 months of age. Trials of AEDs and ACTH were partially effective, but he became encephalopathic and hypotonic. EEG showed diffuse slowing with right posterior epileptiform discharges. A PET scan showed global cortical hypometabolism. Continued on phenobarbital monotherapy, he presented at 10 months with status and respiratory compromise. IV pyridoxine, 100 mg, controlled the seizure within 4 minutes, he was extubated after 1 day, and was maintained on 50 mg pyridoxine daily. Phenobarbital was tapered without relapse. He gradually recovered muscle tone, walked at 15 months, and was seizure-free at 20 months, but speech was delayed. MRI showed diffuse cortical atrophy, especially frontal. (Shih JJ, Kornblum H, Shewmon DA. Global brain dysfunction in an infant with pyridoxine dependency: evaluation with EEG, evoked potentials, MRI, and PET. <u>Neurology</u> Sept 1996;47:824-826). (Reprints: Dr JJ Shih, Neurology Department, University of New Mexico Health Sciences Center, 915 Camino de Salud, NE, Albuquerque, NM 87131).

COMMENT. Pyridoxine-dependent seizures may be complicated by structural and functional brain disease. These abnormalities demonstrated by MRI and PET may result from the metabolic dysfunction secondary to pyridoxine-dependency, but the effects of hypoxia with repeated episodes of status epilepticus and possibly the use of ACTH in treatment of the seizures could have contributed to the cerebral atrophy demonstrated by MRI. The remarkable clinical recovery of this patient, after the diagnosis was made and specific treatment initiated at 10 months, emphasizes the importance of a trial of pyridoxine for intractable epilepsy, even in older infants and children. -Editor. *Ped Neur Briefs* Oct 1996.

PYRIDOXINE-DEPENDENT SEIZURES AND INTELLIGENCE

Clinical manifestations, MRI abnormalities, learning disabilities, and effect of pyridoxine dose on intelligence quotients were studied in 6 definite and 3 possible cases of pyridoxine dependent seizures in children, ages 2.5 to 14 years, seen at Newcastle General Hospital, Newcastle upon Tyne, UK. Additional presenting features included jitteriness, encephalopathy, neonatal dystonia, hepatomegaly, and abdominal distension with bilious vomiting. Abnormal fetal movements, a hammering sensation, were noted in 4. Later complications included break-through seizures with fever, visual agnosia, squint, articulatory apraxia, motor delay and dyspraxia, macrocephaly, and hydrocephalus. MRI showed focal thinning of the posterior third of the corpus callosum, cerebellar hypoplasia, and mild cerebral atrophy. Psychometric tests revealed specific impairments of expressive language with relative preservation of receptive verbal comprehension. IQ scores were below average (Full scale 50 to 73), but showed improvements after pyridoxine dose increases, particularly in the performance subscale. EEG abnormalities disappeared following pyridoxine therapy. (Baxter P, Griffiths P, Kelly T, Gardner-Medwin D. Pyridoxine-dependent seizures: demographic, clinical, MRI and psychometric features, and effect of dose on intelligence quotient. <u>Dev Med Child Neurol</u> Nov 1996;38:998-1006). (Respond: Dr P Baxter, Department of Paediatrics, Northern General Hospital,

Herries Road, Sheffield S5 7AU, UK).

COMMENT. The diagnosis of pyridoxine-dependent seizures is based on clinical features and an absolute response to pyridoxine, recurrence after pyridoxine withdrawal, and immediate control after re-introduction. Language and cognitive disabilities may be partially reversible with optimal dosage. -Editor. *Ped Neur Briefs* Dec 1996.

FAT OVERLOAD FOCAL SEIZURES

Two 9-year-old patients receiving fat emulsion therapy (FET) who presented with focal seizures and other neurologic complications are reported from the Baylor College of Medicine, Neurology Service, Texas Children's Hospital, Houston, TX. FET (Intralipid) was administered during treatment of aplastic anemia by bone marrow transplantation in one and because of poor oral intake in another with cystic fibrosis. Focal seizures were associated with a hemiparesis, weakness, and altered mental status. CT of one child showed bilateral hypodensities, more prominent in one hemisphere. Both patients died of pneumonia. Autopsy findings included cerebral endothelial and intravascular lipid deposition, and multiple areas of necrosis and hemorrhage. (Schulz PE et al. Neurological complications from fat emulsion therapy. <u>Ann Neurol</u> May 1994;35:628-630). (Respond: Dr Schulz, Department of Neurology, NB-302, Baylor College of Medicine, One Baylor Plaza, Houston, TX 77030).

COMMENT. A rapid rise in triglyceride levels may have contributed to the lipid deposition in brain endothelium and onset of seizures. Early recognition of the fat overload syndrome may allow prompt withdrawal of fat emulsion therapy and reversal of neurologic symptoms. -Editor. *Ped Neur Briefs* June 1994.

HYPOCALCEMIC AND HYPOMAGNESEMIC SEIZURES

The clinical findings and neurologic outcome of 15 newborn infants with seizures due to hypocalcemia (HC) and hypomagnesemia (HM) admitted to St Louis Children's Hospital are reported from Washington University, St Louis. Patients with perinatal asphyxia, cerebral hemorrhage, or other cerebral lesion were excluded. Seven infants had associated congenital heart disease, 2 were premature and 2 had hypoparathyroidism. None had nutritional abnormalities. Five died and 2 had neurologic abnormalities at follow-up. Prognosis was related more to associated medical conditions than the seizures. (Lynch BJ, Rust RS. Natural history and outcome of neonatal hypocalcemic and hypomagnesemic seizures. <u>Pediatr Neurol</u> July 1994;11:23-27). (Respond: Dr Rust, Dept Neurology, University of Wisconsin-Madison Medical School, H6/571 Clinical Science Center, 600 Highland Ave, Madison, WI 53792).

COMMENT. The associated congenital heart disease in almost 50% of these patients is remarkable and indicates the need for careful monitoring of serum calcium and magnesium levels before and after open heart surgery. Although hypocalcemic seizures caused by high phosphate content of cow's milk-based infant formula is now a rare event, seizures related to low calcium and magnesium may be experienced in infants with parathyroid disorders, low birth weight, prematurity, fatty diarrhea, gastrointestinal disease, chronic nephropathy, and cardiac disease, in addition to infants with asphyxia, brain hemorrhage, and other cerebral lesions.

In four infants with hypocalcemia treated personally at the Mayo Clinic, a history of cerebral anoxia or intracranial hemorrhage was reported at birth, and in one infant, an intracranial tumor was diagnosed. Seizures did not respond to intravenous calcium gluconate and a *neurogenic* hypocalcemia was postulated. (Millichap JG. <u>Nutrition, Diet, and Child's</u>

<u>Behavior</u>. Springfield, CC Thomas, 1986). -Editor. *Ped Neur Briefs* Sept 1994.

STATUS EPILEPTICUS

PLEOCYTOSIS AFTER STATUS EPILEPTICUS

Cerebrospinal fluid (CSF) findings in 138 of 217 patients with status epilepticus (SE) seen by the Neurology Service in a 3-year period are reported from the Columbia-Prebyterian Medical Center, New York, NY. Pleocytosis, defined as a WBC count of 6×10^6/L or greater or one or more polymorphonuclear leukocytes, was found in 31 (22%) with SE. Those with generalized myoclonic SE and a history of acute CNS infection or trauma were most likely to have pleocytosis. Of 40 patients with epilepsy and no acute brain insult, 4 (10%) had abnormal CSF counts associated with a generalized SE. (Barry E, Hauser WA. Pleocytosis after status epilepticus. <u>Arch Neurol</u> Feb 1994;<u>51</u>:190-193). (Reprints: Dr Elizabeth Barry, Dept Neurology, University of Maryland Hospital, 22 S Greene St, Baltimore, MD 21201).

COMMENT. The authors caution that pleocytosis should not be attributed to SE unless all other causes have been ruled out. -Editor. *Ped Neur Briefs* March 1994.

INTERFERON-INDUCED STATUS EPILEPTICUS

Prolonged, refractory status epilepticus in a 22-month old girl treated with interferon for giant cell hepatitis is reported from the Depts of Neurology and Pediatrics, University of Texas Southwestern Medical School, Dallas, TX. CSF and MRI were normal. Complex partial seizures following recovery from status were associated with right hemisphere slowing and spikes on the EEG. Seizures were controlled with phenytoin and carbamazepine. Her hepatitis became stable, and anticonvulsants were discontinued when seizure free for > 1 year. (Miller VS et al. Interferon-associated refractory status epilepticus. <u>Pediatrics</u> March 1994;<u>93</u>:511-512).

COMMENT. Seizures and other neurologic adverse effects of interferon, including peripheral neuropathy, have been reported. Children receiving interferon should be monitored for possible EEG dysrhythmia and neurotoxicity. -Editor. *Ped Neur Briefs* March 1994.

EEG IN NONCONVULSIVE STATUS EPILEPTICUS

Ictal and interictal EEG findings and the diagnostic utility of iv diazepam in 78 patients with nonconvulsive status epilepticus (NCSE) are reported from the Department of Neurology, University of Virginia Health Sciences Center, Charlottesville, VA. Ictal discharges were generalized in 59 episodes (69%) of NCSE, diffuse with focal predominance in 15 (18%), and focal in 11 (13%). EEG characteristics were heterogeneous. Atypical spike and wave was the predominant pattern, and typical spike and wave of absence seizures was rare. Rhythmic delta with intermittent spikes was most prevalent in the group with diffuse and focal discharges. Response to iv diazepam, 1 or 2 mg every 30-60 sec, occurred at a dose < 8 mg. Focal NCSE was less likely to respond than generalized NCSE. Persistence of interictal focal discharges after diazepam may differentiate generalized from focal onset NCSE. (Granner MA, Lee SI. Nonconvulsive status epilepticus: EEG analysis in a large series. <u>Epilepsia</u> Jan/Feb 1994;<u>35</u>:42-47). (Reprints: Dr SI Lee, Department of Neurology, Box 394, University of Virginia, Health Sciences Center, Charlottesville, VA 22908).

COMMENT. NCSE is characterized by slowness in behavior and mentation, confusion, or stupor, lasting >1 hour and accompanied by EEG epileptiform, continuous activity, either generalized, focal, or focal with secondary generalization.

In a study of 253 adults with SE admitted to the

Medical College of Virginia, Richmond, VA, mortality rates of patients with prolonged (>60 min) compared to nonprolonged (30-59 min) status were significantly different (32% cf 2.7%). Duration of status was a strong prognostic factor, while the type of seizure was not a determinant of mortality. The mortality rate was 30% in 70 patients with partial SE, and 20% in 180 with generalized SE. Anoxia and increasing age were significantly correlated with higher mortality. (Towne AR et al. Determinants of mortality in status epilepticus. <u>Epilepsia</u> Jan/Feb 1994;<u>35</u>:27-34). -Editor. *Ped Neur Briefs* March 1994.

MANAGEMENT OF STATUS EPILEPTICUS

The care given to 8 children with epilepsy admitted with convulsive status epilepticus during 1990 is evaluated at the University Hospital of Wales, Cardiff. All had significant learning disabilities. In 17 admissions, eye-witness accounts of the seizure leading to admission were not recorded in 5, and were poorly described in 11. Of 9 convulsive episodes persisting on admission, 6 had been treated with rectal diazepam in the home. All children were on maintenance therapy for previously diagnosed epilepsy, but only one was recorded as compliant. AED dosage was adjusted after 8 of the episodes, less than half the total. Prevention of further episodes after discharge was not considered in 8 cases. The availability of rectal diazepam in the home was ignored for most admissions, and parents had not been instructed in its optimal usage. Average length of stay was 2 days. (Matthes JWA, Wallace SJ. Convulsive status epilepticus in children treated for epilepsy: an assessment of management. <u>Dev Med Child Neurol</u> 1995;37:226-231). (Respond: Dr SJ Wallace, Department of Child Health, University Hospital of Wales, Heath Park, Cardiff CF4 4XW, Wales, UK).

COMMENT. The importance of epilepsy prevention is stressed both in the US and UK current literature. The release of excitotoxic amino acids such as glutamate and aspartate from discharging neurons, with further cerebral damage as a consequence of uncontrolled seizures is cited as a reason for optimal control. Neurological, psychological and social dysfunction resulting from poorly controlled epilepsy are additional reasons for closer attention to the prevention of seizures and their consequencies. The failure of rectal diazepam administered in the home in 6 patients admitted in status epilepticus might be explained by the inadequate instruction or compliance of parents. -Editor. *Ped Neur Briefs* May 1995.

OUTCOME OF STATUS EPILEPTICUS

Treatment practice and outcome of generalized convulsive status epilepticus (GC-SE) in The Netherlands were studied at the Dr Hans Berger Clinic, Breda and University Hospital, Nijmegen, The Netherlands. SIG, a Dutch documentation center that collects nationwide hospital statistics, showed an average annual GC-SE frequency of 344 in patients aged >15 years, with an annual mortality of 24. Of 346 admissions collected at 12 hospitals and 2 epilepsy centers 236 (68%) had known previous epilepsy.

Analysis showed that factors important in outcome were the underlying cause, noncompliance with AED treatment, and systemic infection. Of 38 patients who died, 44% had received insufficient therapy. This percentage was higher (62%) in patients dying as a result of SE itself. Duration of SE >4 hours caused an increase in morbidity and mortality, especially in those where GC-SE itself was responsible rather than some underlying cause.

Outcome was related to the occurrence of medical complications: respiratory insufficiency and aspiration, cardiac arrhythmias, hypotension, renal and/or hepatic failure, and rhabdomyolysis were associated with a poor prognosis. Inadequate management led to several complications and a worse outcome. (Scholtes FB, Renier WO, Meinardi H. Generalized convulsive status epilepticus: causes, therapy, and outcome in 346 patients. <u>Epilepsia</u> 1995;35:1104-1112). (Reprints: Dr FB Scholtes, Dr Hans Berger

Clinic, PO Box 90108, 4800 RA Breda, The Netherlands).

COMMENT. A poor outcome of convulsive status epilepticus is determined particularly by the underlying cause but also by a duration of SE greater than 4 hours, by the occurrence of one or more medical complications, and by inadequate anticonvulsant therapy. Therapies most frequently employed in the management of convulsive status epilepticus in The Netherlands were clonazepam, diazepam, and phenytoin.

Status Epilepticus and Seizure Recurrence. Shinnar S, Berg AT, and Moshe SL, at the Albert Einstein College of Medicine, Bronx, NY, report a study of the effect of status epilepticus on the long-term outcome of a cohort of 342 children and adolescents prospectively followed for a mean of 72 months from the time of their first idiopathic unprovoked seizure (Dev Med Child Neurol March 1995 (suppl 72);37:116 [abstact]). Status epilepticus was the first seizure in 38 (11%). At follow-up, 127 (37%) had experienced a seizure recurrence, including 42% of those who presented with status and 37% of those who had a briefer first seizure. The occurrence of status epilepticus did not appear to have an adverse effect on outcome in the children in this study. -Editor. *Ped Neur Briefs* May 1995.

LORAZEPAM V DIAZEPAM IN STATUS EPILEPTICUS

A prospective, open, odd and even dates trial of lorazepam compared to diazepam for the treatment of acute convulsions and status epilepticus in 102 children is reported from the Royal Liverpool Children's NHS Trust, UK. Lorazepam (0.05 - 0.1 mg/kg) and diazepam (0.3 - 0.4 mg/kg) controlled convulsions within 20 to 60 seconds in 76% and 51% of patients, respectively, after a single dose administered IV over 15 to 30 seconds. Multiple doses as well as additional AEDs were required in 17 patients who received an initial injection of diazepam compared to only 1 who received lorazepam. Respiratory depression occurred in 7 diazepam treated patients and necessitated admission to intensive care. No patient receiving lorazepam required intensive care. Rectal administration, when venous injection was not possible, was 100% effective with a single dose of lorazepam in 6 patients treated, whereas 13 of 19 patients receiving diazepam rectally required multiple doses, 12 required additional AEDs, 1 had respiratory depression, 2 were admitted to intensive care, and 7 relapsed with recurrence of seizures within 24 hours. (Appleton R et al. Lorazepam versus diazepam in the acute treatment of epileptic seizures and status epilepticus. <u>Dev Med Child Neurol</u> 1995;37:682-688). (Respond: Dr Richard Appleton, Royal Liverpool Children's NHS Trust, Alder Hey, Eaton Road, Liverpool L12 2AP, UK).

COMMENT. Lorazepam appears to be safe, at least as effective as diazepam in the initial control of acute convulsions, including status epilepticus, and more effective in sustaining seizure control. Rectal lorazepam was useful in infants when intravenous injection was impractical. Lorazepam has a longer half life than diazepam, and its duration of action is more prolonged, accounting for the more sustained control. (See <u>Progress in Pediatric Neurology I</u>, 1991, PNB Publishers, pp124-5). -Editor. *Ped Neur Briefs* Dec 1995.

EEG STUDIES

EEG MATURATIONAL CHANGES IN PARTIAL EPILEPSIES

Changes and migration of EEG foci with age in 208 patients with childhood partial epilepsy followed for more than 3 years are reported from the Department of Pediatrics, Toyama Medical and Pharmaceutical University, Toyama City, Japan. Frontal and central foci were frequent before school age and after adolescence. Temporal foci peaked around adolescence, and occipital foci between 3 to 7 years.

Parietal foci were rare at all ages. Migration of EEG foci in 39% of patients was frequent at early school age (anterior to posterior) and preadolescence (posterior to anterior). The migration of EEG foci was not accompanied by changes in seizure patterns or frequency. (Konishi T, Naganuma Y, Hongou K et al. Changes in EEG foci with age in childhood partial epilepsies. <u>Clin Electroencephalogr</u> July 1994;25:104-109). (Reprints: Tohru Konishi MD, Dept of Pediatrics, Faculty of Medicine, Toyama Medical and Pharmaceutical University, 2630 Sugitani, Toyama City 930-01, Japan).

COMMENT. Migration of EEG foci in this study occurred with symptomatic partial epilepsies as well as idiopathic seizures. This phenomenon is not necessarily indicative of a benign epilepsy but reflects maturational changes in the brain, similar to those that characterize the changing patterns of seizures and EEG with infantile spasms and other epileptic syndromes. The authors suggest that this migration is an epiphenomenon on the scalp EEG since changes in clinical seizures were not observed. -Editor. *Ped Neur Briefs* July 1994.

EEG DISCONTINUITY AND NEONATAL ACIDOSIS

The effect of acidosis on cerebral function was evaluated by computerized online EEG monitoring in 14 ventilated preterm infants less than 32 weeks' gestation at the Department of Paediatrics and Neonatal Medicine, Royal Postgraduate Medical School, Hammersmith Hospital, London, UK. All episodes of acidosis were associated with periods of EEG discontinuity (attenuated activity between bursts of EEG activity). In more than half a pH <7.20 was recorded, but EEG changes were noted even with acidosis levels of pH 7.20-7.25. In 21 of 32 episodes, EEG activity returned to pre-acidosis levels after therapy for acidosis. Duration of EEG discontinuity was related to severity of acidosis. Recovery of EEG was quickest for pure-respiratory acidoses that required only simple ventilatory adjustments. (Murdoch Eaton

DG, Dubowitz V et al. Reversible changes in cerebral activity associated with acidosis in preterm neonates. <u>Acta Paediatr</u> May 1994;83:486-92). (Respond: Dr D Murdoch Eaton, Academic Unit of Paediatrics, D Floor, Clarendon Wing, The General Infirmary at Leeds, Belmont Grove, Leeds LS2 9NS, UK).

COMMENT. Increases in the amount of discontinuity in the EEG of infants may reflect disturbances in neonatal cerebral function caused by acidosis, hypoxia, or low cerebral blood flow. These changes are reversible in contrast to EEG suppression associated with hemorrhage that is persistent. EEG discontinuity may be used as a sign of acute neonatal cerebral dysfunction requiring immediate therapeutic intervention. This apears to be the first report of EEG changes in the neonate associated with acidosis. -Editor. *Ped Neur Briefs* July 1994.

EEG BACKGROUND ACTIVITY AND ANTICONVULSANT DRUGS

The effects of antiepileptic drugs (AED) on EEG background activity in 37 newly treated children with epilepsy were examined at the Departments of Pediatrics, Faculty of Medicine, Toyama Medical and Pharmaceutical University, Toyama City, Japan. Compared to 46 age-matched healthy controls, the EEGs in children with epilepsy, before AED therapy, showed significant slowing. Both idiopathic and symptomatic epilepsies were associated with EEG slowing. Following 3 to 6 months of AED therapy, the EEG slowing was increased in 23 taking carbamazepine for partial seizures and reduced in the 14 treated with valproic acid for generalized seizures. Despite continuous treatment with carbamazepine, after 1 year the background activity had slowly increased in frequency with age. (Konishi T et al. Effects of antiepileptic drugs on EEG background activity in children with epilepsy: initial phase of therapy. <u>Clin Electroencephalogr</u> April 1995;26:113-119). (Reprints: Tohru Konishi MD, Department of Pediatrics, Faculty of Medicine, Toyama Medical and

Pharmaceutical University, 2630 Sugitani, Toyama City, 930-01 Japan).

COMMENT. EEG background activity in children with epilepsy may be slowed because of underlying central nervous system dysfunction related to the epilepsy itself as well as the result of treatment with certain anticonvulsant drugs. Patients with partial epilepsy may be more sensitive to slowing than those with generalized seizures, but drugs such as carbamazepine may exacerbate the tendency to EEG slowing while valproic acid decreases delta activity and is associated with increased EEG frequencies. -Editor. *Ped Neur Briefs* May 1995.

DIAGNOSIS AND TREATMENT

PREVENTION OF EPILEPSY AND COMPLICATIONS

Prevention of epilepsy and its consequencies is discussed in a special article from the Department of Neurology, School of Medicine, University of Virginia, Charlottesville. Prevention should apply at various levels: 1. *epileptogenesis* may be prevented by a) avoidance of premature birth, in utero infection, and anoxia; b) prevention of febrile convulsions and their complications; c) avoidance of head trauma by wearing helmets when bicycling and banning of boxing as high school sport; 2. *ictogenesis*, individual epileptic seizures, may be prevented by identifying and controlling precipitating or provocative factors such as drugs and alcohol, sleep deprivation, AED withdrawal or poor compliance, and photic stimulation; 3) *neurologic consequencies* can be prevented by early and optimal treatment of seizures and avoidance of status epilepticus; 4) *psychosocial consequencies* could be lessened by public education, removal of stigmata, and improvement in the quality of life; and 5) *treatment consequencies* involving anticonvulsant side-effects, teratogenicity, and cognitive and other deficits resulting from overzealous surgical resections. (Dreifuss FE. Prevention as it pertains to epilepsy. <u>Arch Neurol</u> April 1995;52:363-366). (Reprints: Dr Dreifuss, Department of Neurology, School of Medicine, University of Virginia, Charlottesville, VA 22908).

COMMENT. Prevention in the management of epilepsy has been sadly neglected, and Dr Dreifuss in his synopsis draws attention to many adverse factors and aspects of etiology and treatment that could be avoided or corrected when addressed appropriately. Additional problems, especially important to the adolescent and young adult, include the permission to drive an automobile and the risk of accidents. Young drivers account for one half those with seizures at the wheel, and a complex partial seizure, usually without aura, is the most common pattern associated with accidents. Those with auras are significantly less likely to lead to accidents. Males, 19 to 30 years, in higher socioeconomic classes, form the majority continuing to drive without adequate seizure control. The monitoring of young male drivers with complex partial seizures should be close and frequent, including serum drug levels to check compliance and adequate AED dosage. (<u>Ped Neur Briefs</u> Oct 1987; see <u>Progress in Pediatric Neurology I,</u> 1991, p129-131).

The stress and anxieties associated with the first year away at college are additional reasons for relapse and recurrence of seizures in the young adult. Seizures may be prevented by counselling and by modification of medications to cover this period. -Editor. *Ped Neur Briefs* May 1995.

TREATMENT DURATION FOR ABSENCE EPILEPSY

The effects of 6 months of treatment followed by a 5- to 6-week withdrawal period of ethosuximide (ESM) in 3 children, ages 5, 10, and 10 years, with new onset absence epilepsy are reported from the Departments of Neurology, State University of New York at Stony Brook, and the Division of Child Neurology, Schneider

Children's Hospital and Albert Einstein College of Medicine, New York. The patients had responded promptly to ESM at levels of 75-90 mcg/ml, and their 24-hour ambulatory EEGs were normal. After this early withdrawal of ESM, 2 patients remained seizure-free and their 24-hour ambulatory EEG was burst free, and one was seizure-free but showed 3/sec spike-wave bursts in the EEG. Optimizing medication until both clinical and electrographic seizure activity are continuously suppressed, as determined by 24-hour ambulatory EEG, allows early withdrawal of treatment without increased risk of relapse. (Amit R, Vitale S, Maytal J. How long to treat childhood onset absence epilepsy. <u>Clin Elecroencephalogr</u> July 1995;26:163-165). (Reprints: Rami Amit MD, Neurology, HSC 12-020, SUNY at Stony Brook, Stony Brook, NY 11794).

COMMENT. In this study, ethosuximide was chosen as the drug of first choice in the treatment of childhood onset absence epilepsy. In my experience, while ethosuximide and valproate are equally effective in controlling clinical absence attacks, valproate appears, in uncontrolled studies, to be superior in the suppression of electrographic 3/sec spike-wave discharges. A comparative trial of these drugs using 24-hour ambulatory EEG monitoring would be of interest. The authors found that a burst-free routine EEG will not guarantee a complete remission of electrographic seizure activity, and a clean 24-hour ambulatory EEG is essential before attempting this recommended early drug withdrawal.

A 2 year seizure free interval is the generally recommended time before antiepileptic drug withdrawal. (Shinnar S, Zacharowicz L, Moshe SL. Initiation and cessation of antiepileptic drug therapy in children and adolescents. <u>Acta Neuropediatr</u> 1995;1(3):153-166). -Editor. *Ped Neur Briefs* July 1995.

PRETREATMENT SEIZURE FREQUENCY, CONTROL AND REMISSION

The effect of the number of seizures before

antiepileptic drug (AED) treatment on the ease of seizure control and remission was studied in a population-based regional cohort of 479 children with epilepsy at the IWK Children's Hospital, Halifax, Nova Scotia, Canada. Only 55 of 99 patients (56%) with more than 10 pretreatment seizures were seizure free for a sufficient time to attempt discontinuation of medicine, compared with 276 of 380 patients (73%) with 10 or fewer seizures. When patients discontinued AED treatment, 232 of 331 patients overall (70%) remained seizure free. For each pretreatment seizure number greater than one, the number of patients successfully discontinuing medication was the same. Of those treated after a single seizure, 57% were seizure free after AED discontinuation, compared to 72% with more than one pretreatment seizure. Patients with more than 10 pretreatment seizures were more likely to have complex partial seizures (59%) than those with 10 or fewer seizures (16%). (Camfield C, Camfield P et al. Does the number of seizures before treatment influence ease of control or remission of childhood epilepsy? Not if the number is 10 or less. <u>Neurology</u> January 1996;46:41-44). (Reprints: Drs Camfield, IWK Children's Hospital, Box 3070, Halifax, Nova Scotia, B3J 3G9, Canada).

COMMENT. These findings tend to disprove the theory that seizures beget seizures, at least in children permitted to have 10 or fewer seizures before treatment with AEDs is begun. The ease of seizure control and frequency of remission are unaltered if medication is delayed for up to 9 recurrences. Children excluded from this study were those with myoclonus, absence, akinetic, and infantile myoclonic seizures, which are too numerous to count. The introduction of antiepileptic treatment after a first or second seizure in children with generalized tonic-clonic or partial seizures requires further evaluation. Each patient must be considered as an individual, and these findings should be weighed in conjunction with past practices when considering advisability of antiepileptic treatment. Some previous studies have found that risk factors for seizure relapse after withdrawal of antiepileptic treatment have included delay in initiation of therapy. See <u>Progress in Pediatric Neurology I</u>, PNB Publishers, 1991, pp100-104. -Editor. *Ped Neur Briefs* Feb 1996.

EARLY TREATMENT OF SEIZURE PREVENTS RECURRENCE

The rate of occurrence of a second seizure after a single unprovoked generalized tonic-clonic seizure was compared in 45 patients who received immediate anticonvulsant therapy and 42 untreated patients followed for 36 months at the Edith Wolfson Medical Center, Holon, and the Sackler Faculty of Medicine, Tel Aviv, Israel. A second epileptic attack occurred in 29 (71%) of the untreated group and in 10 (22%) of the treated group. The risk rates for relapse in untreated patients were 0.33, 0.62, and 0.77 and, in the treated group, 0.1, 0.2, and 0.4, after 12, 24, and 36 months, respectively. Treated men were less susceptible to recurrence than treated women. EEG abnormalities were observed in 20% of both treated and untreated patients, and rate of seizure recurrence was not correlated with EEG epileptiform activity. Treatment consisted of carbamazepine (10 mg/kg/day) in 36 (80%) patients; it had to be changed to valproic acid (600-1200 mg/d) in 9 (20%). (Gilad R, Lampl Y, Gabbay U, Eshel Y, Sarova-Pinhas I. Early treatment of a single generalized tonic-clonic seizure to prevent recurrence. <u>Arch Neurol</u> November 1996;53:1149-1152). (Reprints: Ronit Gilad MD, Department of Neurology, the Edith Wolfson Medical Center, Holon 58100, Israel).

COMMENT. The age range of these patients was 18 to 50, mean 30 years. Studies in children and adolescents might show different results. The benefits of immediate anticonvulsant treatment in these adults is apparent, but the decision to begin treatment after a single seizure must be made on an individual basis, having regard to drug toxicity on the one hand and the adverse consequences of a seizure recurrence on the other. Risk factors for recurrence of seizures, with and without therapy, require further study in children and adult populations. Previous studies have shown seizure recurrence rates varying from 33 to 80%. -Editor. *Ped Neur Briefs* Nov 1996.

PREDICTORS OF INTRACTABLE EPILEPSY

Risk factors for intractable epilepsy at the time of initial diagnosis were determined in a case-control study at Yale University, New Haven, CT. Children with an average of one seizure or more per month over a 2-year period and refractory to at least 3 different AEDs were compared to controls who had been seizure-free for >2 years and had never had intractable epilepsy. Independent predictors of intractability were infantile spasms, early age of onset, remote symptomatic epilepsy, and status epilepticus. (Berg AT et al. Predictors of intractable epilepsy in childhood: a case-control study. Epilepsia 1996;37:24-30). (Reprints: Dr AT Berg, School of Allied Health Professions, Program in Community Health, DeKalb, IL 60115).

COMMENT. Age at onset was the predominant predictor of seizure intractability in this study, even after controlling for infantile spasms as a cause. Prognosis was progressively better with increasing age at onset during childhood and adolescence. For reports of neuropathology associated with intractable epilepsy, see Progress in Pediatric Neurology I, 1991, pp 131-138; and II, 1994, pp 129-141. -Editor. *Ped Neur Briefs* March 1996.

LOCALIZING VALUE OF CLINICAL SEIZURE PATTERNS

The value of ictal clinical manifestations in differentiating frontal and temporal lobe partial epilepsies was determined in a prospective study of 252 patients selected according to imaging, EEG, and focal clinical patterns from records at the National Hospital for Neurology and Neurosurgery, , London, UK. Cluster analysis gave 14 distinctive clinical types of patterns, but these had limited localizing value with the exception of perirolandic seizures. Two seizure types with prominent, early motor manifestations, especially version and posturing, were associated with frontal lobe abnormalities. Very high seizure frequencies were seen more often with frontal lesions. Seizures associated with temporal lobe lesions were characterized by absences and those with subjective onsets such as fear and oroalimentary automatisms. Location of interictal EEG spikes and ictal EEG onsets were generally consistent with lesion sites. Relatively few seizures could be localized reliably on clinical grounds. (Manford M et al. An analysis of clinical seizure patterns and their localizing value in frontal and temporal lobe epilepsies. Brain Feb 1996;119:17-40). (Respond: Dr M Manford, Wessex Neurological Centre, Southampton General Hospital, Tremona Road, Southampton SO16 6YD, UK).

COMMENT. The ILAE classification of seizure types based on electroclinical criteria may be justified for well-defined syndromes, eg benign epilepsy of childhood with centrotemporal spikes, but in the differentiation of frontal and temporal lobe partial epilepsies in adults there is significant clinical/pathological overlap. The authors argue in favor of an anatomical-pathological definition of fronto-temporal seizures, and they disagree with the ILAE classification of 7 different localizable seizure types within the frontal lobes based on electroclinical manifestations. Neuroimaging appears to be the only reliable method of lesion localization for frontal and temporal lobe partial epilepsies.

Magnetoencephalographic analysis of rolandic discharges in benign childhood epilepsy is reported from Kyushi University, Fukuoka, Japan. (Minami T et al. Ann Neurol March 1996;39:326-334). Dipole methods of MEG allow more precise location and quantification of electrically active brain regions compared to the EEG, and the recorded signal reflects intracellular rather than extracellular current flow. Equivalent current dipoles (ECDs) of prominent negative sharp waves of rolandic discharges appeared as tangential dipoles in the rolandic region and showed a limited localization compared with other components. ECDs of preceding small positive waves, positive waves following negative sharp waves, and negative slow waves were located close to negative sharp waves. ECDs of rolandic discharges were localized to the origin of somatosensory evoked magnetic field stimulated at the lower lip on a reconstructed three-dimensional MR image. Rolandic discharges are generated by a similar mechanism to that for the somatosensory evoked responses. -Editor. *Ped Neur Briefs* April 1996.

AED WITHDRAWAL: RISK FACTORS

The results of a prospective cohort study to investigate the effects of withdrawal of AEDs in 264 children with epilepsy after a mean seizure-free interval of 2.9 years are reported from the Montefiore/Einstein Epilepsy Management Center, Bronx, NY. Seizures recurred in 95 (36%); the mean time to recurrence was 9.5 months with a median of 4.3 months, and 90% of recurrences occurred within 25 months after study entry. The mean follow-up period was 58 months.

Etiology was a significant risk factor. In the group with *idiopathic epilepsy*, significant risk factors for recurrence included age at onset > 12 years, family history of epilepsy, history of atypical febrile seizures (defined as seizures with fever and a history of prior afebrile seizures, or complex febrile seizures), EEG slowing, and specific syndromes such as benign rolandic epilepsy and juvenile myoclonic epilepsy.

In the *remote symptomatic* group (includes only children with significant prior cerebral pathologies), significant predictors of seizure recurrence were age at seizure onset > 12 years, moderate to severe mental retardation, history of atypical febrile seizures, and history of absence seizures. (Shinnar S et al. Discontinuing antiepileptic drugs in children with epilepsy: a prospective study. <u>Ann Neurol</u> May 1994;35:534-545). (Respond: Dr Shinnar, Epilepsy Management

Center, Montefiore Medical Center, 111 E 210th Street, Bronx, NY 10467).

COMMENT. The results of this extensive, prospective study agree with previous reports showing that approximately one third of children who have been seizure free for 2 or more years while on AED therapy will relapse when medication is withdrawn. In children with cerebral pathologies and remote symptomatic epilepsy, almost 50% suffered recurrences. The risk factors reported in these study groups provide a valuable guide to a decision to terminate therapy. However, the final decision should consider each child as an individual, taking into account the consequences of a seizure recurrence and the possible adverse effects of continued antiepileptic medications. For further articles on this topic, see Progress in Pediatric Neurology, PNB Pub,1991.

Holmes GL, Children's Hospital, Boston, in an editorial (Ann Neurol 1994;35:509), appears to favor a trial period of withdrawal rather than indefinite continuation of AEDs, even in children with significant risk factors. He cites Lennox and Lennox (1960) who criticized proponents of anticonvulsant continuance for life, and notes the psychological consequences and expense of long term therapy. In contrast to the concerns of Shinnar and colleagues, Holmes down plays AED side effects as a compelling reason to discontinue therapy and finds that cognitive and behavioral impairments are overstated. He takes issue with the provocative statement of our respected colleague, John Freeman, that "antiepileptic drugs are all poisons."(Curr Probl Pediatr April 1994;24:139-48).-Editor. *Ped Neur Briefs* June 1994.

ANTIEPILEPTIC DRUG MONITORING

The appropriateness of antiepileptic drug (AED) level monitoring was assessed in a tertiary care center performing more than 10,000 AED level determinations per year and reported from the Brigham and Women's Hospital, Boston, MA. In a total of 330 inpatients with

AED levels measured a total of 855 times, only 27% of levels had appropriate indications, and only half of these were sampled correctly as trough levels, resulting in an overall appropriate test rate of 14%. Indications were baseline, control levels after starting treatment or after steady state was achieved with a change of dose (13%), after a seizure relapse (8%), suspected drug toxicity (4%), presumed patient noncompliance (1%), and possible drug interaction (1%). The rate of determination was the same for all drugs (phenytoin, carbamazepine, phenobarbital, valproic acid). Of the 73% of levels considered inappropriate, three quarters had been obtained after starting or changing the drug regimen, frequently on a daily basis, and before achieving a steady state; 23 (3.7%) were above the therapeutic range and potentially toxic. The avoidance of inappropriate testing would have resulted in a saving of >$300,000. (Schoenenberger RA et al. Appropriateness of antiepileptic drug level monitoring. <u>JAMA</u> November 22/29 1995;274:1622-1626). (Reprints: David W Bates MD, Division of General Medicine and Primary Care, Brigham and Women's Hospital, 75 Francis St, Boston, MA 02115).

COMMENT. Appropriate indications for AED levels include: 1) seizure recurrence, 2) drug toxicity, 3) patient noncompliance. Blood should be drawn at time of steady state (6 days for phenytoin, 3 days for carbamazepine and valproic acid, and 20 days for phenobarbital), as a baseline, after change of dose, after addition of second drug, or after change in liver or gastrointestinal function. Except after seizure relapse or with suspected toxicity, trough levels should be obtained. More frequent AED level determinations may be indicated during pregnancy and labor, after surgery, and in infants and children.

The authors of this study conclude that appropriate indications and timing of AED level determinations were not followed in 75% of patients in their tertiary care hospital. More careful adherence to appropriate monitoring indications would have resulted in cost reductions without significant risk of ineffective therapy or toxicity. -Editor. *Ped Neur Briefs* Dec 1995.

AGE FACTORS AND ANTIEPILEPTIC DRUG WITHDRAWAL

Age dependent factors concerning the withdrawal of antiepileptic drugs (AED) and seizure relapse rates, after a seizure-free period longer than 3 years, were evaluated in 304 patients with childhood epilepsies treated at the Toyama Medical and Pharmaceutical University, Toyama City, Japan. The incidence of AED withdrawal differed significantly between epileptic syndromes, being higher in idiopathic than in symptomatic epilepsies. Age at withdrawal peaked at preadolescence and early school age. Relapses occurred in 14%, the rate differing between epileptic groups and occurring at a unique age in each epileptic syndrome. Relapse rates were 33% and 20% in symptomatic *generalized* and *partial* epilepsies, respectively, and 5 to 8% in benign infantile convulsions, and idiopathic partial epilepsies. Idiopathic generalized epilepsy syndromes had higher relapse rates: 25% in juvenile absence, 100% in juvenile myoclonic, and 27% in grand mal on awakening epilepsy. Relapses were more frequent in epilepsies of infantile or adolescent onset than in those of school age onset. Age of relapse peaked at ages 7 to 11, mainly benign childhood epilepsy with centrotemporal spikes, and 17 to 19 years, mainly symptomatic partial, juvenile myoclonic, and grand mal.

EEG paroxysmal discharges did not necessarily predict a relapse, but changes in background activity with age showed correlations with rate of seizure recurrence. In patients without relapse, the background showed an increased maturation in mean frequency, with decrease in slow waves and increased alpha activity, during AED control before drug withdrawal. (Murakami M et al. Withdrawal of antiepileptic drug treatment in childhood epilepsy:

factors related to age. <u>J Neurol Neurosurg Psychiatry</u> 1995;59:477-481). (Respond: Dr Miyako Murakami, Department of Pediatrics, Toyama Medical and Pharmaceutical University, 2630 Sugitani, Toyama City 930-01, Japan).

COMMENT. Age dependent factors are important in time of withdrawal of AED and in prognosis after attempted AED withdrawal. Epileptic syndromes have an age dependent onset and course, related to CNS maturation, and varying relapse rates. Most frequent relapse rates occurred in patients undergoing drug withdrawal in preadolescence, eg benign childhood epilepsy with centrotemporal spikes, and early adulthood, eg symptomatic partial epilepsies. The characteristic course of each epileptic syndrome should be considered when attempting AED withdrawal. Background activity in the EEG is also an important factor, the persistence of slow waves and decreased alpha activity indicating an increased risk of relapse. -Editor. *Ped Neur Briefs* Dec 1995.

AED WITHDRAWAL IN CHILDREN WITH CEREBRAL PALSY

The safety of antiepileptic drug (AED) withdrawal in 65 children with cerebral palsy (CP) who had been seizure-free for at least 2 years was investigated in the Neurology Department, Texas Scottish Rite Hospital for Children, Dallas. Seizure relapses occurred in 27 patients (41%). Those with spastic hemiparesis had the highest relapse rate (61%) and spastic diplegia was associated with the lowest rate (14%). Mental subnormality, epileptiform EEG abnormality, type of CT abnormality, family history of epilepsy, mono or polytherapy, and gender were not correlated with risk of seizure relapse. (Delgado MR et al. Discontinuation of antiepileptic drug treatment after two seizure-free years in children with cerebral palsy. <u>Pediatrics</u> February 1996;97:192-197). (Reprints: Dr MR Delgado, Texas Scottish Rite Hospital for Children, 2222 Welborn St, Dallas, TX 75219).

COMMENT. Despite abnormal neurologic examinations, almost two thirds of these CP patients remained free from seizures for periods of at least 2 years after AED withdrawal. Patients with spastic hemiparesis have the highest relapse rate, and drug withdrawal should be discouraged or attempted only with great caution. -Editor. *Ped Neur Briefs* Feb 1996.

FAMILIES' VIEWS ON DISCONTINUING ANTICONVULSANTS

The opinions of families of 76 children with epilepsy (>3 months seizure-free) and their 4 physician epilepsy specialists regarding acceptable risks of seizure recurrence (RSR) after AED withdrawal were investigated by questionnaire at the IWK Children's Hospital, Halifax, Nova Scotia, Canada. Families' responses were very variable: a RSR of 25% was unacceptable to 42% of families, whereas a >75% risk was considered acceptable by 20%. Families responses were dependent on previous seizure frequency, multiple seizure types, school grades repeated, and the *habits of playing the lottery.* The degree of risk acceptable to a particular family was not predicted by their physicians. Physician's opinions of acceptable RSR were more consistent, a median of 40%, but they varied from 0 to 90% for individual children. Families gave the primary responsibility for discontinuing AEDs to the physician in 80% of cases, but 46% reserved a secondary role in the decision for the parents. The majority of families (89%) denied the physician an exclusive role in the decision making. (Gordon K et al. Families are content to discontinue antiepileptic drugs at different risks than their physicians. Epilepsia June 1996;37:557-562). (Reprints: Dr K Gordon, IWK Children's Hospital, 5850 University Ave, Box 3070, Halifax, Nova Scotia, Canada, B3J 3G9).

COMMENT. This center's practice of discontinuing AEDs after a seizure-free 2 year period, with an expected seizure recurrence of 30-40%, results in an unacceptable degree of risk for more than half the families in this study. Withdrawal of AEDs after a 1 year seizure-free period provided a similar high risk of recurrence of 30-40%, in a recent study from the same center (Dooley J, Gordon K et al. <u>Neurology</u> April 1996;46:969-974).

Physicians should be aware of the parents' opinions and attitudes in regard to risk of seizure recurrence, when advising on the time to discontinue treatment of a child with epilepsy, but they cannot allow a "parent's strategy of playing lotteries" to intervene in this important decision. Each child with epilepsy is an individual, and the time for anticonvulsant withdrawal should be determined on an individual basis, having regard to varying predictive factors, not based on a generalized fixed period of 1 or 2 years. An expected seizure recurrence of 30-40% should be unacceptable in current practice, and the consequences of a single seizure relapse, especially in adolescents and young adults, should demand a more conservative and individual approach to this important decision. See <u>Progress in Pediatric Neurology I</u>, PNB Publishers, 1991, pp 100-104, for further references and commentaries on anticonvulsant withdrawal practices. -Editor. *Ped Neur Briefs* June 1996.

VALUE OF EEG IN ANTIEPILEPTIC DRUG WITHDRAWAL

The prognostic value of the EEG in 120 seizure-free epileptic patients, during and after antiepileptic drug withdrawal, was analyzed at the Department of Neurology, University of Bologna, Italy. Of 128 patients studied with mean age of 28 years, 49 had complex partial seizures (CPS), and 20 had simple partial seizures. Patients included had a history of partial epilepsies treated with AEDs for at least 2 years, and were seizure-free for at least 2 but not more than 6 years. Overall, 75 (63%) relapsed within 3 years from complete drug withdrawal, 29 during drug reduction. Of 36 (30%) showing EEG epileptiform abnormalities at the start of the study, 16 showed an increase in EEG abnormality during and after drug withdrawal. Of 84 with normal EEGs initially, 20 showed epileptiform abnormalities with drug withdrawal. The lowest relapse rate occurred in CPS patients (45%) and the highest in those with SPS (100%). The EEG at the start of the study was not predictive of relapse, but EEG worsening during the withdrawal of AEDs was associated with a significantly higher relapse rate. (Tinuper P, Avoni P, Riva R et al. The prognostic value of the electroencephalogram in antiepileptic drug withdrawal in partial epilepsies. <u>Neurology</u> July 1996;47:76-78). (Reprints: Dr Paolo Tinuper, Department of Neurology, via Foscolo 7, I-40123 Bologna, Italy).

COMMENT. In this study of young adults with partial epilepsies, the EEG was predictive of relapse during but not before starting the withdrawal of antiepileptic drugs, especially if abnormalities appeared when previously absent.

Similar studies in children have not included large numbers of partial epilepsies, but some have indicated a higher relapse rate in female, mentally retarded children with focal neurologic signs and partial seizures. For further reports of the EEG and AED withdrawal see <u>Progress in Pediatric Neurology I</u>, PNB Publ, 1991, pp100-104; and <u>Ped Neur Briefs</u> Dec 1995;9:90. In this 1995 Japanese study, Murakami M et al found a relapse rate of 20% in symptomatic partial epilepsies and 8% in idiopathic partial epilepsies in children. Age dependent factors were important in predicting relapse, peaking at 17 to 19 years for symptomatic partial seizures. Background activity in the EEG was also a predictive factor, the risk of relapse being greater with persistence of slow waves and decreased alpha activity. -Editor. *Ped Neur Briefs* Aug 1996.

ANTIEPILEPTIC DRUG EFFICACY

GABAPENTIN *[NEURONTIN®]* EFFICACY IN REFRACTORY EPILEPSIES

Gabapentin (Neurontin®), another newer

anticonvulsant, recently approved and introduced for treatment of partial and secondarily generalized seizures in adults and children older than 12 years, was found to be safe and well-tolerated as monotherapy in a multicenter study. (Hayes A et al. An open-label multicenter study of gabapentin (Neurontin) monotherapy and safety in medically refractory patients with partial seizures. Neurology April 1994;44 Suppl 2):A204).

COMMENT. Adverse effects were minor and psychometric testing revealed no cognitive impairments. In follow-up studies > 1 year, there was no evidence of chronic toxicity. Unlike other anticonvulsants, gabapentin is not metabolized by the liver and is free of interactions with other drugs. (Leppik IE. Epilepsia 1994;35 (Suppl 4):S29-S40). -Editor. *Ped Neur Briefs* May 1994.

GABAPENTIN EFFICACY AND SAFETY

The results of three large, placebo-controlled, multicenter clinical trials of gabapentin as add-on therapy in patients with refractory partial seizures are summarized in a report from the Departments of Neurology and Psychiatry and the International Center for Epilepsy, University of Miami School of Medicine, and the Veterans Affairs Medical Center, Miami, FL. In a total of 705 patients (646 evaluable, mean age 33 years) treated the responder rate (RR) ranged from 18% to 28% in those receiving 600 to 1800 mg gabapentin daily; the median seizure frequency decreased by 17.8 to 31.9% in gabapentin-treated compared with 0.3 to 12.5% in placebo-control patients. Based on the RR (the percentage of patients with >50% decrease in seizure frequency), a dose-response effect was present for simple partial, complex partial, and secondarily generalized tonic-clonic seizures. Adverse effects, primarily mild to moderate in severity and transient, mainly affected the CNS and included somnolence (24%), dizziness (20%), and ataxia (17%). Skin rash in only 0.54% gabapentin-treated patients compared to an average 5 to 10% incidence with traditional AEDs. No significant changes in liver function were noted. (Ramsay RE. Clinical efficacy and safety of gabapentin. Neurology June 1994;44(suppl 5):S23-30). (Reprints: Dr R E Ramsay, 1150 NW 14th St, Suite 410, Miami, FL 33136).

COMMENT. Gabapentin is approved for patients >12 years of age with partial and secondarily generalized seizures. The role of gabapentin in the management of epilepsy is the subject of five papers in the above Neurology supplement. In addition to efficacy and safety addressed by Ramsay RE, the profile of desirable properties of a new AED are outlined by Mattson RH, the mechanism of action of gabapentin is reviewed by Taylor CP, and its lack of drug interaction and advantageous pharmacokinetics are stressed by McLean MJ. The absence of interactions between gabapentin and other AEDs and the rarity of serious adverse effects should encourage the expansion of clinical trials to include children younger than 12 years of age. -Editor. *Ped Neur Briefs* July 1994.

GABAPENTIN IN REFRACTORY PARTIAL SEIZURES

The efficacy of gabapentin as an additional medication in 32 children with refractory partial seizures was studied at the Children's Hospital, Boston, MA. A greater than 50% decrease in seizure frequency was obtained in 34% and a 25% to 50% decrease occurred in 12%. Approximately half the patients were benefited. Doses ranged from 10 to 50 mg/kg/day, and the mean gabapentin serum concentration correlating with seizure control was 3.7 mcg/ml. Hyperactivity, irritability, and agitation, in 15 (46%) children with mental retardation and attention deficits, were the major side effects. Mild behavior changes not requiring drug withdrawal, including impulsivity, irritability, and hyperactivity, were reported in 11 additional children. Personality was improved in 3 children. (Khurana DS, Mikati MA et al. Efficacy of gabapentin therapy in children with refractory partial seizures. <u>J Pediatr</u> June 1996;128:829-33). (Reprints: Mohamad A Mikati MD, Department of Pediatrics, American University Hospital, c/o American University of Beirut New York Office, 850 Third Ave, 18th Floor, New York, NY 10022).

COMMENT. Gabapentin may be an effective adjunctive medication in children with refractory partial seizures. Behavioral side effects were reversible when the drug was discontinued and were most prominent in the mentally retarded. -Editor. *Ped Neur Briefs* July 1996.

FELBAMATE IN INTRACTABLE CHILDHOOD EPILEPSY

Of 51 children with intractable seizures treated for two months with add on felbamate (50-75 mg/kg/day) at the Scottish Rite Children's Hospital, Atlanta, GA, 51% responded with improved seizure control, 22% were unchanged, and 28% had increased seizure frequency. Significant insomnia limited the usefulness of felbamate in 39% of children. Other adverse effects included anorexia, hyperactivity, and choreoathetosis. (Trevathan E et al. Febamate: Short-term efficacy and side effects in 51 children with intractable epilepsy. <u>Neurology</u> April 1994;<u>44</u> (Suppl 2):A273 (abstr)). (Respond: Dr Edwin Trevathan, 5455 Meridian Mark Rd, Ste 530, Atlanta, GA).

COMMENT. Clinically significant weight loss and anorexia were troublesome side effects during a trial of felbamate in 68 children and adults with intractable seizures at Rush-Presbyterian-St Luke's Medical Center, Chicago. (Waicosky K et al. Weight loss in patients taking felbamate. <u>Neurology</u> April 1994;<u>44</u> (Suppl 2):A296). Insomnia was reported in 25% of felbamate-treated patients in a further study of 16 patients (Luciano D et al. <u>Neurology</u> April 1994;<u>44</u> (Suppl 2):A296). -Editor. *Ped Neur Briefs* May 1994.
Felbamate has since lost FDA approval because of hematologic and hepatic side effects.

ABNORMAL EEG IN AUTISM: VALPROATE RESPONSE

Three children, ages 3, 4, and 5 years, with autism and epileptiform EEG discharges showed clinical improvement with valproic acid therapy at Mercy Hospital and Medical Center, Chicago, IL. None had a history of seizures. Within one month of VPA 125 mg tid treatment, language and social skills improved and the DSM-III-R criteria for autism no longer applied. Improvement had been maintained at follow-up 7 to 11 months later. (Plioplys AV. Autism: electroencephalogram abnormalities and clinical improvement with valproic acid. <u>Arch Pediatr Adolesc Med</u> Feb 1994;<u>148</u>:220-222). (Reprints: Dr Plioplys, Division of Neurology, Mercy Hospital and Medical Center, Stevenson Expressway at King Drive, Chicago, IL 60616).

COMMENT. The author stresses the importance of sleep EEGs to uncover epileptiform discharges in young autistic patients without history of clinical seizures. Further trials of antiepileptic drugs in autistic children seem justified. -Editor. *Ped Neur Briefs* March 1994.

SAFETY OF INTRAVENOUS VALPROATE

A multicenter. open-label study of the safety of intravenous sodium valproate in 318 hospitalized patients with epilepsy is reported from the NYU Hospital for Joint Diseases; MINCEP Epilepsy Care and Minnesota Epilepsy Group, MN; University of Texas, Houston; Medical College of Virginia, Richmond; Bowman-Gray School of Medicine, Winston-Salem, NC; and University of Miami, FL. Mean age was 34 years (range, 2-87 years). Valproate aqueous solution (500mg/5 ml), one-fourth daily dose (median dose 375 mg or 5.1 mg/kg), diluted with 50 ml normal saline or 5% dextrose/water, infused over 1 hour, repeated 6 hourly for up to 2 days. Transient severe side effects in 54 (17%) included headache, reaction at injection site, nausea, vomiting, somnolence (2% each), dizziness, and abnormal taste (1% each). Six left the study prematurely due to valproate intolerance: pain at IV site, amylase elevations, headache, nausea and vomiting. Abnormal serum chemistries following treatment in 7 generally returned to normal. (Devinsky O et al. Safety of intravenous valproate. <u>Ann Neurol</u> Oct 1995;38:670-674). (Respond: Dr Devinsky, Department of Neurology, Hospital for Joint Diseases, 301 East 17th Street, New York, NY 10003).

COMMENT. This study demonstrates the relative safety of IV valproate, which is not yet available for general use in the US. Previous studies in Europe, where the IV preparation is available, have demonstrated efficacy in neonatal seizures, and in neurosurgical adult patients with status epilepticus resistant to diazepam. The authors recommend further trials to determine optimal dose, efficacy, and safety. -Editor. *Ped Neur Briefs* Dec 1995.

HIGH-DOSE STEROIDS IN RASMUSSEN'S SYNDROME

Ten of 17 patients with Rasmussen's syndrome receiving IV methylprednisolone and/or oral predisolone, and eight of nine patients receiving immunoglobulins showed some short-term reduction in seizure frequency in a multicenter international report. Side effects included fluid retention, psychotic symptoms and behavior problems. The authors propose a central register and standardized protocol with initial trial of IV immunoglobulin (400 mg/kg/d on 3 successive days) followed by monthly one day treatments if improvement occurs. Steroid therapy (IV methyl-prednisolone, 400 mg/m^2 on 3 alternate days followed by monthly single infusions for one year or longer, and oral predisolone starting at 2 mg/kg/d) is recommended for patients not responding to IVIG. (Hart YM, Cortez M, Andermann F et al. Medical treatment of Rasmussen's syndrome (chronic encephalitis and epilepsy): Effect of high-dose steroids or immunoglobulins in 19 patients. <u>Neurology</u> June 1994;44:1030-1036). (Respond: Dr F Andermann, Montreal

Neurological Institute, 3801 University Street, Montreal, PQ, Canada H3A 2B4).

COMMENT. The patients were treated at the Montreal Neurological and Children's Hospitals; the National Hospital, London; Great Ormond Street Hospital, London; Hospital for Sick Children, Toronto; and Hospital Juan Garrahan, Buenos Aires. The diagnosis was confirmed by biopsy in all but three of the patients. As with infantile spasms, the earlier the therapy the better the results. Since ACTH is usually considered superior to prednisone in the treatment of infantile spasms, it is surprising that only one of the 17 patients with Rasmussen's syndrome received ACTH and ACTH is omitted from the recommended treatment protocol for further trials. If a comparison with infantile spasms is carried further, patients benefited by steroids or ACTH usually respond within 4 to 8 weeks and prolongation of therapy in non-responders is generally ineffective and is accompanied by serious toxicity. The authors recommend frequent monitoring of patients on high-dose steroids when continued for the suggested periods of 1 to 2 years or longer and caution that improvements may be delayed for several months. -Editor. *Ped Neur Briefs* July 1994.

ANTIEPILEPTIC SIDE-EFFECTS

LONG-TERM VALPROATE HEMATOLOGIC SIDE EFFECTS

Hematologic side effects in 60 patients, aged 2-29 years (mean 14 years), receiving valproate (VPA) monotherapy for >4 years in a long-term care facility, are reported from the Department of Pediatrics, East Carolina University School of Medicine, Greenville, North Carolina. Hematologic abnormalities, especially thrombocytopenia, <130,000/mcl (12 patients) and macrocytosis (11), were demonstrated in 20 (33%) patients. With VPA levels >100 mcg/ml in 22 patients, the incidence increased to 55%. Platelet counts were inversely related to VPA levels; thrombocytopenia was corrected when VPA dosage was reduced. Three had anemia, and 3 had leukopenia. Serum B_{12} levels were increased (>1000 mcg/ml) in 51 (86%); folate levels were normal. Blood smears showed increased numbers of bilobed polymorphonucleic cells (Pelger-Huet-like cells), an anomaly commonly associated with VPA-induced macrocytosis. (May RB, Sunder TR. Hematologic manifestations of long-term valproate therapy. Epilepsia Nov/Dec 1993;34:1098-1101). (Reprints: Dr RB May, Craven County Health Department, PO Drawer 12610, New Bern, NC 28561).

COMMENT. The authors recommend close regular surveillance of patients receiving valproate, with continuous attention to blood counts, especially platelets and mean corpuscular volumes. The early recognition of these relatively frequent blood count anomalies may lead to reduction in VPA dosage or drug withdrawal and avoidance of major hematologic toxicity. -Editor. *Ped Neur Briefs* Jan 1994.

VALPROATE-INDUCED THROMBOCYTOPENIA

A 14-year-old mentally retarded boy with seizures who presented with severe thrombocytopenia, macrocytic anemia and allergic dermatitis after treatment with valproate for 12 years is reported from the University of Louvain Medical School, Brussels, Belgium. Serum valproate level was 48 mcg/ml. Bone marrow examination showed myeloblastic abnormalities. Recovery followed withdrawal of valproate. (Brichard B et al. Haematological disturbances during long-term valproate therapy. Eur J Pediatr May 1994;153:378-380). (Respond: Dr B Brichard, Dept Paediatric Haematology, Univ Louvain Med School, Avenue Hippocrate 10, B-1200 Brussels, Belgium).

COMMENT. Thrombocytopenia is a well known side effect of valproate therapy. It is related to antibody-mediated platelet destruction, and tests for serum direct antiplatelet antibodies are positive. This report is unusual in the delayed occurrence of hematologic toxicity, even with relatively low serum levels of valproate. -Editor. *Ped Neur Briefs* June 1994.

VALPROATE-INDUCED LUPUS ERYTHEMATOSUS

A mentally retarded 30-year-old woman with partial trisomy of chromosome 9, suffering from epilepsy since age 11 months, developed systemic lupus erythematosus after one year of treatment with valproate (VPA) and ethosuximide (ESM) at the Clinica Neurologica, Universita di Roma Tor Vergata, Italy. When prednisone 1 mg/kg/day was administered and VPA gradually discontinued, clinical remission occurred within 10 days. The patient was maintained on ESM without relapse. (Gigli GL et al. Valproate-induced systemic lupus erythematosus in a patient with partial trisomy of chromosome 9 and epilepsy. Epilepsia June 1996;37:587-588). (Reprints: Dr GL Gigli, Clinica Neurologica, Universita di Roma Tor Vergata, Ospedale S Eugenio, Piazzale Umanesimo 10, 00144, Rome, Italy).

COMMENT. This was the fourth reported case of VPA-induced systemic lupus erythematosus. It presented with arthralgia, fever, and fatigue, after prolonged treatment. It resolved rapidly after discontinuing the drug. -Editor. *Ped Neur Briefs* June 1996.

VALPROIC ACID AND THROMBOCYTOPENIA

The association of thrombocytopenia (TCP) with valproic acid (VPA) therapy was evaluated retrospectively in 167 children treated with VPA between 1989 and 1993 at the Department of Pediatrics, Henry Ford Medical Center, Detroit, MI. VPA monotherapy in 91 and VPA polytherapy in 76 children were compared with 92 age- and sex-matched controls taking AEDs other than VPA. Thrombocytopenia ($<200 \times 10^3 / mm^3$) occurred in 22% of VPA treated children (in 26% on monotherapy and 16% on polytherapy), and in 5% of controls. Patients with TCP were older, had higher serum VPA levels, and received higher doses of VPA than those without TCP. The degree of TCP was mild, no patient developed bleeding or excess bruising, and VPA was not discontinued because of TCP. (Allarakhia IN, Garofalo EA, Komarynski MA, Robertson PL. Valproic acid and thrombocytopenia in children: a case-controlled retrospective study. Pediatr Neurol May 1996;14:303-7). (Respond: Dr I Allarakhia, Department of Pediatrics, Henry Ford Medical Center, 2799 West Grand Boulevard, Detroit, MI 48202).

COMMENT. Despite this documentation of a 22% incidence of thrombocytopenia in children treated with VPA, severe TPA with bleeding complications did not occur, and the withdrawal of VPA was not required. The authors recommend close monitoring of the platelet count in patients receiving VPA in larger doses and with higher serum levels, and particularly in older children. VPA induced bleeding may sometimes be explained by an underlying familial disease, eg. von Willebrand pseudohemophilia or a dysfibrinogenemia. (see Progress in Pediatric Neurology II, 1994, pp102-103).

Pseudo valproate-induced hypofibrinogenemia is reported in a 6-year-old boy with a ventriculoperitoneal shunt for hydrocephalus and a stone in the ureter requiring surgery at the Departments of Pediatrics and Neurology, Park Nicollet Clinic, Minneapolis, MN. Pre-surgical coagulation studies revealed a prothrombin time of 14.9s (N 9.8-13.2), thrombin time of 73.3s (N 13-20), and fibrinogen levels of < 50 mg/dl (N 145-375). The patient's mother also had a prolonged thrombin time, and a diagnosis of inherited dysfibrinogenemia was presumed in this case. (Breningstall GN, Cich JA. Pediatr Neurol May 1996;14:345). Two previous reports are cited of a valproate dose-related decrease in fibrinogen, and one neonate whose mother was receiving VPA had a symptomatic fibrinogen deficiency. -Editor. *Ped Neur*

Briefs Aug 1996.

VALPROATE-INDUCED HEPATIC FAILURE WITH COX DEFICIT

A fatal hepatic failure in a 3 year-old girl with myoclonic epilepsy after 3 months of treatment with valproate (VPA) is reported from Hopital d'Enfants, Marseilles, and Hopital des Enfants-Malades, Paris, France. Elevated plasma lactate and lactate/pyruvate molar ratios in plasma suggested a defect in oxidative phosphorylation and prompted investigation of respiratory chain activity. Circulating lymphocytes revealed a cytochrome c oxidase (COX) deficiency, later confirmed by post-mortem analysis in liver and cultured skin fibroblasts. Skeletal muscle analysis was normal. (Chabrol B et al. Valproate-induced hepatic failure in a case of cytochrome *c* oxidase deficiency. Eur J Pediatr 1994;153:133-135). (Respond: Dr B Chabrol, Service de Neuropediatrie, Hopital d'Enfants, CHU de la Timone, F-13385 Marseille Cedex 5, France).

COMMENT. Lactate/pyruvate plasma levels are recommended in children with possible mitochondrial disorders and epilepsy when VPA treatment is employed. Valproate associated hepatotoxicity is discussed in previous issues of Ped Neur Briefs Jan, May, and Aug 1993, and June 1987. -Editor. *Ped Neur Briefs* March 1994.

VALPROATE-ASSOCIATED HEPATOTOXICITY UPDATE

Eight new fatalities from valproate (VPA)-related hepatotoxicity, 6 reversible cases, and a review of 132 fatal cases Worldwide are reported from various Universities in Germany. In fatal cases, 65% were developmentally delayed, 75% were taking additional AEDs, and 65% were >2 years old. Early symptoms were nausea, vomiting, apathy, coma, exacerbation of seizures, and febrile infections. Two thirds of fatalities occurred within 6 months of introducing VPA. In reversible cases, VPA had been withdrawn promptly. In addition to Alper's disease, a variety of underlying metabolic defects, especially acyl CoA-dehydrogenase deficiency, has been recognized in some cases of VPA-related hepatotoxicity. (Konig St A, Scheffner D et al. Severe hepatotoxicity during valproate therapy: an update and report of eight new fatalities. <u>Epilepsia</u> Sept/Oct 1994;35:1005-1015). (Reprints: Dr S A Konig, Universitats Kinderklinik, Theodor-Kutzer-Ufer, D-68167 Mannheim, Germany).

COMMENT. Metabolic testing is indicated in children <2 years old with developmental abnormalities when considering VPA therapy. Those patients with recognized metabolic disorders should not receive VPA. Further, VPA should be discontinued promptly and alternative AEDs substituted at the earliest sign of liver failure, if seizures are suddenly exacerbated, and particularly with status epilepticus and febrile infections. -Editor. *Ped Neur Briefs* Dec 1994.

HEPATIC FATALITIES AND VALPROIC ACID

The results of a third retrospective study of the US experience since 1986 with fatal hepatotoxicity associated with valproic acid (VPA) are reported from the Department of Neurology, University of Virginia School of Medicine, Charlottesville, VA. In 29 case fatalities, the most common presenting signs were drowsiness, jaundice, vomiting, hemorrhage, seizure exacerbation, anorexia, and edema. Risk factors included young age, especially below 2 years when the risk was 1:600, polytherapy, developmental delay, and coincident metabolic disorders, especially Alpers' disease. (Bryant AE III, Dreifuss FE. Valproic acid hepatic fatalities. III. US experience since 1986. <u>Neurology</u> Feb 1996;46:465-469). (Reprints: Dr Fritz E Dreifuss, Department of Neurology, Box 394, University of Virginia Health Sciences Center, Charlottesville, VA 22908).

COMMENT. The authors advise avoidance of VPA

in patients who are at greatest risk of developing liver toxicity. Liver transplant had been received by 28% of the patients in this study. -Editor. *Ped Neur Briefs* April 1996.

CARNITINE IN VALPROATE-INDUCED HYPERAMMONEMIA

The effect of carnitine supplementation in valproic acid (VPA) treated patients presenting with hyperammonemia was investigated in 69 children and young adults seen at the Zentrum der Kinderheilkunde, Goethe-Universitat Frankfurt, and Universitat Erlanger, FRG. Plasma total carnitine was low (27 mcmol/l cf normal of 40 mcmol/l) in 48 tested. After supplements of carnitine (1 gm/m2 per day) in 15 patients, the plasma ammonia decreased by 25% after 9 days and 46% after 80 days. The plasma free carnitine was increased by 12%. Plasma ammonia concentrations were significantly correlated with free plasma carnitine %. (Bohles H, Sewell AC, Wenzel D. The effect of carnitine supplementation in valproate-induced hyperammonaemia. <u>Acta Paediatr</u> April 1996;85:446-9). (Respond: Dr H Bohles, Zentrum der Kinderheilkunde, Theodor Stern Kai 7, 60590 Frankfurt/Main, FRG).

COMMENT. Carnitine supplementation was recommended in VPA-treated patients with hyperammonemia. The risk of VPA-induced Reye's-like syndrome could not be determined from this study. -Editor. *Ped Neur Briefs* June 1996.

FETAL VALPROATE SYNDROME IN SIBLINGS

Clinical and neurodevelopmental findings in four children (two sibling pairs) exposed in utero to valproic acid are reported from the Departments of Paediatrics and Human Genetics, University of Witaterstrand, Johannesburg, South Africa. Three were globally developmentally delayed with marked speech disability, characteristic dysmorphic features, and one with autism. The fourth child had dysmorphism and a learning disability. (Christianson AL et al. Fetal valproate syndrome: Clinical and neurodevelopmental features in two sibling pairs. <u>Dev Med & Child Neurol</u> April 1994;<u>36</u>:357-369). (Respond: Dr Arnold L Christianson, Dept of Human Genetics and Developmental Biology, University of Pretoria Faculty of Medicine, PO Box 2034, Pretoria 0001, South Africa).

COMMENT. Future children could be at increased risk of fetal valproate syndrome if valproate is continued during pregnancy. The drug itself, the dosage, the genetic susceptibility, and other environmental factors are involved in the etiology of drug-related birth defects. In addition to adverse effects on the fetus, valproate is reported to cause reproductive disorders, including polycystic ovaries and hyperandrogenism, in women with epilepsy (see <u>Ped Neur Briefs</u> Dec 1993). -Editor. *Ped Neur Briefs* May 1994.

CHOREIFORM MOVEMENTS AND VALPROIC ACID

Three patients, aged 10, 17, and 36 years, who developed chorea during long-term treatment with valproic acid are reported from the Comprehensive Epilepsy Program, Bowman Gray School of Medicine, Winston-Salem, NC. All patients had severe brain damage, one had a vascular lesion in the caudate nucleus, and two were also receiving phenytoin. Chorea developed within 1/2 to 3 hours of valproic acid ingestion and lasted 1/2 to 8 hours. Movements were not relieved by phenytoin withdrawal. Chorea resolved when valproic acid was withdrawn in one patient and replaced by divalproex sodium sprinkles in the other two. (Lancman ME, Asconape JJ, Penry JK. Choreiform movements associated with the use of valproate. <u>Arch Neurol</u> July 1994;51:702-704). (Reprints: Dr Lancman, Department of Neurology, Bowman Gray School of Medicine, Medical Center Boulevard, Winston-Salem, NC 27157).

COMMENT. Valproate-induced chorea in these patients appeared to be dose related, occurring at peak serum concentrations. The use of divalproex sodium sprinkles avoided the excessive fluctuations of serum levels seen with valproic acid and movements were controlled. Choreoathetosis is a known side effect of the majority of antiepileptic drugs. This may be the first recorded case of valproate-induced chorea. -Editor. *Ped Neur Briefs* Aug 1994.

ANTICONVULSANTS AND BONE MINERAL DENSITY: VALPROATE-INDUCED LOSS

The effect of carbamazepine and valproate monotherapy on bone mineral density was measured by dual-energy x-ray absorptiometry in 27 healthy children and 26 children with uncomplicated idiopathic epilepsy treated with an anticonvulsant for longer than 18 months at the Memorial University of Newfoundland, St John's, Canada. Mean serum trough levels for carbamazepine and valproate were 6.88 and 72.04 mcg/ml, respectively. Dietary calcium was similar in treated and control patients. Valproate caused a 10 to 14% reduction in bone mineral density, and the percent reduction was related to treatment duration. Carbamazepine had no significant effect on bone mineral density. (Sheth RD, Bodensteiner JB et al. Effect of carbamazepine and valproate on bone mineral density. <u>J Pediatr</u> August 1995;127:256-262). (Reprints: Raj D Sheth MD, Pediatric Neurology, Box 9180, West Virginia University Health Sciences Center, Morgantown, WV 26506).

COMMENT. Valproate but not carbamazepine causes reduction in mineralization of bone in children and adolescents, aged 8 to 20 (mean 15 years) and may predispose to osteoporotic fractures. The mechanism of decreased mineralization is undetermined. The authors suggest possible preventive measures including calcium dietary supplements, weight-bearing exercises, and avoidance of smoking. -Editor. *Ped Neur Briefs* Sept 1995.

VALPROATE, BRAIN ATROPHY AND REVERSIBLE DEMENTIA

Two children who developed severe cognitive and behavioral deterioration while being treated with sodium valproate for idiopathic epilepsy are reported from the Miami Children's Hospital, Miami, FL. Patient 1 presented at age 5 years with left focal seizures and right central sharp waves on the EEG, consistent with benign rolandic epilepsy (BRE). After his fourth seizure at age 8 years he received sodium valproate (Depakote), with blood levels of 91-106 mg/dl, and methylphenidate (MPH) 20 mg twice daily for an associated ADDH. MPH was replaced by thioridazine (Mellaril) and benztropine (Cogentin) at age 9 years. Impaired motor ability was noted at age 10 years. Activity level, speech, and IQ progressively deteriorated, with ataxia and marked obesity developing by 10 years 8 months. MRI showed enlarged ventricles and cortical sulci. Felbamate was substituted for valproate and his motor activity, speech, gait, weight, and IQ returned to normal within a few weeks. The MRI improved after 3 months and was normal at 1 year. Pemoline (Cylert) was introduced for ADDH without relapse of behavior or seizure recurrence. Patient 2 had an onset of a similar degenerative syndrome within 3 weeks of prescribing valproate for migraine and BRE. The condition resolved 4 to 6 months after substituting phenobarbital. No metabolic changes were uncovered. (Papazian O et al. Reversible dementia and apparent brain atrophy during valproate therapy. <u>Ann Neurol</u> October 1995;38:687-691). (Respond: Dr Papazian, 3200 SW 60th Ct, #302, Miami, FL 33155).

COMMENT. Patients treated with valproate need to be monitored for mental and motor deterioration in addition to liver dysfunction. -Editor. *Ped Neur Briefs* Nov 1995.

VALPROATE INDUCED OBESITY AND POLYCYSTIC OVARIES

Fourteen (64%) of 22 women receiving valproate monotherapy for epilepsy had polycystic ovaries, hyperandrogenism, or both, in a study at the Departments of Neurology, Obstetrics and Gynecology, and Pediatrics, University of Oulu, Finland. They had a progressive obesity associated with hyperinsulinemia and low serum insulin-like growth factor-binding protein 1, leading to hyperandrogenism and polycystic ovaries. The mean duration of treatment was 7 years, and the mean daily dose of valproate was 1070mg. In contrast, polycystic ovaries and hyperandrogenism occurred in 9 (21%) of 43 women receiving carbamazepine monotherapy and 8 (19%) of 43 in a control group. (Isojarvi JIT et al. Obesity and endocrine disorders in women taking valproate for epilepsy. Ann Neurol May 1996;39:579-584). (Respond: Dr Isojarvi, Department of Neurology, University of Oulu, FIN-90220 Oulu, Finland).

COMMENT. Polycystic ovarian syndrome (PCOS), hyperandrogenic chronic anovulation, is characterized clinically by hirsutism and menstrual disorders. Obesity occurs in 30 to 50% of patients affected. It may have multiple etiologies, including genetic, endocrine, metabolic, and neurologic. PCOS induced by valproate medication for epilepsy has been attributed to the coincidental obesity and resultant endocrine abnormalities. An increased incidence of PCOS among untreated epileptic women is greater with left than with right-sided temporal lobe foci. Antiseizure medications other than valproate induce hepatic enzymes that reduce testosterone levels and tend to moderate hyperandogenism. Hertzog AG, at the Harvard Neuroendocrine Unit, Beth Israel Hospital, Boston, MA, suggests that valproate may not be the primary cause of PCOS, citing epileptic and neurologic factors (Ann Neurol May 1996;39:559-560). -Editor. *Ped Neur Briefs* June 1996.

MATERNAL VALPROATE TREATMENT AND NEONATAL BEHAVIOR

The relationship between antiepileptic drug (AED) treatment during pregnancy, neurobehavior of the neonate, and the neurological outcome in later life of 40 children exposed in utero to a single AED (phenobarbital, phenytoin, valproic acid) was studied at Children's Hospital, Virchow Klinikum of the Humboldt University Berlin; Institute of Toxicology and Embryopharmacology, Free University Berlin; and Department of Neuropediatrics, Children's Hospital, University of Heidelberg, Germany. Tonic clonic seizures during pregnancy occurred in 5 (27%) of the phenobarbital-treated women, in 5 (38%) treated with phenytoin, and in 3 (33%) of valproic-acid-treated women. AED exposed neonates had greater neurobehavioral disorders than the controls. Apathy was most pronounced in phenobarbital-exposed neonates, whereas hyperexcitability was more severe after maternal valproic acid (VPA) exposure. Phenytoin-exposed neonates, having the least neurobehavioral side effects, had low serum concentrations, whereas the concentrations of VPA in cord blood were relatively high. VPA concentrations at birth correlated with the degree of neonatal hyperexcitability and neurological dysfunction found at 6 year follow-up. (Koch S et al. Antiepileptic drug treatment in pregnancy: drug side effects in the neonate and neurological outcome. <u>Acta Paediatr</u> June 1996;84:739-46). (Respond: Dr S Koch, Rehabitationszentrum fur Kinder, Dorfstr 16, 14476 Kartzow, Germany).

COMMENT. The authors suggest that the neonatal VPA-induced malformations and neurobehavioral and late neurological side effects may be related to unexpectedly high levels of the drug and its active metabolites during pregnancy, at birth, and in the neonatal period. Mothers taking VPA during pregnancy should have drug levels closely monitored, especially at the time and shortly after conception but also throughout pregnancy. -Editor. *Ped Neur Briefs*

July 1996.

VALPROATE AND CARBAMAZEPINE COMPARATIVE TRIAL

The efficacy and side-effects of sodium valproate (VA) and carbamazepine (CBZ) were compared in 260 children (5 to 16 years of age) with primary generalized epilepsy or partial epilepsy followed for three years at 63 outpatient clinics in the UK and Ireland and results were reported from Addenbrooke's Hospital, Cambridge, the Hospital for Sick Children, Great Ormond Street, London, and the Trial Office at Sanofi Winthrop Ltd, Guildford, Surrey, UK. Patients with newly diagnosed epilepsy and at least two seizures in the previous six months were randomized to receive either sodium valproate (200mg twice daily initially, mean maximum 17mg/kg daily) or carbamazepine (5mg/kg initially, mean maximum 10mg/kg daily). Doses were increased until seizures were controlled or toxicity ensued. VA or CBZ was stopped in 12% and 13%, respectively, because of poor seizure control, and in 15% and 12% because of adverse side-effects. Approximately 50% of patients were completely free of seizures for the first 6 months, and 75% had been free for 12 months and 50% for at least two years, by the end of the trial. Primary generalized seizures responded better than partial seizures. VA and CBZ were equally effective; a higher remission rate for VA treated patients was not statistically significant. Most frequent VA side-effects were appetite and weight increase (11%), somnolence (10%), and alopecia (4%). CBZ cf VA caused a higher incidence of somnolence (20% v 10%), diplopia (4% v 0%), ataxia (4% v 0%), and rash (6% v 3%). (Verity CM, Hosking G, Easter DJ. A multicentre comparative trial of sodium valproate and carbamazepine in paediatric epilepsy. <u>Dev Med Child Neurol</u> Feb 1995;37:97-108). (Respond: Dr DJ Easter, Sanofi Winthrop Ltd, One Onslow St, Guildford, Surrey GU1 4YS, UK).

COMMENT. The incidence and type of side-effects are the main determinants for the choice of anticonvulsant in a particular patient. As with previous reports of comparative trials of phenobarbital, phenytoin, carbamazepine, and sodium valproate in both adults and children, there were no significant differences in efficacy between drugs regardless of seizure type, generalized tonic-clonic or partial. However, side-effects with VA and CBZ were significantly different. Weight gain was particularly troublesome with VA, while somnolence, dizziness, and ataxia required modification of dosage of CBZ. Severe rash noted in 10% of patients taking CBZ in previous adult studies necessitated drug withdrawal in only 3% of children in the present report. Carbamazepine-induced skin rash was reported in 10% of 335 children treated at Toyama Medical University, Japan, and additional reports are cited in <u>Progress in Pediatric Neurology II</u>, PNB Publ, 1994, pp107-109. -Editor. *Ped Neur Briefs* March 1995.

CARBAMAZEPINE TOXICITY WITH GENERIC SUBSTITUTION

Two 6-year-old children with carbamazepine (CBZ) toxicity, reported from the University of Miami School of Medicine, were found to have 22% and 41% increases in serum CBZ levels after substitution of Tegretol with the generic brand, Epitol. Substitution was necessary because of insurance company policies. Adverse effects included lethargy, ataxia, slurred speech, and nystagmus. When dosage was adjusted, symptoms of toxicity resolved. (Gilman JT, Alvarez LA, Duchowny M. Carbamazepine toxicity resulting from generic substitution. <u>Neurology</u> Dec 1993;<u>43</u>:2696-7). (Reprints: Dr Jamie Gilman, Clinical Pharmacology, Miami Children's Hospital, 6125 SW 31st Street, Miami, FL 33155).

COMMENT. Generic substitution of Tegretol has previously been associated with lowered serum levels of CBZ and seizure exacerbation. Reduced bioavailability is also reported with moisture-exposed CBZ, resulting in status epilepticus (Bell WL et al. <u>Epilepsia</u> Nov/Dec 1993;<u>34</u>:1102-4). Gilman et al have documented 2 cases of increased bioavailability with Epitol substitution, one of 4 generic carbamazepine products available in the US. In 1988, 70 million CBZ tablets were recalled because of bioinequivalence and clinical seizure exacerbation (Oles KS, Gal P. Bioequivalency revisited: Epitol versus Tegretol. Editorial. <u>Neurology</u> Dec 1993;<u>43</u>:2435-6).

Factors other than generic substitution may account for significant variations in CBZ concentrations, including interlot variability, exposure of drug to excessive heat or moisture, food and drug interactions, sample timing, and patient compliance. -Editor. *Ped Neur Briefs* Jan 1994.

CARBAMAZEPINE-RELATED STATUS EPILEPTICUS

High serum carbamazepine-epoxide concentrations were correlated with unexpected seizure exacerbation and partial status epilepticus in 6 young adults reported from the Marshfield Clinic, WI, and the Mayo Clinic, MN. All patients were mentally retarded. Ages at epilepsy onset ranged from 1 month to 11 years. Seizure exacerbation coincided with changes in drug combinations other than CBZ: VPA dosage had recently been increased in 4 patients and phenytoin had been discontinued in 1 who also took felbamate. CBZ dosage and serum levels had been therapeutic and stable for 1 to 14 years, whereas CBZ-10,11-epoxide levels exceeded an upper limit of 4 mcg/ml. CBZ-epoxide/CBZ ratios were greater than the accepted 0.2 in patients on polytherapy. Withholding CBZ was followed by seizure control within 2 to 3 days, and CBZ-epoxide toxicity (lethargy and ataxia) resolved. Withdrawal of VPA was also corrective in 1 patient who continued CBZ.(So EL et al. Seizure exacerbation and status epilepticus related to carbamazepine-10,11-epoxide. <u>Ann Neurol</u> June 1994;35:743-746). (Respond: Dr So, Epilepsy Service, Neurology, Mayo Clinic, 200 1st Street SW, Rochester, MN 55905).

COMMENT. CBZ-epoxide serum levels should be measured in carbamazepine-treated patients with unexplained seizure exacerbation or toxicity. Risk factors for CBZ-epoxide induced status and toxicity include high dose CBZ, combination therapies, and patients with mental retardation who often require polytherapy. Valproate, primidone, and felbamate combined with CBZ may increase levels of CBZ-epoxide by altering metabolic conversion or breakdown. In contrast, phenytoin promotes the conversion of the epoxide into an inactive form and reduces risk of CBZ-related toxicity and seizure exacerbation. Gabapentin, an AED having no drug interactions, should reduce the risk of these complications when polytherapy is considered essential. -Editor. *Ped Neur Briefs* July 1994.

RISK OF STEVENS-JOHNSON SYNDROME WITH CARBAMAZEPINE AND OTHER AEDs

An international case-controlled study of medication use and the risk of Stevens-Johnson syndrome or toxic epidermal necrolysis is reported by the Groupe Epidemiologie LY Stevens Johnson (ELYS), Department of Dermatology, and Department of Public Health, Universite Paris XII, Cretcil, France; and centers in Boston, US; Milan, Italy; Freiburg, Germany; Porto, Portugal; and Toronto, Canada. In 245 patients hospitalized for treatment, the relative risks with various drugs were as follows: carbamazepine 90, phenytoin 53, phenobarbital 45, valproic acid 25, compared to 172 for sulfonamide antibiotics, 6.7 for aminopenicillins, and 54 for corticosteroids. For many other drugs in common use, including contraceptive pills, benzodiazepines, and phenothiazines, the risk of serious skin reactions was not increased. (Roujeau JC et al. Medication use and the risk of Stevens-Johnson syndrome or toxic epidermal necrolysis. <u>N Engl J Med</u> Dec 14, 1995;333:1600-7). (Reprints: Dr Roujeau, Service de Dermatologie, Hopital H Mondor, 94010 Creteil, France).

COMMENT. The incidence of toxic epidermal necrolysis is estimated at 0.4 to 1.2 cases per million person-years and of Stevens-Johnson syndrome, at 1 to 6 cases per million person-years. None of the above drugs caused an excess risk greater than 5 cases per million users per week. The excess risks ranged from a low of 0.2 per million for aminopenicillins to a high of 4.5 per million for sulphonamides.

For the anticonvulsants, excess risks of these skin reactions ranged from a low of 0.7 for valproic acid to a high of 2.5 for carbamazepine. Despite the relatively low incidence, these skin syndromes may be fatal or lead to prolonged hospitalization and extreme discomfort. Patients introduced to any of the above anticonvulsants should be warned of the dangers of skin rash, especially within the first two weeks of treatment, and instructed to discontinue medication and report to a physician immediately at the first sign of reaction. Carbamazepine appears to be the worst offender, and valproic acid is not immune. Corticosteroids, a controversial treatment for Stevens-Johnson syndrome, carries a surprisingly increased risk of inducing the disorder. Benzodiazepines, having no excess risk of Stevens-Johnson syndrome, are the obvious agents to substitute when other anticonvulsants are discontinued due to these severe skin reactions.

Carbamazepine-induced skin rash is reviewed in <u>Progress in Pediatric Neurology II</u>, 1994, PNB Publishers, pp 107-109. A personal communication from Ciba-Geigy recorded 30 cases of carbamazepine-induced Stevens-Johnson syndrome, 8 erythema multiforme, and 5 toxic epidermal necrolysis (Lyell's syndrome) reported to the company in an eight year period, 1982-89. The above international study found 13 cases related to carbamazepine, and accounting for 5% of the total drug-induced severe cutaneous reactions, during a four year period, 1989-93. -Editor. *Ped Neur Briefs* Dec 1995.

CBZ AND PHENYTOIN THERAPY IN PREGNANCY AND FETAL THYROID LEVELS

The neonatal screening results of TSH and 17-hydroxyprogesterone (17-OHP) in 34 study neonates born to mothers exposed to AEDs during pregnancy and their matched controls were evaluated at the

Department of Paediatrics, Karolinska Institute, Stockholm, Sweden. The AEDs were carbamazepine 17, phenytoin 10, and polytherapy in 7 patients. In the group as a whole, there were no significant differences in the TSH and 17-OHP values in patients and controls. In a separate analysis of 6 infants exposed to polytherapy of 2 or more AEDs, there was a non-significant tendency to lower TSH and 17-OHP. Thyroid and steroid screening values were not correlated with AED plasma concentrations measured 1 month before delivery. (Wide K et al. Antiepileptic drug treatment during pregnancy and neonatal screening results. <u>Acta Paediatr</u> July 1996;85:870-1). (Respond: Dr K Wide, Department of Paediatrics, Karolinska Hospital, S-171 76 Stockholm, Sweden).

COMMENT. Carbamazepine and phenytoin induce metabolic enzymes and enhance metabolism of steroid and thyroid hormones. Low levels of thyroxine T4 and steroid hormones are reported in young adults treated with CBZ and PHT but not with valproate monotherapy. Serum T3 is unaffected by AEDs. (<u>Prog</u> Ped <u>Neur</u> <u>I</u>, 1991, pp126-7). The above study suggests that CBZ and PHT monotherapy during pregnancy may not alter fetal thyroid and steroid metabolism. Editor. *Ped Neur Briefs* Aug 1996.

LAMOTRIGINE-INDUCED SKIN RASH

Five of 68 consecutive children treated for epilepsy with lamotrigine developed a skin rash, one a Stevens-Johnson syndrome, in a report from Dalhousie University, and IWK Children's Hospital, Halifax, Nova Scotia, Canada. Two patients required intensive care. The interval between introduction of lamotrigine and the rash varied from 2 to 8 weeks. One child in whom the drug was reintroduced after 6 months had a recurrence of the rash within 30 minutes of a single small dose. In 4 patients taking concomitant therapy, the AEDs were continued during and after the lamotrigine-induced rash. (Dooley J, Camfield P et al. Lamotrigine-induced rash in children. <u>Neurology</u> Jan

1996;46:240-242). (Respond: Dr Joseph M Dooley, Neurology Division, IWK Children's Hospital, 5850 University Avenue, Halifax, Nova Scotia, Canada B3J 3G9).

COMMENT. Skin rash, especially Stevens-Johnson syndrome, is one of the most disturbing side-effects of AEDs. The introduction of any anticonvulsant, especially carbamazepine, should be accompanied by a parental warning of possible skin rash, particularly during the first 2 weeks of treatment. In my own view, a drug having once caused a serious skin rash should never be readministered to the sensitive individual. For reviews of carbamazepine-induced skin rash, including use of prednisone in treatment, see Progress in Pediatric Neurology II, PNB Publ, 1994, pp 107-109. -Editor. *Ped Neur Briefs* April 1996.

AEDS AND COGNITIVE FUNCTION

CARBAMAZEPINE, AUDITORY ERPs, AND COGNITIVE FUNCTION

The effects of carbamazepine (CBZ) on cognitive function were evaluated by using measurements of auditory event-related potentials (ERPs) and P300 latencies in 23 patients, aged 7 to 16 years, with benign childhood epilepsy and centrotemporal spikes (BCECT), at the Department of Pediatrics, Toyama Medical and Pharmaceutical University, Toyama, Japan. As the epilepsy was controlled at the initiation of therapy, and with increasing age, the P300 latency was at first shortened. During the course of therapy with CBZ, P300 latency was prolonged, and the age-corrected P300 latency showed a significant correlation with the serum CBZ level. The dose of CBZ ranged from 10-23 mg/kg/day (mean 15.8). The latency became shorter when CBZ was discontinued. (Naganuma Y et al. Auditory event-related potentials in benign childhood epilepsy with centrotemporal spike: The effects of carbamazepine. Clin Electroencephalogr Jan 1994;25:8-12). (Reprints: Yoshihiro Naganuma MD, Department of

Pediatrics, Toyama Medical and Pharmaceutical University, 2630 Sugitani, Toyama 930-01, Japan).

COMMENT. The major positive component of auditory event-related potentials, at a latency of 300 msec (P300) for rare tones (2000 Hz), has been correlated with cognitive function. Abnormalities in ERPs in patients with epilepsy, and particularly prolongation of P300 latency, have been ascribed to the effects of the seizures and to antiepileptic drug therapy. Various epileptic syndromes have shown different degrees of abnormality in the ERPs. In this study, after a transient beneficial response, the cumulative effect of carbamazepine was associated with a chronic impairment of cognitive function, as measured by changes in auditory event-related potentials.

Studies of the effects of carbamazepine on auditory brainstem responses (ABR) in 21 epileptic patients examined at the Institute of Clinical and Experimental Neurology, Thilisi, Republic of Georgia, demonstrated prolongation of ABR peak latencies and interpeak intervals. In addition, CBZ was associated with increases in peak latencies of middle-latency responses and slow cortical potentials. CBZ has suppressive influences on central auditory structures and the acoustic nerve. (Japaridze G et al. <u>Epilepsia</u> Nov/Dec 1993;<u>34</u>:1105-1109). -Editor. *Ped Neur Briefs* Jan 1994.

COGNITIVE EFFECTS OF PHT AND CBZ AFTER BRAIN TRAUMA

The effects of prophylactic anticonvulsant use of phenytoin (PHT) and carbamazepine (CBZ) on the cognitive and emotional status of a total of 80 brain trauma patients are compared and reported from the Division of Neurosurgery and Department of Neurology, St Louis University School of Medicine and School of Public Health. The median ages of the two groups were 40 (PHT patients) and 36 (CBZ) years. Both phenytoin and carbamazepine had some negative effects on performance measured by neuropsychological tests.

Effects generally were small in magnitude and were evident on tasks with motor and speed components. Earlier hypotheses that phenytoin had a more marked effect on higher-level cognitive skills than did carbamazepine were not confirmed. CBZ had a slightly greater negative effect than PHT on verbal fluency, verbal and visual memory, and complex attentional tasks. Patients receiving PHT were possibly more anxious compared to CBZ-treated patients. (Smith KR Jr et al. Neurobehavioral effects of phenytoin and carbamazepine in patients recovering from brain trauma: A comparative study. <u>Arch Neurol</u> July 1994;51:653-660).(Reprints: Dr Smith, Division of Neurosurgery, St Louis University, Box 15250, 3635 Vista at Grand, St Louis, MO 63110).

COMMENT. The neurobehavioral effects of phenytoin and carbamazepine were small and of limited functional significance. Most of the patients had no clinically detectable deficits while receiving either drug. Substantial variability was noted in drug serum concentrations at test sessions in individual patients, and between drug levels and test scores from subject to subject. Individual differences among patients and possible idiosyncratic responses to drugs are factors to be considered in the use or choice and evaluation of AEDs in brain trauma patients.

A previous randomized, double-blind study has shown that phenytoin prevents posttraumatic seizures only during the first week after severe head injury. (Temkin NR et al. <u>N Engl J Med</u> 1990;323:497). Some authorities have concluded that prophylactic drugs should be withheld, or administered only in a single loading dose, after severe head injury, minimizing the risk of idiosyncratic side-effects, especially exfoliative dermatitis. (<u>Progress in Pediatric Neurology</u>. Millichap JG, Ed, Chicago, PNB Publishers, 1991, pp 54-56). -Editor. *Ped Neur Briefs* Aug 1994.

CARBAMAZEPINE, BAEPS, AND COGNITION

The effects on brainstem auditory evoked

potentials (BAEPs) of carbamazepine in 18 and of valproate in 10 epileptic children were determined after 13 months of therapy at Istanbul University, Turkey. Blood levels were therapeutic and not associated with side effects. The peak latencies of waves I, II, and V, and interpeak intervals I-III and I-V were significantly prolonged following carbamazepine. Valproate monotherapy caused similar changes in BAEP but prolongation was not significant nor consistent. Carbamazepine suppresses auditory pathways peripherally, at the cochlea and/or auditory nerve and centrally, at the brainstem. (Yuksel A et al. Effects of carbamazepine and valproate on brainstem auditory evoked potentials in epileptic children. <u>Child's Nerv Syst</u> August 1995;11:474-477). (Respond: Dr Adnan Yuksel, Cingirakli Bostan Sok. 44/3, Deniz Apt., Aksaray, Istanbul, Turkey).

COMMENT. Similar findings have been reported in 21 epileptic patients treated with carbamazepine and studied at the Institute of Clinical and Experimental Neurology, Thilisi, Republic of Georgia. (Japaridze G et al. 1993; see <u>Ped Neur Briefs</u> January 1994). Carbamazepine suppressed both central auditory structures and the acoustic nerve. Chronic impairment of cognitive function, as measured by changes in auditory event-related potentials, was also reported in 23 patients treated with carbamazepine at Toyama Medical University, Japan (Naganuma Y et al, 1994; see <u>Ped Neur Briefs</u> Jan 1994). -Editor. *Ped Neur Briefs* Sept 1995.

CARBAMAZEPINE: A THERAPY FOR ADHD

The efficacy of carbamazepine (CBZ) in treatment of ADHD has been determined by meta-analysis of 10 reports from the international literature reviewed at Columbia University, St Luke's-Roosevelt Hospital Center, and New York University Medical Center. In 7 open studies involving a total of 189 patients with features of motor overactivity, impulsivity, and distractibility, 70% showed a marked improvement in target symptoms following treatment with CBZ for periods varying from 1 week to 8 years. Outcome was significantly correlated with duration of treatment; the longer the treatment the better the outcome. In 3 placebo-controlled, double-blind studies, 71% of 53 patients treated with CBZ were benefited whereas only 26% of 52 receiving placebo showed similar improvement in attentiveness and behavior. The difference was significant (p=.018). The most frequent side effects were sedation and skin rash occurring in 7.5% and 5.7% of CBZ-treated patients, respectively. (Silva RR et al. Carbamazepine use in children and adolescents with features of attention-deficit hyperactivity disorder: a meta-analysis. <u>J Am Acad Child Adolesc Psychiatry</u> March 1996;35:352-358). (Reprints: Dr Silva, St Luke's/Roosevelt Hospital Center, Division of Child and Adolescent Psychiatry, 411 W114th Street, Suite 3A, New York, NY 10025).

COMMENT. The authors concluded that carbamazepine may be an effective alternate treatment for ADHD. A response rate of 70% in both open and controlled studies is about the equivalent effectiveness of stimulant medication.

From a neurologist's perspective, the obvious questions would relate to the incidence of epilepsy and epileptiform EEG's in these patients selected for treatment with an anticonvulsant medication. Unfortunately, these data were not discussed and were tabulated for the entire sample and not the subsample with ADHD. My own meta-analysis of these data show that abnormal EEGs occurred in 69% of 57 patients in the controlled studies and in 82% of 50 patients in the one open study providing EEG data. Seizures were mentioned in 4 of the studies, affecting 13 plus patients, but the total number of patients affected was not given. The frequency of abnormal EEGs in these patients is considerably higher than that usually reported for ADHD. It seems that CBZ might be indicated for the treatment of ADHD symptoms in some patients with abnormal EEGs and/or a history of seizures. On a negative note, see <u>Progress in Pediatric Neurology II</u>, 1994, pp188-190, for references to cognitive impairment and impulsivity caused by CBZ treatment of epilepsy.

The cognitive effects of carbamazepine, phenobarbital, and valproate were compared in 73 children with newly diagnosed epilepsy studied at the National Cheng Kung University; Chi Nei Hospital; and Tainan Municipal Hospital, Tainan, Taiwan, ROC. (Chen Y-J, Kang W-M, Chin-Min So W, <u>Epilepsia</u> 1996;37:81-86). Only children treated with phenobarbital showed increased P300 latencies on auditory event-related potentials, which was inversely related to IQ scores after treatment for 6 to 12 months. WISC-R IQs and Bender-Gestalt scores were not significantly different in any of the groups before or after treatment. P300 latency was a more sensitive indicator of AED effects on cognitive function than the WISC-R and Bender-Gestalt.

Behavioral side effects of Gabapentin are reported in 7 children with base-line ADHD and developmental delays who were followed in the epilepsy program and in the Department of Child Psychiatry, Emory University, Atlanta, GA. (Lee DO et al. <u>Epilepsia</u> 1996;37:87-90). Tantrums, aggression, hyperactivity, and defiance were the most troublesome symptoms. The majority (64%) of intensified behaviors were similar to baseline ADHD symptoms; 21% were ODD and 8% were CD symptoms. New behaviors, not exhibited before gabapentin therapy, were ODD or CD. Behavioral side effects resolved after decrease or withdrawal of gabapentin. -Editor. *Ped Neur Briefs* March 1996.

COGNITIVE EFFECTS OF PHENOBARBITAL

Neurocognitive behavior in 9 children with various epilepsies was evaluated before and at 6 months after discontinuing phenobarbital monotherapy at the Department of Child Neurology, Instituto Nazionale Neurologico "Carlo Besta;" Milano, Italy. The patients had been seizure-free for at least 2 years. All of the scores on the WISC improved and the mean

Performance IQ was significantly higher after phenobarbital was withdrawn. Other tests showing significant improvement included the general information subtest on the Verbal IQ, picture arrangement on the Performance IQ, visual spatial memory, and visual-motoric and attentional skills, as measured by coding and the Trail Making test. (Riva D, Devoti M. Discontinuation of phenobarbital in children: Effects on neurocognitive behavior. <u>Pediatr Neurol</u> 1996;14:36-60). (Respond: Dr Riva, Department of Child Neurology, Instituto Neurologico "Carlo Besta;" 11 Via Celorio, 20133 Milano, Italy).

COMMENT. In this small number of children treated, phenobarbital appeared to have impaired attention, spatial memory, and visual/motor skills. The deficits were reversible and disappeared when phenobarbital was discontinued.

Drowsiness secondary to chronic antiepileptic drug therapy was assessed in 30 patients, using an EEG-based Awake Maintenance Task (AMT) measure, and reported from the Portland Veterans Affairs Medical Center, and Oregon Health Sciences University, Portland, Oregon. (Salinsky MC et al. <u>Epilepsia</u> 1996;37:181-187). Ability to maintain wakefulness was determined during a 6-min unstimulated trial. One third of AED-treated patients had >120 s of drowsiness in contrast to only 1 of 63 controls. Objective EEG drowsiness did not correlate with AED levels or performance measures. Untreated seizure patients had more complaints of lack of vigor despite absence of objective drowsiness on the AMT. Subjective reports of AED-related drowsiness may be unreliable. -Editor. *Ped Neur Briefs* April 1996.

COGNITIVE FUNCTION AND VALPROATE MONOTHERAPY

A test battery to assess neuropsychological and behavioral changes associated with anticonvulsant, particularly valproate, therapy in children is proposed from the Departments of Pediatrics (Neurology), and

Clinical Health and Psychology, University of Florida, Gainesville, FL. This includes 1) intellectual functioning (WISC-III, WPPSI-R), 2) verbal memory, sentence recall, story recall, and verbal learning (Wide Range Assessment of Memory and Learning-WRAML, 3) nonverbal memory, picture memory and visual learning-WRAML, 4) attention, digit span, continuous performance task-Paced Auditory Serial Addition Task-PASAT, 5) motor speed-finger tapping test, verbal fluency-Controlled Oral Word Association, and 6) problem behaviors- Child Behavior Check List. These tests were found to be sensitive to AED-induced cognitive changes, and some tests are repeatable to allow for frequent monitoring. (Legarda SB et al. Altered cognitive functioning in children with idiopathic epilepsy receiving valproate monotherapy. <u>J Child Neurol</u> July 1996;11:321-330). (Respond: Dr Stella B Legarda, Division of Neurology, Department of Pediatrics, University of Florida College of Medicine, PO Box 100296, JHM Health Center, Gainesville, FL 32610).

COMMENT. The authors comment that the cognitive effects of valproate reported in normal adult volunteers and adults with epilepsy cannot reliably be applied to children. There is a relative paucity of well-controlled studies assessing memory and attentional differences in pediatric epilepsy patients treated with valproate monotherapy. Reports that cognitively impaired children on valproate therapy improve with L-acetylcarnitine supplements requires further study.

In one study involving children with epilepsy previously untreated, significant positive correlations were found between serum levels of valproate and the sum of 5 memory tests at 1 month and at 6 months after starting valproate monotherapy. Phenytoin had no adverse effects, whereas carbamazepine serum levels showed a negative correlation with memory and reading scores. (Forsythe I et al. <u>Dev Med Child Neurol</u> 1991;33:524). For reviews of Cognitive Effects of Antiepileptic Drugs, see <u>Progress in Pediatric Neurology II,</u> Chicago, PNB Publ, 1994. -Editor. *Ped Neur*

Briefs Sept 1996.

CARBAMAZEPINE VS VALPROATE AND COGNITIVE FUNCTION

Effects of carbamazepine vs valproate on cognitive functioning in patients with previously unmedicated epilepsy were evaluated in a prospective, randomized, double-blind Veterans Affairs multicenter study. Patients with seizures showed deficits relative to a normal control group prior to AED therapy. No significant decline from baseline levels of neuropsychological performance was detected over 6- or 12-month treatment intervals for either drug. Patients with high serum VPA levels (mean, 94 mcg/mL) performed less well than controls on measures of concentration and memory. Subtle compromises of cognitive functioning following treatment with VPA or CBZ were suggested by absence of practice effects. (Prevey ML, Delaney RC, Cramer JA et al. Effect of valproate on cognitive functioning. Comparison with carbamazepine. <u>Arch Neurol</u> Oct 1996;53:1008-1016). (Reprints: Mary L Prevey PhD, Neurology 127, VA Medical Center, West Haven, CT 06516).

COMMENT. Carbamazepine and valproate monotherapies may have subtle effects on cognitive functioning. -Editor. *Ped Neur Briefs* Oct 1996.

MISCELLANEOUS AED SIDE-EFFECTS

CEREBELLAR ATROPHY WITH PHENYTOIN AND EPILEPSY

Cerebellar size measured by MRI was studied in a group of 36 adults (21 to 54 years, mean age 34 years) with intractable partial epilepsy treated with phenytoin longer than 4 years at the Epilepsy Center of the Long Island Jewish Medical Center, New Hyde Park, NY. Patients with IQ < 70, ethanol abuse, status epilepticus, and neurodegenerative disorders were excluded. Measurements were compared to a group of control patients examined because of headache or dizziness. Mean duration of phenytoin exposure was 14 years (range, 4 to 30 years). Mean maximum dosage was 450 mg daily (range, 300 to 700 mg). All patients had received various AEDs other than phenytoin. Moderate to severe cerebellar atrophy was found in 9 (25%) patients and mild atrophy in 12 (33%). The MRI was normal in 15 (42%) phenytoin exposed patients and in 33 (94%) controls. A correlation between cerebellar atrophy ratings and variables reflective of seizure severity or degree of phenytoin exposure could not be demonstrated. (Ney GC et al. Cerebellar atrophy in patients with long-term phenytoin exposure and epilepsy. <u>Arch Neurol</u> Aug 1994;51:767-771). (Reprints: Dr Ney, Dept Neurology, EEG Laboratory, Long Island Jewish Medical Center, New Hyde Park, NY 11042).

COMMENT. The exact cause of the cerebellar atrophy was not determined. The partial seizures, the phenytoin, or both factors were involved. Other known causes of cerebellar atrophy had been excluded. Monitoring the serum phenytoin may have provided a correlation between MRI ratings of atrophy and the possible effects of a chronic level of toxicity. Long-term treatment with phenytoin is generally safe provided optimal therapeutic levels are maintained. Current emphasis on monotherapy may lead to dosage increments above acceptable levels, with the attendant risk of a chronic subtle ataxia, especially in patients with refractory epilepsies. -Editor. *Ped Neur Briefs* Sept 1994.

APLASTIC ANEMIA WITH ETHOSUXIMIDE

An 8-year-old girl who developed aplastic anemia after 8 months ethosuximide therapy for absence seizures is reported from the Children's Medical College of Virginia, Richmond, VA. Blood counts and liver enzymes had been monitored 3 months before admission and were normal. She presented with fatigue, headache, streptococcal pharyngitis, hematuria, bruising, and petechiae. Allogeneic bone marrow transplantation was required and the child recovered. Without further AED therapy she has only occasional "staring spells" and the EEG is normal. A total of 8 cases of ethosuximide-associated aplastic anemia have been reported, and 5 died. (Massey GV, Myer EC et al. Aplastic anemia following therapy for absence seizures with ethosuximide. <u>Pediatr Neurol</u> July 1994;11:59-61). (Respond: Dr Massey, PO Box 980121, MCV Station, Richmond, VA 23298).

COMMENT. Ethosuximide-related aplastic anemia is rare but has a high mortality. Monthly blood counts have been recommended, but their predictive value is questioned by the authors. Fever, rash, bruising, and petechiae should certainly require immediate investigation. -Editor. *Ped Neur Briefs* Sept 1994.

SERUM LIPIDS AND LONG-TERM ANTIEPILEPTIC THERAPY

Serum levels of total cholesterol (TC), high-density lipoprotein cholesterol (HDL-C), low-density lipoprotein cholesterol (LDL-C), very LDL-C, and triglycerides (TGs) were determined in 119 children with epilepsy treated with AEDs for 7 months to 10 years (mean, 5.8 years) and in 125 healthy controls at the Hospital General de Galicia, Clinico Universitario, Santiago de Compostela, Spain. In patients receiving carbamazepine (58) or phenobarbital (22), mean TC, HDL-C, and LDL-C levels were significantly higher than in the control group. Serum TC exceeded the accepted safe level of 200 mg/dl in 41% of carbamazepine-treated children and in 50% of those receiving phenobarbital, compared to only 12% of controls. In those on valproic acid (39), mean TC and LDL-C levels and mean TC/HDL-C and LDL-C/HDL-C ratios were significantly lower than controls. (Eiris JM et al. Effects of long-term treatment with antiepileptic drugs on serum lipid levels in children with epilepsy. <u>Neurology</u> June 1995;45:1155-1157). (Reprints: Dr M Castr-Gago, Department of Pediatrics, Division of Pediatric Neurology, Hospital General de Galicia, 15705 Santiago de Compostela, Spain).

COMMENT. Serum cholesterol levels may need to be monitored in children treated with carbamazepine or phenobarbital for epilepsy. -Editor. *Ped Neur Briefs* July 1995.

CHOREOATHETOSIS WITH GABAPENTIN

A 37-year-old man with severe mental retardation since birth and intractable epilepsy treated with AED polytherapy developed choreoathetosis and orofacial dyskinesia within 5 days of introducing gabapentin (GBP) at the Department of Neurology, West Virginia University, Morgantown, WV. Diphenhydramine 25 mg IV resulted in improvement and movements resolved within 2 days of discontinuing GBP. Other AEDs were continued and dosages were unchanged. (Buetefisch CM et al. Choreoathetotic movements: a possible side effect of gabapentin. <u>Neurology</u> March 1996;46:851-852). (Reprints: Dr Catherin M Buetefisch, Department of Neurology, Robert C Byrd Health Sciences Center, West Virginia University, Morgantown, WV 26506).

COMMENT. AED-induced movement disorder is rare, but is described with phenytoin, carbamazepine, ethosuximide, and with felbamate. This is the first reported case with gabapentin.

Exacerbation of seizures in Lennox-Gastaut syndrome by gabapentin is described in a 14-year old boy from the Epilepsy Center, Swedish Medical Center, Seattle, WA. (Vossler DG. <u>Neurology</u> March 1996;46:852). Gabapentin (GBP), 300 - 600 mg tid, was added to valproate and methsuximide therapy, and absence and myoclonic seizures were markedly exacerbated. A generalized tonic-clonic seizure also occurred for the first time since undergoing corpus callosotomy at age 9 years. When GPA was discontinued over 4 days and phenytoin was added, no seizures recurred in the subsequent 7 months follow-up. -Editor. *Ped Neur Briefs* April 1996.

AED/ORAL CONTRACEPTIVE INTERACTIONS

A national survey to determine obstetricians' and neurologists' awareness of oral contraceptive (OC) and antiepileptic drug (AED) interactions and the risk of birth defects in infants of AED-treated women with epilepsy was conducted by mailed questionnaire at the Departments of Neurology and Psychiatry, Johns Hopkins University, Baltimore, MD. Responses were received from 160 (16%) neurologists and 147 (15%) obstetricians in 47 states. Most neurologists (80%) knew that phenytoin, carbamazepine, and phenobarbital interfered with OCs, but only 38% knew that valproic acid does not interfere with OCs. Most obstetricians knew that phenytoin interfered with OCs (77%), but fewer were aware of interactions with other AEDs and only 29% knew that valproic acid was non-reactive. Both specialties were generally ignorant of the effects on OCs of ethosuximide, gabapentin, and felbamate. OC failure and accidental pregnancies in patients taking AEDs were reported by 27% of neurologists and 21% of obstetricians. Fewer than half of neurologists (41%) and obstetricians (41%) had their patients adjust OC doses when taking AEDs. Neurologists (44%) often underestimated the risk for AED-induced birth defects (actual risk 4-6%), whereas the risk estimate for most obstetricians varied from 1 to 10%. Some respondents guessed the risk was 50%. Only 3% of neurologists and 5% of obstetricians counselled women taking AEDs to avoid pregnancy. (Krauss GL et al. Antiepileptic medication and oral contraceptive interactions: a national survey of neurologists and obstetricians. <u>Neurology</u> June 1996;46:1534-1539). (Reprints: Dr Gregory L Krauss, Johns Hopkins Hospital, Meyer 2-147, 600 N Wolfe Street, Baltimore, MD 21287).

COMMENT. The authors conclude that many women in the US suffering from epilepsy are at risk for unplanned pregnancies because their physicians are not sufficiently aware of the interactions of antiepileptic drugs and oral contraceptives. They admit that the survey may have overestimated the lack of physician awareness of AED/OC interactions because of the small number of respondents and a possible response bias. Enzyme-inducing AEDs, including carbamazepine, phenytoin, phenobarbital, primidone, and ethosuximide, decrease the effectiveness of OCs by increasing metabolism of synthetic estrogens and lowering synthetic sex hormone levels. Valproic acid, gabapentin, and vigabatrin do not induce hepatic metabolism and are unlikely to interfere with OCs. Valproic acid has not been asociated with accidental pregnancies when administered as monotherapy. Irregular or breakthrough menstrual bleeding was used as a sign to increase OC doses in women taking enzyme-inducing AEDs. -Editor. *Ped Neur Briefs* July 1996.

SURGERY IN EPILEPSY

SURGERY FOR PARTIAL SEIZURES AND CORTICAL DYSPLASIA

The role of ictal or continuous epileptogenic discharges (I/CEDs), recorded during intraoperative electrocorticography (ECoG), in the planning of surgical resection for patients with cortical dysplastic lesions (CDyLs) and intractable partial seizures was evaluated at the Montreal Neurological Institute, the Epilepsy Surgery Program, Porto-Alegre, Brazil, and the Chonbuk National Hospital, Chonju, Korea. I/CEDs, consisting of repetitive electrographic seizures, repetitive bursting discharges, or continuous rhythmic spiking, were present in 23 of 34 patients (67%) with seizures associated with CDyLs, and in 1 of 40 (2.5%) whose partial epilepsy was associated with other types of structural leasions. A favorable surgical outcome was obtained in 75% of patients when the cortical dysplastic tissue showing I/CEDs was completely excised, whereas the outcome was poor if areas containing I/CEDs remained in situ. The authors advocate the removal as much as possible of the cortical dysplastic lesion that is visible and also those areas showing I/CEDs on acute

ECoG. (Palmini A, Gambardella A, Andermann F et al. Intrinsic epileptogenicity of human dysplastic cortex as suggested by corticography and surgical results. <u>Ann Neurol</u> April 1995;37:476-487). (Respond: Dr Palmini, Servico de Neurologia, Hospital Sao Lucas-PUCRS, Av Ipiranga 6690, Porto Alegre RS, Brasil CEP 90610-000).

COMMENT. The extent of surgical excision for optimal seizure control in these patients was determined by the intraoperative electrocorticographic as well as visual identification of intrinsically epileptogenic dysplastic cortical tissue. Completeness of excision of tissue showing I/CEDs was important for seizure control. The authors found that dysplastic cortex was more epileptogenic than other structural lesions, and patients with cortical dysplasia have a greater tendency to intractable seizures and a higher incidence of status epilepticus than those with other lesions. Previous reports from Montreal have found status epilepticus in 30% of patients with cortical dysplasia compared to 3% with epilepsy caused by supratentorial tumors. Life-threatening focal status epilepticus due to occult cortical dysplasia, not revealed by MRI, was successfully treated by surgical excision in 4 patients (Desbiens R, Andermann F et al, 1993; see <u>Progress in Pediatric Neurology II</u>, 1994, p292). -Editor. *Ped Neur Briefs* May 1995.

VAGAL NERVE STIMULATION FOR REFRACTORY EPILEPSY

The tolerance and efficacy of periodic left vagal nerve (VN) stimulation in 12 children with medically intractable epilepsies are reported from the Sections of Neurology and Neurosurgery, Children's Mercy Hospital, Kansas City, MO. At 2 to 14 months follow-up, 5 patients had a better than 90% reduction in number of monthly seizures, and the overall status of the child was improved on global evaluation ratings. Antiepileptic drugs were reduced after VN stimulation in 4 patients. No serious adverse effects were noted. Several patients experienced transient coughing with initial activation of the stimulator, and some had vocal hoarseness. Credit card inactivation occurs when the activating magnet is stored in the same pocket with the card. The therapeutic response to VNS appeared to be superior and was achieved more rapidly in children than in adults. (Murphy JV et al. Left vagal nerve stimulation in children with refractory epilepsy. Preliminary observations. Arch Neurol September 1995;52:886-889). (Reprints: Dr Murphy, Section of Neurology, Children's Mercy Hospital, 2401 Gilham Rd, Kansas City, MO 64108).

COMMENT. The advantages of vagal nerve stimulation compared to AEDs in children with refractory seizures were listed as follows: 1) no deterioration of response, 2) no allergic rashes, 3) no cognitive deficits, 4) no drug interactions, and 5) complete compliance. The device was well tolerated and free of serious complications. See Progress in Pediatric Neurology II, 1994, pp132-3, for further reports on vagal nerve stimulation for control of epilepsy. -Editor. *Ped Neur Briefs* Oct 1995.

RASMUSSEN ENCEPHALITIS: SURGICAL BENEFITS

Social communication, language, and PET glucose utilization were studied before and after right hemispherectomy in four children with Rasmussen encephalitis (RE) at the University of California, Los Angeles. Improved social communication and language following surgery was related to age at onset, duration of illness, and reversibility of the hypometabolism in the nonresected prefrontal cortex. Improvements in communication and language were not accompanied by improved IQ scores. Early surgical treatment might lessen the degree of deficit in communication and language skills. Onset of RE after age 11 years is associated with less social communication deficit. (Caplan R, Curtiss S, Chugani HI, Vinters HV. Pediatric Rasmussen encephalitis: social communication. language, PET, and pathology before and after hemispherectomy. Brain Cogn Oct 1996;32:45-66).

(Reprints: Dr R Caplan, Neuropsychiatric Institute, 760 Westwood Plaza, Los Angeles, CA 90024).

COMMENT. Right hemisphere damage is associated with delays in language development. Surgery performed early to control seizures prevents further deterioration in intellectual functioning and results in improved language and communication skills. -Editor. *Ped Neur Briefs* Nov 1996.

NON-EPILEPTIC PAROXYSMAL DISORDERS

BREATH-HOLDING SPELLS

The clinical characteristics, types, diagnosis, and management of breath-holding spells are reviewed from The Department of Pediatrics (Neurology), Park Nicollet Medical Center, Minneapolis, MN. There are two forms, pallid and cyanotic. *Pallid breath-holding spells* (BHS) result from vagal hyperresponsiveness, following a sudden, unexpected, unpleasant stimulus, usually a mild head injury. Cardiac monitoring reveals prolonged asystoles, which can also be induced by ocular compression, and is accompanied by syncope or an anoxic seizure. Vagal cardiac inhibition with cerebral anoxia is the pathophysiology of pallid BHS. *Cyanotic breath-holding spells* result from a complex interplay of hyperventilation followed by apnea in expiration, and increased intrathoracic pressure. Whereas pallid BHS occur after injury, cyanotic BHS are precipitated by anger. Diagnosis may be confirmed by EEG with ocular compression and cardiac monitoring. A pallid spell is associated with cardiac asystole and EEG hypersynchronous slowing. Cyanotic spells have similar EEG changes without bradycardia or asystole. Prolonged QT syndrome is a rare but serious cause of anoxic seizure, induced by exercise, injury, or fright. Cerebral hypoxia may result from ventricular tachycardia. More protracted loss of consciousness with hypotension may indicate a cardiac pathology. A more protracted seizure following a BHS may represent an anoxic-epilepsy, requiring anticonvulsant therapy. Spontaneous remission of BHSs is to be expected, but parents require frequent reassurance about the benign nature of the spells. (Breningstall GN. Breath-holding spells. <u>Pediatr Neurol</u> Feb 1996;14:91-97). (Respond: Dr Breningstall, Pediatric Subspecialties, Park Nicollet Medical Center, 910 East 26th St, Suite 325, Minneapolis, MN 55404).

COMMENT. Although anticonvulsant therapy is sometimes advisable when the convulsive episode is prolonged and represents an anoxic-epilepsy, traditional therapy will not generally prevent the breath-holding spell. Perhaps some of the newer antiepileptic medications should be tried in children with numerous attacks. The therapeutic nihilistic approach to BHS practiced by many physicians is often difficult for a parent to accept. An iron deficiency anemia may be an underlying causative factor in about 20% of cases of breath-holding (Holowach J, Thurston DL. <u>N Eng J Med</u> 1963;268:21). Neurologic deficits with iron deficiency anemia are discussed in <u>Progress in Pediatric Neurology</u> 1991, PNB Publ, pp397-8.

Apnea and bradycardia during epileptic seizures were studied at the Telemetry Unit, National Hospital for Neurology and Neurosurgery, Queen Square, London. (Nashef L et al. <u>J Neurol Neurosurg Psychiatry</u> March 1996;60:297-300). Apnea occurred in 20 of 47 clinical seizures and 10 of 17 patients; it was generally central, but obstructive apnea occurred in 3 patients. Oxyhemoglobin saturation dropped to <85%, and tachycardia was common. Bradycardia/sinus arrest was documented with a change in respiration in 4 patients. Similar mechanisms involving cardiorespiratory reflexes are suggested in relation to cases of sudden death in epilepsy. -Editor. *Ped Neur Briefs* May 1996.

CHAPTER **2**

MIGRAINE AND OTHER HEADACHES

OVERVIEW OF RECENT ADVANCES

Joseph Maytal, M.D.
Schneider Children's Hospital, New Hyde Park, NY.

During the past three years, the most significant progress in the understanding and treatment of migraine headaches in children has been made in the following areas: migraine definition in children, prevalence of migraine and other headaches in children, brain imaging and EEG evaluation of headaches, and finally the introduction of sumatriptan as a novel anti-migraine medication.

The utility of the International Headache Society (IHS) criteria for the definition of migraine in children has been challenged because of the lack of agreement between expert clinical and IHS diagnoses in some studies. These studies have reported levels of agreement ranging from 44 to 61% (Gallai et al.

Headache 1995;35:143-153; Seshia et al. Dev Med Child Neurol 1994;36:419-428; Maytal et al. Neurology in press). The apparently restrictive nature of the IHS criteria decreases their utility in clinical practice, where a clinician must assign a diagnosis as a prelude to treatment. Clinical reports continue to indicate that in many children migraine headaches are shorter than in adults. These results led many to argue that the minimal headache duration required for the diagnosis of migraine in children should be reduced (Gallae et al. Headache 1995;35:143-153; Wober-Bingal et al. Cephalalgia 1995;15:13-21; Winner et al. Headache 1995;35:407-410; Maytal et al. Neurology in press).

A number of population-based studies of headache prevalence in children have been published over the last three years (Abu-Arefeh and Russel. BMJ 1994;309:765-769; Sillanpaa. Headache Classif & Epidemiol 1994;273-281). Stewart et al. (J Clin Epidemiol 1995;48:269-280) conducted a meta-analysis of the prevalence of migraine reported in the literature. Of the 58 published reports on migraine prevalence, the authors identified 24 which met final criteria for inclusion in their study. This review suggested that much of the variation among studies is determined by the age and gender of the sample and the case definition that the study uses. Abu-Arefeh et al found that migraine is a common cause of headache among school children in Aberdeen, Scotland, with prevalence of 11%. This is more than twice the prevalence reported in previous pediatric studies. Raieli et al (Cephalalgia 1995;15:5-12) assessed the prevalence of migraine headache in an epidemiologic survey of 11 to 14 year-old students; overall, migraine prevalence was 3%. It is not clear why Raieli's estimates are lower than those of other studies in this age group.

Several studies done in the 1980s suggested that migraine prevalence may be increasing in adults. Two identical cross-sectional studies of migraine prevalence in school children showed that the prevalence of migraine in seven-year-olds had increased from 1.9% in 1974 to 5.7% in 1992, both in boys and in girls. The highest increases occurred among children exposed to social instability and stress (Sillanpaa. <u>Headache</u> 1996;36:466-470). A putative cause would have to influence both children and adults in the US and Finland over the past two decades. Though the causes are not clear, given the enormous burden of headaches, these findings mandate additional studies. (see p 187-90)

The utility of brain imaging (CT and MRI) in the evaluation of children with headaches was evaluated by Maytal et al (<u>Pediatrics</u> 1995;96:413-416) and others. It was concluded that brain imaging has very limited value in the evaluation of childhood headaches in the absence of clinical signs of structural brain lesions. MRI is warranted in those with atypical recurrent headaches, in those with recent changes in the character of the headaches, in patients with abnormal neurological findings, and in the younger age groups. Headache as the sole manifestation of brain tumor is a rare event, and the risk of an adverse reaction to contrast medium with CT, or with heavy sedation for MRI, in the young child must be weighed against the benefits of the study. (see p 186).

Two articles published during the last two years evaluated the clinical utility of the EEG in children with headaches (Gronseth and Greenberg. <u>Neurology</u> 1995;45:1263-1267; Kramer et al. <u>Brain Dev</u> 1994;16:304-308). Both studies concluded that EEG is not indicated in routine evaluation of pediatric patients with headaches. EEG may be helpful in a small subgroup of patients with headaches and symptoms suggestive of seizures. (p 183).

In the treatment of migraine, the most important progress over the last three years was the FDA approval of sumatriptan. Sumatriptan is a potent selective serotonin receptor (5HT1) agonist. Administered orally or via subcutaneous or intranasal routes, the drug has proved highly effective in adults with migraine (Sargent. <u>Neurology</u> 1995;45(8 suppl 7):510-514). Significant adverse reactions and limitations to its clinical efficacy include the occurrence of chest symptoms suggesting cardiac ischemia. The safety and effectiveness of sumatriptan in children has not been established, since most clinical trials excluded patients less than 18 years of age. In two open labeled studies of sumatriptan administered subcutaneously to patients <18 years, the response was high (Linder. <u>Headache</u> 1996;36:417-422; MacDonald. <u>Headache</u> 1994;34:582); the studies employed different criteria to define efficacy and the doses used differed by ten-fold. Further studies, preferably double-blind, placebo-controlled, are needed to ascertain the efficacy and tolerability of sumatriptan in children. *Joseph Maytal, M.D.*

DEFINITION AND DIAGNOSIS

INTERNATIONAL HEADACHE SOCIETY CRITERIA

A prospective study involving 72 children with recurrent headache, designed to determine whether the diagnosis of headache type made intuitively by each of 4 neurologists would have met the IHS diagnostic criteria, is reported from the Department of Pediatrics and Child Health, Children's Hospital and University of Manitoba, Winnipeg, and the Division of Pediatric Neurology, Children's Hospital, Calgary, Canada. The intuitive clinical diagnoses were as follows: migraine without aura (44 cases), migraine with aura (11), migraine and tension-type (11), tension-type (3), post-traumatic (2), and sinus (1). Features considered were location (unilateral or bilateral), quality (pulsating or pressing), intensity, exercise aggravation, nausea, vomiting, photophobia, phonophobia, and age. Dietary triggers were recognized in 8 of 44 children with migraine without aura, in 2 of 11 with migraine with aura, in 3 of 11 with combined migraine and tension headache, and in none with tension headaches. Family history of migraine in a first-degree relative occurred in 26 of 44 with migraine without aura, and 5 of 11 with migraine with aura. The intuitive diagnosis was completely concordant with the IHS criterion diagnosis in 61%, partially concordant in 31% and at complete variance in 8%. (Seshia SS et al. International headache society criteria and childhood headache. <u>Dev Med Child Neurol</u> May 1994;36:419-428). (Respond: Professor Shashi S Seshia, AE 208, Children's Hospital, 840 Sherbrook St, Winnipeg, Manitoba R3A 1S1, Canada).

COMMENT. The authors concluded that the IHS criteria (1988), intended mainly for adults, can also be applied to children with recurrent headaches, but with some reservations. Revisions to the criteria should take into consideration the inability of children to describe the qualities and location of pain precisely. Children's reports of the quality of headache pain are variable and may be exaggerated in the 9 to 11 age group and minimized in the 6 to 8 year olds (see <u>Ped Neur Briefs</u> April 1991). Prevalence of migraine diagnosis by IHS criteria also favored Caucasian over African-American children, 61% to 35%, in a more recent study. Minority children were less likely to present with vomiting, lateralized pain, or food as a precipitant of headache. (<u>Ped Neur Briefs</u> Nov 1993). The IHS criteria should be modified to increase their sensitivity to children and adolescents and also to racial differences in symptomatology. (<u>Progress in Pediatric Neurology II</u>, Chicago, PNB Publ, 1994). -Editor. *Ped Neur Briefs* June 1994.

INTER-OBSERVER AGREEMENT IN HEADACHE DIAGNOSIS

Inter-observer agreement among 4 pediatric neurologists in the diagnosis of recurrent headaches in 40 children, ages 4 to 17 years (mean 10 years), was prospectively assessed at the University of Manitoba, Winnipeg, Canada. Referring to letters containing reports of the child's symptoms, history and examination, the headache diagnoses were checked off on a data sheet, listing up to 12 types. Agreement in headache diagnoses between pairs of neurologists ranged from 45% to 78%. Agreement was 76% when both neurologists in a pair diagnosed single headache types, but only 4% when multiple diagnoses were applied. (Wolstein JR, Seshia SS et al. Inter-observer agreement in the diagnosis of childhood headache. <u>Headache</u> Sept 1994;34:467-470). (Respond: SS Seshia MD, Section of Pediatric Neurosciences, AE-208 Children's Hospital, 840 Sherbrook St, Winnipeg, MB, R3A 1S1, Canada).

COMMENT. Agreement among pediatric neurologists was relatively good provided that a single headache type was diagnosed. The International Headache Society recommendations for classification of all headache types in a single patient may lower inter-observer agreement on diagnoses in children. For purpose of evaluation of pharmacological, dietary, or psychosocial treatment regimens, selection of patients with a single headache diagnosis is important. The validity of the classification criteria for childhood headache may need to be re-examined. -Editor. *Ped Neur Briefs* Oct 1994.

ASPARTAME-INDUCED HEADACHE

A double-blind crossover study in 32 subjects with self-identified aspartame-induced headache is reported from the University of Washington School of Medicine, Seattle, WA. Volunteers were randomized to receive aspartame (30 mg/kg/d) and placebo in a 2-treatment, 4-period crossover design. Each period was 7 days. Subjects reported significantly more headaches during aspartame treatment (on 33% of the days) compared with placebo (24%). Headache triggered by aspartame was particularly frequent [p < 0.001] in subjects who were "very sure" that aspartame had caused them headaches previously. One-fourth of the subjects withdrew from the study, complaining of too frequent or severe headaches or sleep disturbance. A number of individuals had declined inclusion in the study because of the severity of their reaction to aspartame. (Van Den Eeden SK et al. Aspartame ingestion and headaches: A randomized crossover trial. <u>Neurology</u> Oct 1994;44:1787-1793). (Dr SK Van Den Eeden, Division of Research, Kaiser Permanente Medical Care Program, 3505 Broadway, Oakland, CA 94611).

COMMENT. The authors conclude that aspartame causes headaches in a subset of adults with self-identified aspartame-induced headaches. An underestimation of the adverse effect of aspartame in some studies may reflect differences in subject susceptibility, exclusion of specific responders, and concomitant ingestion of other food or drink. Children with migraine may be more responsive to dietary triggers than adults. (<u>Progress in Pediatric Neurology I & II</u>, Chicago, PNB Publ, 1991, 1994). -Editor. *Ped Neur Briefs* Nov 1994.

BENIGN NOCTURNAL ALTERNATING HEMIPLEGIA

Two brothers who developed recurrent attacks of alternating hemiplegia arising out of sleep, distinguishable from classical alternating hemiplegia of childhood (AHC), are reported from Montreal Neurological and Children's Hospitals, and Children's Hospital of Western Ontario, London, ON, Canada. Both infants awoke screaming 1 1/2 hrs after falling asleep and were paralyzed on one side. After returning to sleep and awakening in the morning, they had recovered. Similar episodes recurred with increasing frequency. Features such as hypotonia, dystonia, and eye movements, characteristic of AHC, were absent. Development remained normal. Both parents had migraine. (Andermann E et al. Benign familial nocturnal alternating hemiplegia of childhood. <u>Neurology</u> Oct 1994;44:1812-1814). (Respond: Dr Eva Andermann, Division of Neurogenetics, Montreal Neurological Hospital, 3801 University Street, Montreal, PQ, Canada H3A 2B4).

COMMENT. This apparently benign, familial form of alternating hemiplegia adds one more variety to the growing list of alternating hemiplegias of childhood. It is distinguished from the more common sporadic, classic form of AHC with a poor prognosis. The disorder is usually classified as a migraine variant. (see <u>Progress</u>

in Pediatric Neurology II, 1994, pp150-1, for a previous report and comment). -Editor. *Ped Neur Briefs* Nov 1994.

HEMICRANIA CONTINUA

Ten new patients and 24 previous reports of hemicrania continua are reviewed from the Albert Einstein College of Medicine, and the Montefiore Medical Center, Bronx, NY. A 20-year-old man presented with an 8-year history of unilateral, right-sided headaches occurring in discrete bouts of continuous pain each lasting 6 months, approximately once yearly. The pain was constant and moderate in severity, with superimposed exacerbations of more severe pain, recurring two to three times daily, and associated with ipsilateral conjunctival injection, ptosis, lacrimation, and rhinorrhea. The patient would rock in a chair, pace, or hit his head against a wall in an effort to allay the pain. Treatments with carbamazepine, propanolol, verapamil, and lithium were of no benefit, whereas indomethacin 25 mg TID resulted in immediate and complete relief. Headaches recurred within 2 days on two occasions when treatment was discontinued during the 6-month pain cycle. Most patients were adults, but the onset was at 12 years of age in one and 18 years in one other. (Newman LC, Lipton RB, Solomon S. Hemicrania continua: Ten new cases and a review of the literature. Neurology Nov 1994;44:2111-2114). (Reprints: Dr Lawrence C Newman, Department of Neurology, Montefiore Medical Center, 111 East 210th Street, Bronx, NY 10467).

COMMENT. Hemicrania continua (HC) is distinguished from cluster headache by the continuous, moderate background pain, and when present, the relatively mild autonomic features. The authors described three types of HC: 1) a remitting or noncontinuous form (15%); 2) an unremitting form evolved from the remitting form (32%); and 3) an unremitting form with continuous headache lasting for years (53%). The majority (85%) have typically continuous, unremitting attacks. The diagnosis is important because of the remarkable response to indomethacin. -Editor. *Ped Neur Briefs* Dec 1994.

PERSISTENT VISUAL PHENOMENA IN MIGRAINE

Ten patients with migraine and persistent positive visual phenomena lasting months to years are reported from the University of Pennsylvania, Scheie Eye Institute, the Children's Hospital of Philadelphia, University of Miami Bascom Palmer Eye Institute, and the Cleveland Clinic, OH. Ages ranged from 9 to 67 years but visual phenomena were very similar in their simplicity, quality, and involvement of the entire visual field. They consisted of diffuse small particles, such as TV static, snow, lines of ants, dots, and rain. Treatment with various medications was of no benefit. (Liu GT et al. Persistent positive visual phenomena in migraine. Neurology April 1995;45:664-668). (Reprints: Dr GT Liu, Division of Neuro-Ophthalmology, Department of Neurology, Hospital of the University of Pennsylvania, 3400 Spruce Street, Philadelphia, PA 19104).

COMMENT. Visual processing in 12 migraineurs has been studied at the Mass General Hospital (Wray SH et al. Brain Feb 1995;118:25-35). An inherited abnormal threshold to visual stimuli is suggested. The high speed of the migraineur's brain in discerning a single target in low-level visual tasks is consistent with an oversensitivity to visual stimuli. -Editor. *Ped Neur Briefs* May 1995.

CEREBRAL VEIN THROMBOSIS, SYSTEMIC LUPUS, AND HEADACHE

Three girls, ages 11, 14, and 17, with systemic lupus erythematosus, who had headache and were diagosed with cerebral vein thrombosis are reported from the Hospital for Sick Children, University of Toronto, and the Children's Hospital, McMaster University, Hamilton, Canada. Diagnosis was established by CT and MRI without need of angiography. Cerebral infarct occurred in one patient when diagnosis was delayed. All patients received low-dose oral anticoagulation and treatment for lupus and none had further thrombotic events during 10-18 month follow-up. (Uziel Y et al. Cerebral vein thrombosis in childhood systemic lupus erythematosus. J Pediatr May 1995;126:722-727). (Reprints: ED Silverman MD, Division of Rheumatology, The Hospital for Sick Children, 555 University Ave, Toronto, Ontario, Canada M5G 1X8).

COMMENT. Headache is the chief presenting symptom of cerebral venous thrombosis. These are of the tension or vascular type in 25%, but migraine headache and those associated with increased intracranial pressure also occur. Associated seizures, papilledema, and hemiparesis are also suggestive. A severe, persistent, throbbing headache, unresponsive to analgesics, points to a possible cerebral vein thrombosis, and is an indication for CT examination. -Editor. *Ped Neur Briefs* June 1995.

MIGRAINE AND ISCHEMIC STROKE

The relation between migraine and ischemic stroke in 72 young women aged under 45 and 173 controls was investigated at five hospital in Paris and suburbs. A questionnaire based on the International Headache Society's criteria for headache and migraine was used in telephone interviews. Migraine and ischemic stroke were strongly associated. Migraine was diagnosed in 60% of patients with stroke compared to 30% of controls. Women with migraine had a more than threefold increased risk of ischemic stroke (19 per 100,000 per year) compared with women without migraine (6 per 100,000 per year). The risk of stroke was higher in cases with aura than in those without aura. It was increased for migrainous women who used oral contraceptives or who were heavy smokers (>20 cigarettes/day). (Tzourio C et al. Case-control study of migraine and risk of ischaemic stroke in young women. BMJ 1 April 1995;310:830-833). (Respond: Dr Tzourio,

INSERM U 360, Recherches Epidemiol en Neurologie et Psychopathologie, Cedex 94807 Villejuif, France).

COMMENT. The authors concluded that despite a relatively small risk of ischemic stroke, smoking and the use of oral contraceptives should be discouraged or limited in young women with migraine. It was not known whether the increased risk of stroke related to all young migrainous women or only to a subgroup that remains to be defined. -Editor. *Ped Neur Briefs* June 1995.

HEADACHE AND GINSENG-RELATED CERBRAL ARTERITIS

A 28-year-old woman who had a severe headache after ingesting a large quantity of ethanol-extracted ginseng was diagnosed with cerebral arteritis in the Department of Neurology, Chang Gung Memorial Hospital, Keelung, Taiwan. Ginseng root 25 gm stewed in rice wine was taken for fatigue associated with sore throat. An explosive headache with nausea and vomiting developed 8 hours later and was temporarily relieved by acetaminophen. Smaller quantities of ginseng had never caused headache. CT showed increased density over the falx, suggestive of subarachnoid hemorrhage. Cerebral angiograms revealed multiple areas of alternating focal constriction and dilatation (beading) in anterior and posterior cerebral arteries and superior cerebellar artery, consistent with arteritis. The headache gradually resolved within 10 days. (Ryu S-J, Chien Y-Y. Ginseng-associated cerebral arteritis. <u>Neurology</u> April 1995;45:829-830). (Reprints: Dr Shan-Jin Ryu, Department of Neurology, Chang Gung Memorial Hospital, 199, Tung Hwa North Road, Taipei 105, Taiwan).

COMMENT. The temporal association between the ingestion of the ethanolic ginseng extract and the onset of a severe headache was strongly suggestive of a causal relationship. The use of cocaine, amphetamine, phenylpropanolamine, and other sympathomimetic drugs was denied. Most ginseng users are not medically supervised, and adolescents and adults may be experimenting with doses larger than those generally recommended in Chinese practice (0.5 to 2 gm). The expected benefits are listed as prevention of aging or tiredness, improved stamina or concentration, and increased resistance to stress or disease. -Editor. *Ped Neur Briefs* June 1995.

MIGRAINE ASSOCIATED SYMPTOMS: PREVALENCE AND PRECIPITANTS

A review of associated symptoms of migraine determined by telephone survey of 500 self-reported migraine sufferers is reported from Temple University School of Medicine and the Comprehensive Headache Center, Germantown Hospital, Philadelphia, PA. Female to male preponderance was 443 to 57; 5.6% were younger than 25 years old. Seventy-one percent took abortive medication, and 26,5% received both abortive and prophylactic medication. Precipitating factors included stress (79%), changes in weather (44%), pre-menstruation (37%), changes in light (34%), and eating certain foods (30%). Symptoms associated with migraine attacks were headache (96%), nausea/vomiting (32%), photophobia (83%), noise sensitivity (60%), dizziness (65%), eye pain, and neck pain (79%). Nausea occurred in one half of attacks in >90% of respondents, and vomiting in one third of attacks in 70%, interfering with oral medication in 30% and 42%, respectively. Many childhood migraineurs have a history of cyclical vomiting, a recognized precursor of migraine. (Silberstein SD. Migraine symptoms: Results of a survey of self-reported migraineurs. <u>Headache</u> July/August 1995;35:387-396). (Respond: Dr Stephen D Silberstein, The Comprehensive Headache Center, Germantown Hospital, One Penn Blvd, Philadelphia, PA 19144).

COMMENT. The authors emphasize the significance of nausea and vomiting as associated symptoms affecting the degree of disability of migraine sufferers. Drugs used to treat migraine often cause nausea and may exacerbate associated symptoms while relieving headache. The treatment or avoidance of nausea may be as important as the relief of headache. The route of administration of migraine medication can alter the prevalence of side-effects. Nausea and/or vomiting occur more frequently with oral administration of ergotamine or sumatriptan than with injection therapy.

Revisions to the International Headache Society classification proposed for pediatric migraine proved more sensitive than existing criteria in a study of 45 children and adolescents at the Palm Beach Headache Center, Florida. For pediatric migraine without aura, the revisions included headache attacks as short as 30 minutes and a bilateral location in addition to unilateral headache. For those pediatric migraines with aura, the only proposed revision was a decrease in duration of headache from 2 - 48 hours to one half - 48 hours. Diagnostic rates increased from 53% to 80%, using the revised criteria. (Winner P et al. Classification of pediatric migraine: Proposed revisions to the IHS criteria. <u>Headache</u> July/August 1995;35:407-410). -Editor. *Ped Neur Briefs* Aug 1995.

HEADACHE AND STOMACH-ACHE CO-OCCURRENCE SYNDROME

Psychosocial risk factors for headache and stomache-ache and their co-occurrence were investigated in a longitudinal study of Norwegian children aged 4-10 years at the Department of Health and Society, National Institute of Public Health, Oslo, Norway. Children with headache only were well behaved as preschoolers, high achievers, and their mothers were employed outside the home. The stomache-ache alone group had an earlier onset of symptoms than those with headache, they were well-adapted emotionally, and their mothers were less educated. Childhood emotional problems and low maternal emotional support differentiated the co-occurrence group from the headache and stomach-ache only groups. School factors were not associated with the co-occurrence syndrome. (Borge AIH, Nordhagen R. Development of stomach-ache and headache during middle childhood: co-occurrence and psychosocial risk factors. <u>Acta Paediatr</u> July 1995;84:795-802). (Respond: Dr AIH Borge, National Institute of Public Health, Geitmyrsveien 75, 0462 Oslo, Norway).

COMMENT. The co-occurrence of headache and stomach-ache in young children appears to constitute a distinct syndrome with psychosocial implications that may need to be addressed early to prevent later childhood incapacity. In the absence of central nervous or abdominal pathology, an interactive pediatric and psychological approach involving the mother and child is advised.

The absence of increased psychological or psychosocial disability in children with recurrent abdominal pain or in their families compared to controls, noted in the above study, is also alluded to in a letter to the editor (Feldman W. Recurrent abdominal pain in childhood. <u>Acta Paediatr</u> July 1995;84:834).

A study of esophogeal, gastric and duodenal biopsies in 31 children with migraine found twenty nine with an underlying inflammatory lesion of the gastrointestinal tract that could explain the associated symptoms of nausea (93% of patients), vomiting (42%), and abdominal pain (55%). The authors suggest that the findings support a causal link between recurrent abdominal pain and migraine. (Mavromichalis I et al. Migraine of gastrointestinal origin. <u>Eur J Pediatr</u> May 1995;154:406-410). -Editor. *Ped Neur Briefs* Aug 1995.

TRANSIENT HEADACHE AND CSF LYMPHOCYTOSIS

A transient syndrome of migrainous headache with neurologic deficits and CSF lymphocytic pleocytosis is described in 7 young adult patients examined at the Strong Memorial Hospital, University of Rochester Medical Center, Rochester, NY. The clinical characteristics of 33 similar cases, 13 in children and adolescents, previously reported in the literature are also analysed. The diagnostic criteria for this syndrome include severe headache, temporary (<4 days) neurologic deficit, CSF lymphocytosis (16-350 WBC/mm3), and self-limited course (range 1-84 days, mean 21 days). The neurologic signs and symptoms were usually transient hemiparesis or sensory changes, confusional episodes, and aphasia. CSF protein was increased in 91% of cases, CSF pressure increased in 73%, focal, nonepileptiform EEG irregularities were recorded in 72%, and a viral illness or fever preceded the headaches in 50%. Apart from 2 patients showing unidentified bright objects on MRI, neuroimaging studies were negative. The headaches had characteristics of migraine with aura, unilateral location, pulsating quality, nausea, and photophobia, but unlike typical migraine, the headache syndrome was not chronic. The syndrome resolved within 3 months. The cause is undetermined. (Berg MJ, Williams LS. The transient syndrome of headache with neurologic deficits and CSF lymphocytosis. <u>Neurology</u> September 1995;45:1648-1654). (Reprints: Dr Michel J Berg, Box 673, Department of Neurology, University of Rochester Medical Center, 60 Elmwood Avenue, Rochester, NY 14642).

COMMENT. The differential diagnoses listed by the authors for this syndrome include Lyme neuroborreliosis, neurosyphilis, neurobrucellosis, mycoplasma infection, granulomatous meningitis, neoplastic meningitis, autoimmune disease, HIV meningitis, and a side effect of cerebral angiography. Other illnesses with similar features are hemiplegic migraine, seizure disorder, and recurrent aseptic meningitis (Mollaret's meningitis). The syndrome is self limited, and a viral etiology seems likely. -Editor. *Ped Neur Briefs* Oct 1995.

FAMILIAL MIGRAINE WITH VERTIGO AND TREMOR

A family with dominantly inherited migraine headaches, episodic vertigo, and essential tremor is reported from the UCLA School of Medicine, Los

Angeles, CA. Episodes were triggered by stress, exercise, or lack of sleep. Tremor began in adolescence or early adulthood. Treatment with acetazolamide in 5 patients relieved visual auras, headaches, and vertigo, and diminished the tremor. Linkage analysis excluded linkage to markers on chromosome 19p, involved in families with hemiplegic migraine and ataxia syndrome. (Baloh RW et al. Familial migraine with vertigo and essential tremor. <u>Neurology</u> Feb 1996;46:458-460). (Reprints: Dr Robert W Baloh, Department of Neurology, UCLA School of Medicine, Los Angeles, CA 90095).

COMMENT. Several studies have shown a beneficial effect of acetazolamide in essential tremor. In the present report, both tremor and headache were relieved by acetazolamide. Of 15 family members with migraine, 8 also had essential tremor, whereas none of unaffected members had tremor. It seemed likely that the migraine and tremor were genetically connected. Migraine is expressed in various clinical forms and appears to be genetically heterogeneous.

An 11-year-old boy with **basilar migraine aura without headache** and ictal fast EEG activity is reported from the Pediatric Institute, Ferrara University, Italy (Soriani S et al. <u>Eur J Pediatr</u> Feb 1996;155:126-129). Anisocoria, ataxia, dysarthria, and confusional state were predominant manifestations. Beta activity in the EEG has been described previously with attacks of basilar migraine.

Familial hemiplegic migraine and autosomal dominant arteriopathy with leukoencephalopathy (CADASIL) is described from St Vincent's Hospital, Dublin, Ireland. (Hutchinson M et al. <u>Ann Neurol</u> Nov 1995;38:817-824). Four subjects with CADSIL (cerebral autosomal dominant arteriopathy with subcortical infarcts and leukoencephalopathy) had a history of familial hemiplegic migraine dating back to childhood. The disorder typically presents in adulthood but the MRI may show evidence of leukoencephalopathy before symptoms develop. This family is the first with both hemiplegic migraine and migraine as presenting symptoms of CADSIL. -Editor. *Ped Neur Briefs* July 1996.

ACUTE CONFUSIONAL MIGRAINE

Of 76 children admitted with migraine between 1982 and 1990, 13 had a discharge diagnosis of confusional migraine at British Columbia Children's Hospital, Vancouver, Canada. A retrospective analysis of cases showed a preponderance of males to females (11:2), age range of 6 to 15 years (mean, 10 years), all having headache followed by a period of confusion, lasting 2-24 hours, and 4 having recurrent episodes. Mild head trauma preceded the headache in 4 patients. In addition to confusion, agitation occurred in 8 patients, past history of headache in 7, and a family history of migraine in 10. One of 11 patients with CT scans had an arachnoid cyst. EEG was mildly abnormal in 2 of 4 patients with recordings. CSF was normal in 2 patients studied. (Shaabat A. Confusional migraine in childhood. <u>Pediatr Neurol</u> July 1996;15:23-25). (Respond: Dr Shaabat, Dept Pediatrics, College of Medicine and Allied Health Sciences, King Abdulaziz University, PO Box 6615, Jeddah 21452, Saudi Arabia).

COMMENT. A diagnosis of migraine should be considered in children with episodes of acute confusion and agitation, lasting from 1 to 24 hours, preceded by headache and sometimes, mild head trauma, and a positive family history of migraine. It is interesting that CT scans uncovered an arachnoid cyst in one patient, a space-occupying lesion, usually developmental in origin, and known to be complicated by headaches and seizures in some. Further studies of the EEG, obtained in only 4 of the above patients, and response to therapy would be of interest. -Editor. *Ped Neur Briefs* Oct 1996.

JUVENILE IDIOPATHIC STABBING HEADACHE

A series of 83 juvenile patients with idiopathic stabbing headache, 3.3% of all juvenile patients referred because of recurrent headache, is reported from the Paediatric Neurology Services of the University of Ferrara and the University of Padua, Italy. Mean age at onset was 7 +/-3 years, and sexes were equally affected. The pain lasted a fraction of a second to a few minutes. The frequency was more than once a week in 52%, once a week in 21%, and once a month in 27%. Intensity was severe in 30%, and mild in 40%. Localization was frontal in 69% and occipital in 23%; bilateral in 48% and alternating in 22%. Headache associated symptoms in 47% included photophobia (15%), nausea (7%), and vertigo (8%). A psychogenic precipitant was recognized in 22%. A history of periodic syndrome, mainly cyclic vomiting and recurrent abdominal pain, preceded the onset of headache illness in 47%. Family history of migraine was present in 58%. Only 14% of patients had other types of headache in addition; 10% had migraine and 4% tension headache. Neurologic exam, imaging in 32 patients, and EEG in 67 were normal. At 1 to 5 year follow-up, 70% were free of symptoms. (Soriani S, Battistella PA, Arnaldi C et al. Juvenile idiopathic stabbing headache. <u>Headache</u> Oct 1996;36:565-567). (Respond: Dr S Soriani, Paediatric Institute, Ferrara Univ, via Savonarola 9, 44100 Ferrara, Italy).

COMMENT. A small group of juvenile headache patients with characteristically very brief attacks of stabbing pain, with onset around 7 years, and spontaneous remission usually within 1 to 5 years, may deserve greater recognition as a childhood headache syndrome with a relatively favorable prognosis. A previous report cited by the authors found a 25% incidence of EEG abnormalities among patients with this syndrome. (Kramer JW et al. The value of the EEG in children with chronic headache. <u>Brain Dev</u> 1994;16:304-308). Others have shown a high incidence of EEG abnormalities in migraine patients and a beneficial response to the anticonvulsant, phenytoin. (Millichap JG. <u>Child's Brain</u> 1978;4:95-105). The use of valproate in headache patients is reviewed in the following article.

-Editor. *Ped Neur Briefs* Dec 1996.

EEG IN CHRONIC HEADACHE EVALUATION

A retrospective analysis of records of 312 children with chronic headache and review of EEGs in 257 are reported from the Tel Aviv Medical Center and University, Israel. Headache was classified as migraine in 143 (55%); classic migraine in 12 and common migraine in 121. The mean age at time of EEG was 9 years. The EEG was normal in 80%. Epileptiform activity occurred in 12% and slowing in 8%. Response was higher to hyperventilation in non-migraine patients and to photic stimulation in those with migraine. The incidence of epileptic EEGs was 11% in both migraine and tension type headaches; it was 26% and significantly higher in 15 children with chronic headache described as "very brief," occurring predominantly in girls, several times a week, and without family history for migraine. Prevalence of epilepsy in families of patients with epileptic EEGs did not differ from the total group. Of six children with epileptiform EEGs who were treated with AEDs, 4 responded and had no further headaches and 2 were not benefited. Of 17 children with focal EEG abnormalities, 9 had head CTs, 1 had an arachnoid cyst, and 3 had sinusitis. The authors conclude that the EEG may be of value in some children with migraine and "very brief" headaches, but epileptiform EEG activity does not prove an epileptic origin for headache and its significance in diagnosis and treatment is minimal. (Kramer U, Harel S et al. The value of EEG in children with chronic headaches. <u>Brain Dev</u> July/Aug 1994;16:304-8). (Respond: Dr S Harel, Institute for Child Development and Pediatric Unit, Beit Habriut Strauss, 7 Balfour St, Tel Aviv 65211, Israel).

COMMENT. See <u>Progress in Pediatric Neurology II</u> (PNB Publ, 1994, p 156) for a report of the EEG findings in children with chronic recurrent headaches and response to phenytoin. Grade III epileptiform EEGs were found in 18% of the total and with the same incidence in migraine patients. Migraine was controlled in 77% but a positive response did not correlate with EEG abnormalities; those with normal EEGs were benefited equally. (Millichap JG. Recurrent headaches in 100 children. Electroencephalographic abnormalities and response to phenytoin (Dilantin). <u>Child's Brain</u> 1978;4:95-104). The significance of the EEG in chronic headache evaluation and the mechanism of the anti-migraine effect of phenytoin and other antiepileptic drugs (eg. valproate) need further investigation. -Editor. *Ped Neur Briefs* Sept 1994.

EEG IN HEADACHE EVALUATION

A literature review of articles published between 1941 and 1994 was used to determine the utility of the electroencephalogram in the evaluation of patients with headache and the results are reported from the Departments of Neurology, Lackland AFB, TX, and Andrews AFB, MD. EEG findings that occurred more frequently in headache patients than in controls were as follows: generalized or focal slowing, hyperventilation-induced high-voltage slowing, excessive fast activity, epileptiform discharges, prominent photic driving, and differences in symmetry and frequencies of alpha rhythm. Two studies showed an increased prevalence of 14 & 6 positive spikes in the EEGs of children with migraine. One author suggested that headaches of children whose EEGs demonstrated epileptiform activity would respond best to anticonvulsants. In well controlled studies, a prominent photic driving response at high flash rates (the "H-response") was the only abnormality distinguishing headache patients from those without headache and migraine from other headache types. Clinical criteria were of greater diagnostic value than the EEG in identifying headache subtypes, including those with structural lesions. (Gronseth GS, Greenberg MK. The utility of the electroencephalogram in the evaluation of patients presenting with headache: A review of the literature. <u>Neurology</u> July 1995;45:1263-1267). (Reprints: Lt Col Gary S Gronseth, Department of

Neurology (PSMN), Wilford Hall Medical Center (AETC), 2200 Bergquist Drive STE 1, Lackland AFB, TX 78236).

COMMENT. The authors conclude that the EEG is not indicated in routine evaluations of patients presenting with headache. However, they do recommend an EEG in patients with headache and symptoms suggestive of seizures and in those with atypical migrainous auras or episodic loss of consciousness.

In one article not cited by the authors, 77 percent of 30 children with migraine benefited from treatment with the anticonvulsant, phenytoin. Response to phenytoin was not correlated with an abnormal EEG. In 13 with abnormal and 17 with normal EEGs, the beneficial response rates were 61% and 88%, respectively. (Millichap JG. Recurrent headaches in 100 children. Electroencephalographic abnormalities and response to phenytoin (Dilantin). <u>Child's Brain</u> 1978;4:95-104). -Editor. *Ped Neur Briefs* Aug 1995.

BRAIN IMAGING INDICATIONS FOR HEADACHES

Charts of all children referred to the pediatric neurology clinic, Schneider Children's Hospital, New Hyde Park, NY, for evaluation of headaches over a 2-year period were reviewed retrospectively for headache characteristics, indications for performing CT and MRI studies, and imaging results. Of 133 patients ages 3 to 18 years, 52% had migrainous headaches, 21% chronic tension headaches, and 19% were unclassified. The indications for brain imaging in 78 patients examined (MRI 45, CT 27, both 6) were not specified in 17, atypical headache pattern in 12, parental concern 12, physician concern about cerebral tumor 11, systemic symptoms of fatigue and weight loss in 11, focal symptoms or signs during headaches in 7, neurologic or ocular abnormalities 6, and increasing severity or frequency of headaches in 5. None of the scans showed brain tumor, vascular abnormality, or hydrocephalus that required neurosurgical intervention. Abnormal scans in 11 patients included evidence of chronic sinusitis in 7, a neuroepithelial cyst adjacent to the foramen of Monroe treated conservatively in 1, right temporal arachnoid cyst in 1, left cerebral hemiatrophy in 1, and Dandy-Walker malformation in 1. (Maytal J et al. The value of brain imaging in children with headaches. <u>Pediatrics</u> September 1995;96:413-416). (Reprints: Joseph Maytal MD, Division of Pediatric Neurology, Schneider Children's Hospital, Long Island Jewish Medical Center, New Hyde Park, NY 11040).

COMMENT. The authors' conclusion that brain imaging has very limited value in the management of childhood headaches is based on negative findings in 86%. Although none of 11 (14%) positive scans was considered indicative of a treatable disease at the time, the abnormalities uncovered might potentially have proved significant. The MRI indications proposed by the authors include atypical recurrent headaches, a recent change in the character of the headache, persistent vomiting, abnormal neurologic findings, and occurrence in younger age groups. Children with symptoms suggestive of seizures and in association with an abnormal EEG should also be considered for neuroimaging studies. Cases of ADHD complicated by headache were recently diagnosed with temporal lobe arachnoid cysts; MRI studies which uncovered the cysts were prompted by focal abnormalities in the EEG. (Millichap JG. <u>Neurology</u> in press).

Headache, without localizing neurologic abnormalities or signs of increased intracranial pressure, may be an uncommon presenting symptom of brain tumor. However, the subtle neurological abnormalities associated with ADHD may attain greater significance when complicated by headache. The luxury of follow-up evaluation and observation over time may not be available to the neurologist who examines a patient in consultation, and the deferral of imaging may not be practical or judicious. For further commentary on the indications for imaging in headache and the value of an EEG as a preliminary test in diagnosis, see <u>Progress in Pediatric Neurology II</u>, PNB Publishers, 1994, pp164-6). -Editor. *Ped Neur Briefs* Oct 1995.

PREVALENCE OF HEADACHE

PREVALENCE OF MIGRAINE IN SCHOOLCHILDREN

The prevalence of migraine in a random sample of the childhood population of the city of Aberdeen, Scotland, was evaluated in the Department of Medical Paediatrics, Royal Aberdeen Children's Hospital, employing the International Headache Society Diagnostic Criteria and validating questionnaire responses with clinical interviews. Among 206 children diagnosed at interview, the causes of severe headache and their prevalence rates (-%) were as follows: migraine in 159 (10.6%). migraine-like headache (<2 hours) in 10 (0.7%), tension headache in 14 (0.9%), non-specific in 20 (1.3%), and sinusitis or other specific diagnosis in 3 (0.2%). The prevalence of migraine increased with age, with male preponderance in children <12 years, and female preponderance >12 years of age. Children with migraine lost a mean of 8 school days a year (3 due to headache) as compared to 3 lost by controls. (Abu-Arefeh I, Russell G. Prevalence of headache and migraine in schoolchildren. <u>BMJ</u> 24 Sept 1994;309:765-769). (Respond: Dr I Abu-Arefeh, Department of Child Health, University of Aberdeen, Aberdeen AB9 2ZD, UK).

COMMENT. Migraine is a common cause of headache among schoolchildren in Aberdeen, with a prevalence of about 11%. This is more than twice the prevalence reported in some previous pediatric studies, comparable to the cited increased prevalence of migraine from 25 to 40% in an adult population in the US in recent years. Environmental factors are thought to be responsible. -Editor. *Ped Neur Briefs* Oct 1994.

FAMILY AND SCHOOL FACTORS AND

HEADACHE PREVALENCE

The prevalence of headache in children aged 7-16 years, representing districts of the city of Goteborg with socioeconomic, family, and school variables, is reported from Sahlgrenska Hospital, Goteborg, Sweden. Data obtained by questionnaires from 1297 pupils, representative of the city population, showed 26% with "headache once a month" and 6% at daily intervals or several times a week "frequent headache." The prevalence of "headache once a month or more" increased with age and school grade, from 16% in first grade to 42% in grade 9. The prevalence of "frequent" headache, presumably of tension-type, increased from 3% in second grade to 10% in third grade. Girls in grades 7-9 were affected more than boys with respect to both types of headache. The risk of frequent headache correlated with class size, increasing with larger classes in lower school, grades 1-3. In intermediate classes, grades 4-6, headache frequency was higher in districts with high unemployment. (Carlsson J. Prevalence of headache in schoolchildren: relation to family and school factors. <u>Acta Paediatr</u> June 1996;85:692-6). (Respond: Dr J Carlsson, Department of Clinical Neuroscience, Neurology Section, Sahlgrenska Hospital, S-41345, Goteborg, Sweden).

COMMENT. The increase in headache frequency in third grade was thought to be related to the larger classes and more targeted schoolwork. The increased prevalence in higher school levels was related to the higher frequency among girls, possibly due to hormonal changes and greater sensitivity to interpersonal conflicts and family stress. Parental separation or divorce and marital problems have been related to recurrent headache in children and adolescents, but these were not risk factors in the present study. -Editor. *Ped Neur Briefs* July 1996.

PREVALENCE OF HEADACHE IN SCHOOL CHILDREN

The prevalence of migraine and other headaches

in 7-year-old children, in 1974 and 1992, was determined by school physicians at the time of medical examinations, using the identical study design and a similar urban child population of the same age group, and the data analysed in the Department of Child Neurology, University of Turku, Finland. The prevalence of "present" headache at age 7 years, defined as headache occurring in the preceding 6 months, increased from 14.4% in 1974 to 51.5% in 1992. Boys and girls were affected similarly. "Past" headache, having occurred at any time prior to present headache, also showed a significantly increased prevalence from 23.4% of children affected in the 1974 study to 71.1% in 1992. In both present and past headache categories, those having headaches infrequently. less than once a month or yearly, showed the greatest increase in prevalence. Precipitating factors, fever, fatigue, and head trauma, were equally prevalent in 1974 and 1992. Migraine headache had also increased from 1.9% affected in 1974 to 5.7% in 1992. Migraine prevalence was especially high in city areas with high percentages of council houses and family relocations. (Sillanpaa M, Anttila P. Increasing prevalence of headache in 7-year-old schoolchildren. <u>Headache</u> Sept 1996;36:466-470). (Respond: Dr Matti Sillanpaa, University of Turku Hospital, TYKS, 20520 Turku, Finland).

COMMENT. The prevalence of headache, including migraine, has increased significantly in school age children living in an urban area in Finland, in an 18 year period from 1974 to 1992. Highest increases occur among children exposed to social instability and stress. Similar increases in headache prevalence are known to have occurred in adults in the United States in the 1980s. (see <u>Progress in Pediatric Neurology II</u>, PNB Publ, 1994, pp153-155).

The Children's Headache Assessment Scale (CHAS), a parent questionnaire focusing on situations and events surrounding the headaches, emphasizes stress antecedents and coping responses rather than symptom details, and is of value in following responses to behavioral therapy. Environmental factors, including nutrition, are important in the etiology and management of childhood headache and warrant further study. (see <u>Progress in Pediatric Neurology I</u>, 1991, pp141-150). -Editor. *Ped Neur Briefs* Oct 1996.

TREATMENT OF HEADACHE

CLUSTER HEADACHES RELIEVED BY INDOMETHACIN

The clinical features and treatment of cluster headaches are reported in two patients, a boy aged 8 and a girl 10 years, evaluated at the Department of Neurology, University of North Carolina at Chapel Hill. Indomethacin 25 mg bid produced immediate and complete relief. The headaches were sharp, unilateral, localized to the temporal region, and associated with lacrimation, nasal congestion, and photophobia. They occurred several times a day for 3 to 4 weeks, sometimes early morning, and lasted 10 minutes to 1 to 2 hours. Clusters were followed by a 2- to 3-week headache-free period. Trials of propanolol, amitryptyline, and biofeedback were unsuccessful. (D'Cruz OF. Cluster headaches in childhood. <u>Clin Pediatr</u> April 1994;33:241-242). (Respond: Dr D'Cruz, Univ of N Carolina, Burnett-Womack Bldg, CB #7025, Chapel Hill, NC 27599).

COMMENT. Cluster headaches are rare in children and are frequently atypical. Although remarkably effective in the two patients reported, indomethacin toxicity may limit chronic usage. Dietary factors in etiology might be considered. -Editor. *Ped Neur Briefs* June 1994.

DIVALPROEX SODIUM IN HEADACHE

An approach to treating migraine with the anticonvulsant, divalproex sodium, is reviewed from the Comprehensive Headache Center, Germantown Hospital, Philadelphia, PA. Four double-blind, placebo-controlled studies have confirmed the efficacy of valproate in treatment of migraine. The frequency of attacks as well as the duration and intensity were reduced. The most frequent adverse effects included nausea, asthenia, dyspepsia, dizziness, somnolence, and diarrhea. The use of valproate for headache prevention in children under 10 years should be avoided, except in exceptional cases. (Silberstein SD. Divalproex sodium in headache: literature review and clinical guidelines. Headache Oct 1996;36:547-555). (Respond: Dr Stephen D Silberstein, Germantown Hospital, One Penn Boulevard, Philadelphia, PA 19144).

COMMENT. The occurrence of liver toxicity in children treated with valproate, between 1:500 to 1:9000, prompts caution since the reaction may be fatal. Attention to possible dietary factors in the cause of migraine, and the initiation of less toxic medications or alternative treatments should be investigated thoroughly before resorting to valproate therapy.

The acute treatment of migraine with Rizatriptan vs Sumatriptan has been studied in 10 US and 4 Dutch investigator centers, involving 449 patients, and is reported from the Department of Neurology, Leiden University Hospital, the Netherlands. (Visser WH, Ferrari MD et al. Arch Neurol Nov 1996;53:1132-1137). The antimigraine effect of 10 and 20 mg rizatriptan was superior to placebo, and equal to 100 mg sumatriptan succinate; 40 mg rizatriptan was superior to 100 mg sumatriptan succinate in efficacy but caused frequent side effects. -Editor. *Ped Neur Briefs* Dec 1996.

PSYCHOSOCIAL THERAPIES FOR CHRONIC HEADACHE

Psychosocial interventions in the management of recurrent headache disorders are reviewed from Ohio University, Athens, OH, and University of Mississippi Medical Center, Jackson, MS. The most frequently used interventions in adult patients are: 1) relaxation training, 2) biofeedback, 3) stress-management (cognitive-behavioral) therapy, and 4) dietary modification. Three types of relaxation training are employed: a) progressive muscle relaxation-alternately tensing and relaxing selected muscle groups, b) autogenic training-use of self-instructions of warmth and heaviness to promote relaxation, and c) meditation - use of a silently repeated word or sound to promote mental relaxation. Cognitive-behavioral interventions teach patients to identify stressful precipitants and strategies for coping with stress. Behavioral interventions yielded outcomes roughly equivalent to those obtained with propanolol in 60 clinical trials and 2400 patients with migraine. More than 50% improvement was obtained with either relaxation/biofeedback training or propanolol, compared to 14% with placebo and 3% if untreated. (Holroyd KA, Penzien DB. Psychosocial interventions in the management of recurrent headache disorders 1: Overview and effectiveness. <u>Behav Med</u> Summer 1994;20:53-62). (Reprints: Kenneth A Holroyd PhD, Dept of Psychology and Institute of Health and Behavioral Sciences, Ohio University, Athens, OH 45701).

COMMENT. The management of headache in children is different from that of adults and requires an assessment of cognitive and affective development and a knowledge of children's concepts of illness and pain. The use of long-term investigational medications in children is often undesirable and relaxation techniques and dietary modification may be more effective and appropriate. (<u>Ped Neur Briefs</u> April 1991; <u>Progress in Pediatric Neurology II</u>, 1994, p 170). -Editor. *Ped Neur Briefs* Oct 1994.

PROGNOSIS AND TREATMENT OF HEADACHES

The prognosis and methods of coping with headaches were studied by telephone interview in 98 children followed for 10 years after diagnosis at the Department of Pediatrics, Dalhousie University and Children's Hospital, Halifax, Canada. Of 77 contacted, 18

(23%) were diagnosed initially with tension-type headaches, 49 (64%) with common migraine, and 5 (6%) had classical migraine with aura. Headaches had persisted in 73% but were improved in 81%. Prognosis was related to the type of headache at initial diagnosis: only 18% of those with migraine were symptom free after 10 years whereas 50% of those with tension headaches had obtained relief. Headache types changed with time: 11% of children with initial tension headaches had migraine at follow-up, whereas 22% with common migraine had developed headaches of tension-type after 10 years. At diagnosis the mean headache frequency was 11/month compared to 2/month at 10 year follow-up. Treatment at follow-up consisted of 1) a period of sleep in 17%; 2) relaxation therapy in 10%; and 3) avoidance of precipitants in 5%. Food was a precipitant in 5 patients. One-third required no treatment for headaches; 41% were using nonprescription medications: and only 3% had recently seen a physician for prescription medication. Associated symptoms included motion sickness in 26% somnambulism in 14%, "Alice in Wonderland" hallucinations of size in 10%, and hallucinations of motion and time ("The Rushes") in 17%. (Dooley J, Bagnell A. The prognosis and treatment of headaches in children - a ten year follow-up. <u>Can J Neurol Sci</u> February 1995;22:47-49). (Reprints: Dr JM Dooley, Neurology Division, The IWK Children's Hospital, 5850 University Avenue, Halifax, Nova Scotia, Canada B3J 3G9).

COMMENT. In this group of children, no patient was prescribed medication at diagnosis and only two required prescription drugs at follow-up. Nonprescription medications had been employed by 30-40%, but rest and relaxation techniques were encouraged as alternatives to drugs when possible.

Biofeedback Treatment. Treatment of childhood migraine with autogenic relaxation and skin temperature biofeedback was analysed in 30 patients, ages 7 to 18 years, using a controlled group outcome design, at the Department of Psychology, University of

South Alabama, Mobile, AL (Labbe EE. <u>Headache</u> Jan 1995;35:10-13). Headache frequency and duration, but not headache intensity, improved in the treatment groups as compared to the waiting list controls; 80% of the biofeedback group, 50% of the autogenics group, and none of the controls were symptom-free. In this study, biofeedback and relaxation therapies were practical and effective in the management of childhood migraine and were free from adverse side-effects.

In a previous report from the University of Ottawa, Canada, McGrath et al found that relaxation training was no more effective than brief reassurance and self-control suggestion techniques in treating pediatric migraine (see <u>Progress in Pediatric Neurology I</u>, Chicago, PNB Publ, 1991, pp 144-5). Perhaps certain foods may have been observed to play a greater role in precipitating headaches in the Halifax study if the influence of diet had been stressed at the time of initial diagnosis. -Editor. *Ped Neur Briefs* Feb 1995.

CHAPTER **3**

ATTENTION DEFICIT HYPERACTIVITY DISORDER

INTRODUCTION

HISTORICAL OVERVIEW

The symptoms of attention deficit hyperactivity disorder include hyperactivity, impulsivity, inattention, and distractibility. The most prominent and troublesome of these symptoms is the hyperactivity, leading to the term, "The Hyperactive Child" syndrome.

Hyperactivity or "hyperkinesia" has long been recognized as a sign of brain damage, particularly to the frontal lobes of the brain. This in turn provided evidence in favor of the term, "Brain Damage" syndrome, later to be followed by the "Brain Dysfunction" or "Minimal Brain Dysfunction" syndrome.

Postencephalitic behavior disorder

(Hohman, 1922) was one of the earliest references to a hyperactive behavior syndrome that followed an injury to the brain caused by von Economo's encephalitis. This World War 1 epidemic of encephalitis resulted in behavior disorders in children and Parkinsonism in adults. In addition to hyperactivity, the children exhibited impulsiveness, irritability, antisocial behavior, and emotional lability, but no significant cognitive impairment.

This description of behavioral sequelae to a clearly demonstrable central nervous system disease or injury was followed by a variety of reports of behavioral syndromes having similar characteristics that were linked to brain damage or dysfunction. Some emphasized the hyperactive behavior, others stressed the associated perceptual dysfunction, language or cognitive disorders, and some described the so called "soft" or subtle neurological abnormalities found in the child with incoordination and associated movement disorders. The specialty of the observer sometimes determined the emphasis of symptoms and the terminology used to describe this hyperactive behavior syndrome.

The **Brain-injured child** concept was postulated and developed by Strauss and Lehtinen and others (1947). The so-called **Strauss syndrome**, a term coined by Stevens and Birch (1957), provided an alternative explanation for the learning and behavior problems of children previously described as emotionally disturbed, badly behaved, or lazy. The blame for the child's shortcomings was shifted from a parent's mismanagement to an organic brain disorder, requiring special educational, psychological, and medical investigation and treatment. A heterogeneous group of behaviorally disturbed and learning disabled children was now perceived as a homogeneous entity consisting of exceptional children needing specialized educational attention.

The term **"learning disabilities,"** o r "learning diasabled child," was coined by Samuel Kirk (1963) at the first meeting of the Association for Children with Learning Disabilities, an organization of concerned parents and various professionals interested in the recognition and management of the hyperactive child with educational difficulties. Psychologists preferred the term **"perceptually handicapped"** child (Kephart, 1963), emphasizing the visual-motor and spatial imperceptions, a characteristic that had been included in the Strauss syndrome. Frostig (1964) also stressed visual perception handicaps in brain injured hyperactive children, and she developed methods for the training and remediation of the perceptual and eye-hand coordination disorders.

Clements (1966) and others coined the term **"minimal brain dysfunction"** syndrome, commonly known as **MBD.** MBD was thought to best describe the child of normal intelligence who had learning and behavioral disabilities that were thought to be associated with or a consequence of dysfunction of the central nervous system. Brain dysfunction syndromes differentiated those with minimal or mild symptoms and signs (MBD) from such severe or major disabilities as cerebral palsy, epilepsy, mental retardation, blindness, deafness,and aphasias. This classification was embraced by the pediatric neurologists who recognized the frequent occurrence of "soft" or subtle neurologic abnormalities in children with hyperactivity and learning disabilities.

An organic etiology of MBD was supported by a history of prenatal and perinatal complications, including prematurity, birth asphyxia, exposure of the fetus to alcohol, drugs, lead and other toxins, and head injury, especially involving the frontal lobes of the brain. Electroencephalographic abnormalities and CT and MR neuroimaging have sometimes uncovered structural cerebral lesions as a basis for the behavioral and learning disability. A new syndrome of *"temporal lobe arachnoid cyst-attention deficit disorder"* has recently deen described in three children who presented with ADHD complicated by headaches, episodes suggestive of seizures, or tremors. Focal epileptiform discharges in the EEG prompted MRI studies which uncovered the arachnoid cyst in the temporal lobe. A causal association with the ADHD seemed plausible because of coincidental learning and language disabilities, explained by temporal lobe and sylvian region pathology. (Millichap JG. 1997).

Despite the evidence for a neurobiological, environmental and organic etiology for the hyperactive child syndrome, the American Psychiatric Association, in their Diagnostic and Statistical Manuals, have chosen to discount the brain injury, MBD, or neurogenic causal classification, preferring to use diagnostic terms that identify symptomatic consequences or causally-related criteria. In 1968, DSM-II, the syndrome was described as **"hyperkinetic reaction of childhood or adolescence."** In 1980, DSM-III, the term **"attention deficit disorder" (ADD)** was introduced, with subtypes, ADD *with hyperactivity,* and ADD *without hyperactivity.*

In 1987, DSM-III-R, the terminology was again changed to **"attention deficit hyperactivity disorder" (ADHD);** and in 1994, DSM-IV, lists of criteria were introduced to distinguish an **ADHD-AD,** an *inattentive* subtype, **ADHD-HI,** a *hyperactive-impulsive* subtype, and **ADHD-CT,** a *combined type.* The original Strauss syndrome and subsequent MBD diagnostic criteria of hyperactivity, inattention, distractibility, and poor organizational skills have been retained in the DSM-IV classification of ADHD, but any reference to poor motor performance, clumsiness, and neurological abnormalities is omitted. It appears that the DSM definitions of the syndrome attempt to deemphasize the role of cerebral disease, and the concept of an etiological-related, organic syndrome has been rejected. *-J. Gordon Millichap, M.D.,* Editor.

ORGANIC THEORY OF ADHD

The evidence for a neurobiological basis for hyperkinesia, distractibility, inattention, and learning disabilities is based on numerous experimental studies of cortical ablation and subcortical lesions in animals, clinical studies of brain-damaged children and adults, batteries of neuropsychological tests, and EEG, MRI, and PET studies of the electrical activity, structure, and metabolism of brain regions.

Neurophysiologists, Langworthy and Richter (1939), reported increased spontaneous activity produced by frontal cerebral lesions in cats. Kennard and colleagues (1941) produced hyperactivity in monkeys following lesions of the frontal lobes, bilateral removal of prefrontal and frontal areas causing the greatest total increase in activity. Ruch and Shenkin (1943) demonstrated the specific relation of area 13 on the orbital surface of the frontal lobes to hyperactivity and hyperphagia in monkeys.

Livingston, Fulton and colleagues (1948), and Mettler (1967), studied the effects of stimulation and regional ablation of the frontal and other areas of the brain on motor activity. Parietal lobe lesions produced hyperactivity of a lesser degree than frontal lobe lesions. Two type of hyperactivity were distinguished: *overreactivity,* related to external stimulation or distractibility, caused by frontal lobe injury; and *essential overactivity,* a disinhibitive hyperkinesia due to striatal lesions and release from fronto-cortical-reticular inhibition of ascending systems. Magoun (1963) considers persistent exploratory behavior and distractibility as release phenomena.

Our own studies at Children's Memorial Hospital and Northwestern University Medical School, Chicago (1973, 1975), have demonstrated the paradoxical quietening effects of CNS stimulants on hyperkinetic behavior, and the relation of the response to the degree of activity and brain damage. Prefrontal destructive lesions caused increased locomotor activity, greater in animals with bilateral lesions than in those with unilateral prefrontal lobe ablation. The quietening effect of methylphenidate was most marked in animals with highest levels of activity induced by bilateral lesions. Our clinical studies of children with ADHD also showed the greatest benefit from methylphenidate in those with the highest pre-medication levels of hyperactivity and in the children with the greatest number of neurological abnormal signs. Our report of the syndrome of ADHD, temporal abnormalities in the EEG, and MRI evidence of temporal lobe arachnoid cyst

(Millichap, 1997) provides further support for an organic etiology of ADHD.

Zametkin and Rapoport, at the National Institutes of Health (1987), reviewed the advances in our concept of the neurobiology of ADHD during the previous 50 years. They postulate that different sites of dysfunction in the cortical-striatal "circuit" might account for the varying symptoms and heterogeneous nature of the ADHD syndrome. These authors have also reported PET studies and changes in cerebral glucose metabolism in the frontal lobes of adults with hyperactivity of childhood onset. Further studies of the neurobiological organic basis of ADHD are needed, and an etiological classification of ADHD would be preferred.

J. Gordon Millichap, M.D., F.R.C.P., Editor
Children's Memorial Hospital, Chicago, Illinois

BIBLIOGRAPHY

American Psychiatric Association. Diagnostic and Statistical Manual of Mental Disorders. 2nd, 3rd, 3-Revised, and 4th eds. Washington, DC, American Psychiatric Association, 1968, 1980, 1987, and 1994.

Clements, SD. Minimal Brain Dysfunction in Children. NINDS Monograph no. 3, Public Health Service Bulletin no. 1415, Washington, DC, US Dep Health, Educ. and Welfare, 1966.

Frostig M, Horne D. The Frostig Program for the Development of Visual Perception. Chicago, Follett, 1964.

Holman LB. Post-encephalitic behavior disorders in children. Johns Hopkins Hospital Bulletin. 1922;380:372-375.

Kennard MA, Spencer S, Fountain G Jr. Hyperactivity in monkeys following lesions of the frontal lobes. J Neurophysiol. 1941;4:512.

Kephart NC. The Brain-Injured Child in the Classroom. Chicago, National Society for Crippled Children and Adults, 1963.

Kirk SA. Behavioral diagnosis and remediation of learning disabilities. In Conference on exploration into the problems of the perceptually handicapped child. Evanston, Ill. 1963;1-7. Quoted in Lerner JW. Children with Learning Disabilities. 2nd ed. Boston, Houghton Mifflin, 1976.

Langworthy OR, Richter CP. Increased spontaneous

activity produced by frontal lesions in cats. Amer J Physiol. 1939;126:158-161.

Livingston RB, Fulton JF, Delgado JMR et al. Stimulation and regional ablation of orbital surface of frontal lobe. In: The Frontal Lobes, Res Publ Ass Nerv Ment Dis. 1948:27:405.

Magoun HW. The Waking Brain. 2nd ed, Springfield, Ill, Charles C Thomas, 1963.

Mettler FA. Cortical subcortical relations in abnormal motor functions. In: Neurophysiological Basis of Normal and Abnormal Motor Activities. Yahr MD, Purpura DP (eds), New York, Raven Press, 1967.

Millichap JG. Drugs in management of MBD. NY Acad Sci. 1973;205:321-334; Int J Neurol. 1975;10:241-251.

Millichap JG. Temporal lobe arachnoid cyst - Attention deficit disorder syndrome. Neurology, 1997; in press.

Ruch TC, Shenkin HA. The relation of area 13 on orbital surface of frontal lobes to hyperactivity and hyperphagia in monkeys. J Neurophysiol. 1943;6:349.

Stevens GD, Birch JW. A proposal for clarification of the terminology used to describe brain-injured children. Exceptional Children. May 1957;23:346-349.

Strauss AA, Lehtinen LE. Psychopathology and Education of the Brain-Injured Child. NY, Grune Stratton, 1947.

Zametkin AJ, Rapoport JL. Neurobiology of ADHD. J Am Acad Child Adolesc Psychiatry. 1987;26:676-686.

DIAGNOSIS OF ADHD

ADHD DEFINITION AND CLASSIFICATION

Issues relating to the definition and classification of ADHD are outlined from the Departments of Pediatrics, Neurology, and Child Study, Yale University School of Medicine, New Haven, CT. In *DSM-III-R* (1987) attention deficit disorder with hyperactivity was referred to as ADHD, and ADD without hyperactivity was called undifferentiated ADD. In *DSM-IV* (1994) the categories of ADHD are 1) inattention only, 2) hyperactive only, or 3) combined inattention-hyperactive type. "Attention," the psychological construct as measured in the laboratory, should not be confused with "*behavior* attention deficit," the disorder evaluated by rating scales. Despite the *DSM* definitions of types, children with ADHD represent a heterogeneous population that varies with 1) the degree of cognitive and behavioral overlap, 2) the relative predominance of inattention or hyperactive-impulsive behavior, and 3) the specialty interest of the professional who diagnoses and treats the patient - pediatrician, child neurologist, psychiatrist, psychologist, educator, or speech-language pathologist. Samplings from mental health settings have different characteristics compared to those from pediatric neurology clinics. Patients with comorbid behavioral disorders such as oppositional and conduct disorders would be referred to psychiatrists and clinical psychologists, while those with ADHD complicated by learning disabilities are more likely to be seen by the pediatric neurologist and educational psychologist. A systematic classification of subtypes of ADHD should lead to more precise definitions of etiology, treatment, and prognosis. (Shaywitz BA, Fletcher JM, Shaywitz SE. Defining and classifying learning disabilities and attention-deficit/hyperactivity disorder. <u>J Child Neurol</u> 1995;10 (suppl 1):S50-S57). (Respond: Dr Bennett A Shaywitz, Department of Pediatrics, Yale University School of Medicine, PO Box 208064, New Haven, CT 06520).

COMMENT. The neurologic and psychiatry examinations, psychologic evaluations, and EEG and evoked potentials are important in the differentiation and treatment of subgroups of ADHD children and adolescents. (see Millichap JG, Ed, <u>Progress in Pediatric Neurology I</u>, Chicago, PNB Publ, 1991; and <u>Ped Neur Briefs</u> March 1995;9:20). Abnormalities of CNS maturation and function revealed by longitudinal auditory evoked responses and EEGs were found to characterize non-delinquent ADHD subjects, while delinquent hyperactive subjects showed normal CNS maturation. ADHD boys with neurologic abnormalities had a better outcome than those with normal CNS function who later exhibited delinquent behavior secondary to environmental social factors, (Satterfield JH et al. Electroenceph Clin Neurophysiol 1987;67:531; see PPN I, pp159-160). -Editor. *Ped Neur Briefs* July 1995.

DSM-III-R   cf   DSM-IV   DIAGNOSTIC CRITERIA FOR ADHD

Teacher-reported prevalence rates for attention-deficit hyperactivity disorder (ADHD) using DSM-IV and DSM-III-R criteria were compared in a middle Tennessee county during the 1993-94 academic year and analysed by subtypes at Vanderbilt University, Nashville, TN. Rating scales for 8258 children were completed by 398 teachers. Prevalence rates were 7.3% for ADHD using DSM-III-R diagnostic criteria; 5.4% for ADHD, inattentive type (AD); 2.4% for hyperactive-impulsive type(HI); and 3.6% for combined type (CT) using DSM-IV criteria. Boys outnumbered girls with a 4:1 ratio for ADHD-HI and 2:1 for ADHD-AD. The number of children meeting criteria for the total of all three DSM-IV subtypes (11.4%) was 57% greater than those with ADHD DSM-III-R criteria. Children with ADHD-CT had the highest rate of comorbid conditions, 55% having ODD, 29% CD, and 29% ANX/DEP. ADHD-AD was associated with much lower rates of ODD and CD than other subtypes. Anxiety or depression rates were highest for ADHD-CT types and lowest with ADHD-HI. Behavioral problems predominate in ADHD-HI types and academic problems predominate in ADHD-AD. The use of DSM-IV in place of DSM-III-R criteria increased the prevalence of the diagnosis of ADHD in this community, and the new subtypes better characterized the heterogeneity of the disorder. (Wolraich ML et al. Comparison of diagnostic criteria for attention-deficit hyperactivity disorder in a county-wide sample. J Am Acad Child Adolesc Psychiatry March 1996;35:319-324). (Reprints:Dr Wolraich, Vanderbilt Child Development Center, 2100 Pierce Avenue, Nashville, TN 37232).

COMMENT. The new diagnostic criteria in DSM-IV which include two new subtypes are likely to increase the prevalence of ADHD when compared to DSM-III-R criteria. The ADHD inattentive subtype (AD) is characteristic of children with predominant academic problems and fewer behavioral complaints, and it occurs more frequently in females than do other subtypes. ADHD hyperactive-impulsive type (HI) is characterized by behavioral problems, with fewer academic problems, and a low rate of anxiety or depression. ADHD combined type (CT) criteria are close to the the original DSM-III ADD with hyperactivity. **Validity of DSM-IV ADHD subtype diagnoses in relation to previous DSM III and DSM-III-R diagnoses.** ADHD-AD and ADHD-CT diagnoses corresponded with DSM-III ADD/WO and ADD/H diagnoses, respectively, in a study at the University of Georgia, Athens, GA. (Morgan AE et al. <u>J Am Acad Child Adolesc Psychiatry</u> March 1996;35:325-333). For the ADHD-AD, predominantly inattentive type, diagnosis the child must have 6 of 9 inattentive symptoms but less than the specified number of HI symptoms. These frequent and sometimes premature modifications of the DSM criteria for diagnosis of ADHD are certainly leading to confusion and have prompted a rash of articles and studies attempting to clarify the dilemma. -Editor. *Ped Neur Briefs* March 1996.

ADHD AND MOTOR PERCEPTION DYSFUNCTION COMORBIDITY

The epidemiology, co-morbidity and overlap of attention deficit hyperactivity disorder (ADHD) and deficits in attention, motor control and perception (DAMP), as defined in Scandinavia, were assessed in a total population of 589 6-year-old children screened for neurodevelopmental and neuropsychiatric disorders at the Skovde Central Hospital, and the University of Goteborg, Sweden. Among 63 children (10.7%) with identified disorders, the prevalence rates for ADHD and DAMP were 2.4-4% and 5.3-6.9%, respectively. One in four to three in four of children with DAMP had ADHD. Attention problems were more pronounced in the ADHD group, but overactivity and impulsivity did not distinguish ADHD from DAMP. Children with DAMP had, by definition, more deficits in perception and motor function. (Landgren M, Pettersson R, Kjellman B, Gillberg C. ADHD, DAMP and other neurodevelopmental/psychiatric disorders in 6-year-old children: epidemiology and co-morbidity. <u>Dev Med Child Neurol</u> Oct 1996;38:891-906). (Respond: Dr Magnus Landgren, Department of Paediatrics, Skovde Central Hospital, S-541 85 Skovde, Sweden).

COMMENT. The Scandinavian syndrome of DAMP emphasizes the association of neurological signs of motor dysfunction, perceptual dysfunction, and attention deficits, whereas the current American DSM criteria for ADHD include only symptoms of inattentiveness, hyperactivity, and impulsivity, excluding reference to tests for neurological and perceptual dysfunction. The overlap of these syndromes and the higher prevalence of DAMP compared to ADHD suggests that the neurological examination and tests for perceptual dysfunction should form an integral part of the criteria for diagnosis of the attention deficit disorders (ADIID). A return to the former minimal brain dysfunction (MBD) criteria, in addition to symptoms of ADHD, would allow a more objective diagnosis and earlier recognition and remediation of associated motor incoordination and perceptual deficits.

Conflicting parent and teacher reports of problem behaviors were noted in children with reading disabilities and/or ADHD in a study at the University of Houston. (Pisecco S et al. <u>J Am Acad Child Adolesc Psychiatry</u> Nov 1996;35:1477-1484). In evaluating a child for ADHD, it is important to obtain both teacher and parent reports. -Editor. *Ped Neur Briefs* Nov 1996.

INFRARED MOTION ANALYSIS OF HYPERACTIVE CHILDREN

Movement patterns of 18 boys with ADHD and 11 normal controls were recorded using an infrared video and motion analysis system during a continuous performance task (CPT) at the Department of Psychiatry, Harvard Medical School, Boston, and the McLean Hospital, Belmont, MA. Compared to controls, subjects with ADHD moved their extremities and head more than twice as often, they covered a 3.4-fold greater distance and a 4-fold greater area. Whole body movements were also 3 to 4 times more frequent and covered a greater distance. Their responses on the CPT were slower and more variable. The less complex and more linear movement patterns of ADHD children correlated with teacher ratings of overactivity-inattention. (Teicher MH et al. Objective measurement of hyperactivity and attentional problems in ADHD. <u>J Am Acad Child Adolesc Psychiatry</u> March 1996;35:334-342). (Reprints: Dr Teicher, McLean Hospital, 115 Mill Street, Belmont, MA 02178).

COMMENT. In addition to the infrared motion analysis of overactivity in ADHD children, the authors used a wristwatch sized "actigraph"worn on a belt to measure activity levels (results to be published separately). Previous publications describing similar objective measurements of hyperactivity were apparently overlooked.

Schulman JL and Reisman JM, at Children's Memorial Hospital, Chicago, devised an "actometer," an automatically winding calender wristwatch with the pendulum connected directly to the hands of the watch, to measure movements of the arms and legs (<u>Amer J Ment Defic</u> 1959;64:455).

Millichap JG et al, also at Children's Memorial and Northwestern Univ Med School, employed the actometer to demonstrate significant lessening of overactivity in hyperactive children treated with methylphenidate (<u>Am J Dis Child</u> 1968;116:235). The "actometer" was worn on the wrist of the nondominant arm during neuropsychological test periods, and activity was measured in units of hours and minutes. The effect of methylphenidate was related to the level of motor activity before treatment; the more active patients were benefited the most by stimulant medication. This simple objective measure of motor activity could be of value, not only in experimental situations but also, in confirming the diagnosis of ADHD when parent and teacher impressions are in disagreement. -Editor. *Ped Neur Briefs* March 1996.

ATTITUDES OF PEDIATRICIANS TO ADHD DIAGNOSIS

Pediatricians' perceptions of ADD and ADHD diagnosis, child and family communication concerning diagnosis and treatment, and treatment issues were examined in a cross-sectional survey involving 380 members of the American Academy of Pediatrics and conducted by the Department of Psychology, University of California-Riverside and Loma Linda University Medical Center, CA. Two thirds of respondents enjoyed treating children with ADD/ADHD, but 40% complained of the time involved, and 87% obtained inadequate insurance compensation. Only 18% were likely to refer patients with ADHD to other specialists, including psychiatrists, psychologists, social workers, educators, or neurologists. Most found schools cooperative in providing information of help in diagnosis and in administering medications. The relative frequencies of medications prescribed were as follows: methylphenidate 98%, slow-release methylphenidate 80%, pemoline (Cylert) 51%, amphetamines 27%, clonidine 6%, and tricyclics 4%. Medications were given daily (57%), weekdays only (44%), and during school year only (60%). Side effects reported by parents included: insomnia (18%), change in mood or affect (15%), headaches (10%). Parental views of ADHD included: diet related (20%), due to poor discipline (10%), poor parenting (12%), classroom inadequacies (21%), boredom at school (13%), medicine is addicting (49%), medicine makes child zombielike (19%), and drugs inhibit growth (8%). (Kwasman A et al. Pediatricians' knowledge and attitudes concerning diagnosis and treatment of attention deficit and hyperactivity disorders. A national survey approach. <u>Arch Pediatr Adolesc Med</u> Nov 1995;149:1211-1216).

(Reprints: Dr Tinsley, Department of Psychology, University of California, Riverside, CA 92521).

COMMENT. The authors recommend further studies to elucidate relationships among pediatrician, parent, and patient beliefs about ADD/ADHD diagnosis and treatment. The low pediatrician referral rate to other specialists in the field might be explained in part by 50% of parents having consulted a psychologist before requesting medical treatment. The lack of educational testing in 50% of patients before receiving medication was disturbing, since many have associated learning disabilities. The pediatricians' attitudes and knowledge of comorbid psychiatric and neurologic disorders and their management would have been of interest, since only 18% referred patients to other specialists. -Editor. *Ped Neur Briefs* Dec 1995.

AUDITORY EVOKED POTENTIALS IN ADD

Brainstem auditory evoked potentials (BAEPs) were performed on 114 children with attention deficit disorder (ADD) referred to the Assaf Harofeh Medical Center, and Sackler Faculty of Medicine, Tel Aviv University, Israel. The latencies of waves III and V and brainstem transmission time interval of waves I-III and I-V were longer in the study group compared to controls. Recordings of the latencies performed for each ear separately showed asymmetries of wave III in children with ADD. The results point to brainstem dysfunction in ADD.(Lahat E et al. BAEP studies in children with attention deficit disorder. <u>Dev Med Child Neurol</u> Feb 1995;37:119-123). (Respond: Dr Eli Lahat, Child Neurology Unit, Assaf Harofeh Medical Center, Zerifin 70300, Israel).

COMMENT. BAEP performed in children with ADD/ADHD during inactivity shows abnormalities and asymmetries that may be used as an objective diagnostic test for ADD. Previous studies have demonstrated the value of BAEP in the differentiation of subgroups of hyperactive children, non-delinquent versus delinquent types. (Satterfield JH et al. 1987; see <u>Progress in Pediatric Neurology I,</u> 1991, pp159-160). -Editor. *Ped Neur Briefs* March 1995.

ETIOLOGY OF ADHD

ETIOLOGY OF ADHD REVIEWED

The various proposed etiologies of attention deficit hyperactivity disorder (ADHD) are reviewed from the Department of Neurology, New York University Medical Center, New York. These include:
1) *genetics, familial environmental factors;*
2) *pregnancy related risk factors*: smoking, maternal anemia, breech delivery, chorioamnionitis, small head circumference, prematurity, low birth weight, birth asphyxia, cocaine, and alcohol (fetal alcohol syndrome),
3) *childhood illness sequelae*: meningitis, encephalitis, Reyes syndrome, otitis media, anemia, cardiac disease, thyroid disease, epilepsy, autoimmune disorders, and metabolic disorders,
4) *head injury,* especially involving frontal lobes,
5) *toxins and drugs*: lead, theophylline, anticonvulsants.
(Nass R. Etiologies of attention deficit hyperactivity disorder:Facts and myths. <u>Int Pediatr</u> 1995:10:236-241).(Reprints: Dr Ruth Nass, NYU Medical Center, 440 East 34th Street, Room 311, New York, NY 10016).

COMMENT. The recognition of risk factors for ADHD can lead to early intervention and improved prognosis.

Diet and nutrition enthusiasts would add the effects of food additives, food allergies and sucrose to the above list of potential etiological factors in ADHD. The relation of fatty acids to ADHD and dyslexia has also received renewed attention. Mitchell EA et al, University of Auckland, New Zealand, found that docosahexaenoic, dihomogrammalmolenic, and arachidonic acid serum levels were significantly lower in 44 hyperactive children compared to 45 age- and sex-matched controls. (<u>Clin Pediat</u> 1987;26:406-411). Stordy BJ, University of Surrey, Guildford, UK, reported that docosahexaenoic acid (DHA) supplements improved dark adaptation (scotopic vision) in 5 adults with dyslexia. (<u>Lancet</u> Aug 5, 1995;346:385). She later proposed DHA as a treatment for ADD and poor short term memory problems. For a review of recent articles concerning pros and cons of dietary factors in ADHD and learning disorders, see <u>Progress in Pediatric Neurology I and II</u>, 1991 and 1994, Chicago, PNB Publishers. -Editor. *Ped Neur Briefs* Nov 1995.

SEASON OF BIRTH: ADHD RISK FACTOR

Seasonal variations in the birth patterns of 140 ADHD boys compared to 120 controls were studied at the Massachusetts General Hospital, Boston, with particular reference to issues of psychiatric and cognitive comorbidity and familiality. Statistically significant peaks for September births were noted in ADHD children with comorbid learning disabilities and in those without psychiatric comorbidity. A trend toward an increase in winter births was also evident. A first-trimester viral hypothesis for ADHD is suggested. (Mick E, Biederman J, Faraone SV. Is season of birth a risk factor for attention-deficit hyperactivity disorder? <u>J Am Acad Child Adolesc Psychiatry</u> Nov 1996;35:1470-1476). (Reprints: Dr Biederman, Pediatric Psychopharmacology Unit (ACC 725), Massachusetts General Hospital, Fruit Street, Boston, MA 02114).

COMMENT. Exposure to viral infections during winter months in the first trimester of fetal life or at the time of birth may be a predisposing factor in 10% of ADHD subjects having comorbid learning disabilities. Prenatal or perinatal infection as a possible cause of ADHD requires further evaluation.

Familial transmission of ADHD is supported by a prospective four-year follow-up study of siblings of ADHD children, one fourth having developed ADHD and one half showing evidence of school failure.

(Faraone SV, Biederman J et al. <u>J Am Acad Child Adolesc Psychiatry</u> Nov 1996;35:1449-1459). -Editor. *Ped Neur Briefs* Nov 1996.

ETIOLOGY OF ADHD: PERINATAL HYPOXIC ENCEPHALOPATHY

Recent evidence pointing to a disturbance of function of the striatum in attention deficit hyperactivity disorder (ADHD) is reviwed from the Department of Pediatric Neurology, The John F Kennedy Institute Glostrup, Denmark. Concomitant involvement of the cingulo-striato-thalamo-cortical loop which subserves awareness results in impulsivity, inattention and hyperactivity. Perinatal hypoxic-ischemic encephalopathy, common in prematurity, a known antecedent of ADHD, results in release of excitatory amino acids, especially glutamate, which cause neuronal swelling and cell death. The anatomy of the striatum, with its convergent glutaminergic afferent synaptic transmission from the cortex, contributes to its vulnerability in ischemia-induced glutamate release. The increased survival of premature infants has led to a higher incidence of ADHD in this patient group. (Lou HC. Etiology and pathogenesis of attention-deficit hyperactivity disorder (ADHD): significance of prematurity and perinatal hypoxic-haemodynamic encephalopathy. <u>Acta Paediatr</u> Nov 1996;85:1266-1271). (Respond: Dr HC Lou, Department of Pediatric Neurology, The John F Kennedy Institute, Gl Landevej 7 DK-2600 Glostrup, Denmark).

COMMENT. ADHD is a heterogeneous disorder with a number of presumed etiologic factors. This author emphasizes the role of prematurity and hypoxic-ischemic events in damage to the striatum and its connections in the pathophysiology of ADHD. Several studies are cited showing up to one third of premature infants with birthweight <1500 gm have ADHD when examined at 5 to 7 years. -Editor. *Ped Neur Briefs* Dec 1996.

STRUCTURAL CEREBRAL ANOMALIES

CORPUS CALLOSUM UNDERDEVELOPMENT
The need for subtyping is stressed by reports of brain structural changes in a group of 15 children with ADHD examined by MRI at the Massachusetts General Hospital.The splenial area of the corpus callosum was smaller in ADHD children compared to normal controls. Age was not a factor. (Semrud-Clikeman M et al. Attention-deficit hyperactivity disorder: Magnetic resonance imaging morphometric analysis of the corpus callosum. <u>J Am Acad Child Adolesc Psychiatry</u> July/Aug 1994;33:875-881). -Editor. *Ped Neur Briefs* July 1994. Also, see Chap. 5 for further reference to corpus callosum size in ADHD and Tourette's syndrome.

QUANTITATIVE MRI CHANGES IN ADHD
Anatomic brain MRIs for 57 boys with ADHD and 55 healthy matched controls, aged 5 to 18 years, were compared at the National Institute of Mental Health, Bethesda, MD. ADHD subjects had a 4.7% smaller total cerebral volume, a significant loss of normal right>left asymmetry in the caudate nucleus, smaller right globus pallidus, smaller right anterior frontal region, smaller cerebellum, and reversal of normal (L>R) lateral ventricular asymmetry. Whereas ventricular volume increased significantly with age for normal subjects, no age-related changes were found in ADHD subjects. Within the ADHD group, Full-Scale WISC-R IQ score correlated with total cerebral volume. Decreased normal caudate asymmetry was associated with increasing perinatal risk only in the ADHD boys. (Castellanos FX, Rapoport JL et al. Quantitative brain magnetic resonance imaging in attention-deficit hyperactivity disorder. <u>Arch Gen Psychiatry</u> July 1996;53:607-616). (Reprints: F. Xavier Castellanos MD, Child Psychiatry Branch, National Institute of Mental Health, Building 10, Room 6N240, 10 Center Dr, MSC 1600, Bethesda, MD 20892).

COMMENT. Evidence that a lack of normal asymmetry of regional brain structures is involved in the pathophysiology of ADHD is further supported by this study. Decreased volume of the prefrontal cortex, caudate nucleus, and globus pallidus on the right side point to a dysfunction of right-sided prefrontal-striatal systems in ADHD. A decrease in size of the splenium of the corpus callosum, previously reported in ADHD children (see <u>Ped Neur Briefs</u> July 1994;8:55), was not observed. -Editor. *Ped Neur Briefs* Aug 1996.

SUGAR AND OTHER DIETARY FACTORS

BRAIN GLUCOSE METABOLISM: PET STUDY

Differences in brain glucose metabolism in girls with ADHD compared to boys are reported in PET studies at the National Institute of Mental Health, Bethesda, MD. Global cerebral glucose metabolism in 5 ADHD girls was 15% lower than in 6 normal girls, but was unchanged in ADHD boys compared to normal boys; it was 20% lower in ADHD girls compared to ADHD boys. Adolescents showed no changes in cerebral glucose metabolism. (Ernst M et al. Reduced brain metabolism in hyperactive girls. <u>J Am Acad Child Adolesc Psychiatry</u> July/Aug 1994;33:858-868). Editor. *Ped Neur Briefs* July 1994.

MECHANISM OF SUGAR-INDUCED BEHAVIORAL EFFECTS

The adrenomedullary response to a standard oral glucose load (1.75 gm/kg; maximum, 120 gm) and susceptibility to neuroglycopenia (assessed by the hypoglycemic clamp and measurements of P300 auditory evoked potentials [AEP]) were studied in 25 healthy children (8 - 16 years of age) compared to 23 young adults at the Children's Clinical Research Center, Yale University School of Medicine, New Haven, CT. Baseline and oral glucose-stimulated plasma glucose and insulin levels were similar in children and adult groups. A late fall in plasma glucose level at 3 - 5 hours after glucose ingestion stimulated a rise in plasma epinephrine, twice as high in children compared to adults. Hypoglycemic symptoms (shaky, sweaty, weak, or tachycardia) increased in children but not in adults, in association with the late fall in plasma glucose. P300 amplitude, a measure of cognitive function, was significantly reduced when glucose concentration was lowered to 75 mg/dl in children, but was preserved until the level fell to 54 mg/dl in adults. Children are more vulnerable to effects of hypoglycemia on cognitive function than are adults. (Jones TW et al. Enhanced adrenomedullary response and increased susceptibility to neuroglycopenia: Mechanisms underlying the adverse effects of sugar ingestion in healthy children. <u>J Pediatr</u> February 1995;126:171-7). (Reprints: William V Tamborlane MD, Department of Pediatrics, Yale University School of Medicine, 333 Cedar St, New Haven, CT 06510).

COMMENT. This study shows that consumption of glucose by healthy children may be followed by a fall in plasma glucose sufficient to induce hormonal changes and adverse behavioral and cognitive effects. The authors stress that their data do not prove a causative role for dietary sugar in children with hyperactivity. However, a balanced diet of protein, fat, and complex carbohydrate, to limit postprandial falls in glucose levels, should avoid symptoms associated with the enhanced adrenomedullary responsiveness demonstrated in healthy children.

Mild hypoglycemia (60 mg/dl) caused a significant decline in performance on a battery of cognitive tests in a study of adolescents with insulin-dependent diabetes mellitus at the University of Pittsburgh School of Medicine. Neither hyperglycemia, nor the rapid drop from acute hyperglycemia to euglycemia, affected symptoms, cognitive function, or counterregulatory hormone secretion. (Gschwend S et al. Effects of acute hyperglycemia on mental efficiency and counterregulatory hormones in adolescents with insulin-dependent diabetes mellitus. <u>J Pediatr</u> Feb

1995;126:178-84). -Editor. *Ped Neur Briefs* Feb 1995.

EFFECT OF SUGAR ON BEHAVIOR AND COGNITION

Meta-analysis of 16 published studies conducted over a period of 12 years from 1982 to 1994 was used to examine the effects of sugar, mainly sucrose, on the behavior or cognition of children with attention deficit disorder and reported from the Department of Pediatrics, Vanderbilt University, Nashville, TN. In studies selected, subjects had consumed a known quantity of sugar; a placebo (artificial sweetener) control had been used; subjects, parents and researchers were blind to the conditions; and statistics had been used to compute the dependent measures effect sizes. Most investigators had used doses per kgm body wt ranging from 1.25 to 5.6 g. Aspartame was used as placebo in 13. No effect of sugar on behavior or cognitive performance of these children could be demonstrated by meta-analysis of the data. A small effect of sugar in the total group or effects on subsets of ADHD children could not be ruled out. (Wolraich ML et al. The effect of sugar on behavior or cognition in children. A meta-analysis. <u>JAMA</u> Nov 22/29, 1995;274:1617-1621). (Reprints: Dr Wolraich, Department of Pediatrics, Vanderbilt University, Child Development Center, 2100 Pierce Ave, 426 MCS, Nashville, TN 37232).

COMMENT. The controversy regarding sugar and behavior and cognition continues. Despite this and other studies negating an adverse effect of sugar, parents and some physicians cite sucrose as a frequent trigger of hyperactive behavior and inattention in children. The authors admit that a small adverse effect may be overlooked in a meta-analysis involving few controlled studies with selected patients. (see <u>Progress in Pediatric Neurology II</u>, 1994. pp 516-19, for other articles on diet and behavior). -Editor. *Ped Neur Briefs* Dec 1995.

ASPARTAME, BEHAVIOR, AND COGNITION IN ADD

The effects of aspartame (34 mg/kg/day for 2 weeks) on the cognition, behavior, and monoamine metabolism of 15 children with a history of ADD were evaluated at the Yale University School of Medicine, using a randomized, double-blind, placebo-controlled crossover study design. Various measures including Conners Behavior ratings, Children's Checking Task, Airplane Test, and Wisconsin Card Sorting Test revealed no significant differences between aspartame and placebo. The Multigrade Inventory for Teachers showed a significant increase in activity level following aspartame treatments. Phenylalanine and tyrosine levels in plasma were significantly elevated at 1 and 2 hours after aspartame ingestion. (Shaywitz BA et al. Aspartame, behavior, and cognitive function in children with attention deficit disorder. <u>Pediatrics</u> Jan 1994;<u>93</u>:70-75). (Reprints: B A Shaywitz MD, Dept of Pediatrics, Yale University Sch of Med, New Haven, CT 06510).

COMMENT. The authors conclude from this study of 15 ADD children receiving single morning doses before school for 2 weeks that aspartame has no clinically significant effect on behavior and cognition, and does not affect urinary excretion rates of monoamines and metabolites.

Studies of aspartame in children with neuropsychiatric problems are limited, but one well controlled evaluation in 10 children with absence seizures has shown that aspartame exacerbates EEG spike-wave discharges. (Camfield PR et al. <u>Neurology</u> 1992;<u>42</u>:1000). The ingestion of aspartame in children with seizures should be limited or avoided until effects on seizure control are investigated further.(<u>Ped Neur Briefs</u> June 1992;<u>6</u>:46-47). Migraine has been exacerbated by aspartame in controlled studies of adult patients. -Editor. *Ped Neur Briefs* Jan 1994.

FOOD COLORING AND BEHAVIOR

The association between the ingestion of tartrazine synthetic food coloring and behavioral change in children referred for assessment of hyperactivity was investigated at the Royal Children's Hospital, University of Melbourne, Australia. Two hundred hyperactive children whose parents had noted changes in behavior with diet were included in a 6-week open trial of a diet free of synthetic colorings. The parents of 150 reported behavioral improvement with the diet, and deterioration when foods containing synthetic colorings were introduced. A 30-item inventory with 5 behavior clusters (irritability, sleeplessness, restlessness, aggression, and inattention) discriminated between dye ingestion and placebo. A double-blind, placebo-controlled, 21-day study of 34 reactive children, using each child as his or her own control, identified 24 atopic children as clear reactors to tartrazine at all six dose levels, between 1 and 50 mg. They were irritable and restless and had sleep disturbance. A dose response was obtained and the effect was prolonged with doses >10 mg. (Rowe KS, Rowe KJ. Synthetic food coloring and behavior: a dose response effect in a double-blind, placebo-controlled, repeated-measures study. <u>J Pediatr</u> Nov 1994;125:691-698). (Reprints: Katherine S Rowe MBBS, Department of Pediatrics, University of Melbourne, Royal Children's Hospital, Parkville, Victoria 3052, Australia).

COMMENT. The authors appear to have demonstrated a relation between tartrazine ingestion and behavior in 24 atopic children, aged 2 to 14 years. Parents were found to be reliable observers and raters of their children's behavior. The strict criteria of ADDH, and a score of >15 on the Conners Abbreviated Parent-Teacher Questionnaire, required for inclusion in many previous studies of diet and hyperactivity may have missed some reactors, accounting for inconclusive results. Further, the Conner's scale places little emphasis on irritability and sleeplessness, symptoms that were prominent in the reactors in the University of Melbourne study. The number of reactors to tartrazine identified in this study contrasts markedly with those of previous studies, and may have been related to the method used for selection of subjects. In Australia, the Feingold hypothesis is still alive. -Editor. *Ped Neur Briefs* Dec 1994.

ZINC-DEPRIVATION, MOTOR ACTIVITY AND ATTENTION

The effects of moderate dietary zinc deprivation (2 mcg/gm diet) compared to an adequate zinc intake (50 mcg/gm) were compared using 24-hour activity patterns and an attention task performance in 10 adolescent female monkeys (18-33 months of age) at the California Regional Primate Research Center, University of California, Davis, CA. Zinc deprivation caused a progressive decrease in daytime activity levels and impaired attention followed by growth retardation. (Golub MS, Takeuchi PT, Keen CL, Hendricks AG, Gershwin ME. Activity and attention in zinc-deprived adolescent monkeys. <u>Am J Clin Nutr</u> Dec 1996;64:908-915). (Reprints: Dr Mari S Golub, California Regional Primate Research Center, University of California, Davis, CA 95616).

COMMENT. Motor activity levels and attention may be decreased during early stages of zinc deprivation and before the onset of growth retardation. The authors cite references to estimates of zinc deficiency in 50% of US children, and especially in adolescent girls, 80% of whom consume less than the recommended dietary allowance of 12 mg/day. Behavioral effects of zinc malnutrition may be observed before the more obvious onset of growth retardation. Children who eat primarily cereal proteins and little meat may be susceptible to zinc deficiency syndrome. (Millichap JG. Environmental Poisons in Our Food. Chicago, PNB;1993:62). ADD without hyperactivity is more prevalent than ADHD in girls compared to boys, and zinc deficiency should be considered as a factor in the etiology of inattentiveness, especially in girls. -Editor. *Ped Neur Briefs* Dec 1996.

METABOLIC AND ENDOCRINE FACTORS

CATECHOLAMINES IN ADHD

A multistage hypothesis emphasizing the interaction of norepinephrine (NE), epinephrine (EPI), and dopamine in the modulation of attention and impulse control is presented by the Department of Psychiatry, University of Texas Health Science Center, San Antonio, TX. A neurochemical deficit in ADHD is frequently proposed, and a "catecholamine hypothesis" is supported by the effectiveness of stimulant medications which act as dopaminergic and noradrenergic agonists. The noradrenergic system consists of 1) a central NE system and 2) a peripheral NE system. Dextroamphetamine and methylphenidate which block the reuptake of NE lead to increases in plasma NE and urinary EPI in children with ADHD. The anterior cingulate and frontal lobe connections which govern inhibitory control of visual attention are influenced by both dopamine and noradrenergic systems. The frontal lobes are normally rich in dopamine, and patients with medio-orbital prefrontal lesions who are characteristically impulsive, having deficits in inhibitory control, may show presynaptic dopamine deficiencies. ADHD has been explained as "a primary deficit in inhibitory control." Stimulants enhance available dopamine at central synapses, suggesting a "dopamine hypothesis" for ADHD. A multistage hypothesis for ADHD involving interacting catecholamine systems is proposed. (Pliszka SR, McCracken JT, Maas JW. Catecholamines in attention-deficit hyperactivity disorder: current perspectives. <u>J Am Acad Child Adolesc Psychiatry</u> March 1996;35:264-272). (Reprints: Dr Pliszka, Department of Psychiatry, UTHSCSA, San Antonio, TX 78284). Paper presented as a memorial tribute to Dr Maas.

COMMENT. No single neurotransmitter imbalance is the answer to ADHD, and the interaction of norepinephrine, epinephrine, and dopamine appears to play a role in the control of impulse and attention.

PHENYLALANINE METABOLISM AND ADHD. Deficits in selective and sustained attention in children with phenylketonuria (PKU) were correlated with serum phenylalanine concentrations in a study of 20 patient at the Department of Paediatrics,University of Munster, Germany (Weglage J et al. Eur J Pediatr March 1996;155:200-204). These patients were treated early and had normal IQs. The attention deficits were attributed to an impairment of frontal lobe function and could probably be avoided by a stricter dietary control of the PKU. Phenylalanine inhibits the synthesis of dopamine and serotonin as well as the uptake of tyrosine and tryptophan. -Editor. *Ped Neur Briefs* March 1996.

THYROID FUNCTION AND ADHD

Routine thyroid function studies in a community referred sample of boys with ADHD were examined for evidence of generalized resistance to thyroid hormone at the National Institute of Mental Health, Bethesda, MD. TSH, T3, and T4 values in 53 subjects were not in the range suggestive of global or pituitary thyroid hormone resistance, and variability of values was not greater in ADHD subjects compared to 41 normal controls. Motor activity measured by an actometer was increased as T4 values increased (P=.06). (Elia J, Rapoport JL et al. Thyroid function and attention-deficit hyperactivity disorder. J Am Acad Child Adolesc Psychiatry Feb 1994;33:169-172). (Reprints: Dr Rapoport, Child Psychiatry Branch, National Institute of Mental Health, Bldg 10, Rm 6N240, 9000 Rockville Pike, Bethesda, MD 20892).

COMMENT. The authors conclude that a generalized resistance to thyroid hormone (GRTH) is rare, and thyroid function should not be measured routinely in nonfamilial ADHD. In another recent study from the National Institutes of Health, endocrinologists had shown that 70% of children with GRTH met criteria for ADHD. (Hauser et al, 1993; see Ped Neur Briefs April 1993;7:25).

Impairments of cognition, attention, and behavior may occur with hyperthyroidism. The correlation between motor activity and serum T4 values in the above study is of interest and deserves further study, if not routine examination in ADHD. -Editor. *Ped Neur Briefs* Feb 1994.

ADD AND CONGENITAL HYPOTHYROIDISM

The ability to sustain attention was studied using continuous performance tasks in 48 children with early treated congenital hypothyroidism (CH) and 35 healthy controls at the University of Groningen, The Netherlands. In 38 patients with T4 levels <50 nmol/l as neonates, performance of a computer-paced task declined over time, suggesting impairment of sustained attention. In a self-paced task, an initial performance decline was followed by an improvement in the final stages, this pattern being most pronounced in the low T4 group, reflecting a greater performance variability over time and a problem with sustained attention. The performance of the 10 children with intermediate T4 levels (-/> 50 nmol/l as neonates) fell between the control group and the low T4 group. The performance declines were correlated with intelligence, but the difference in performance decline between the low T4 group and controls was not related to intelligence. No correlation was found between onset of treatment for CH and sustained attention. A suboptimal motor system may have been a factor underlying the sustained attention deficit in CH children. (Kooistra L et al. Sustained attention problems in children with early treated congenital hypothyroidism. <u>Acta Paediatr</u> April 1996;85:425-9). (Respond: Dr L Kooistra, University of Groningen, Laboratory of Experimental Clinical Psychology, Grote Kruisstraat 2/1, 9712 TS Groningen, The Netherlands).

COMMENT. Motor, cognitive, and motivational factors may influence scores on continuous performance tasks. All three factors can be important influences on sustained attention in children with congenital hypothyroidism. Editor. *Ped Neur Briefs*

June 1996.

ATTENTION DEFICITS AND THYROID FUNCTION

The relation between attention and thyroid function was examined in 85, 7-year-old, children with congenital hypothyroidism (CH) at the Hospital for Sick Children, Toronto, Canada. Children were assigned to subgroups on the basis of concurrent T4 and TSH levels. Almost 10% of children with CH had abnormally high levels of T4 and TSH. Those with this abnormal thyroid profile did not differ from other CH children in intelligence but they did perform more poorly on a measure of cognitive attention, while rating more favorably on parent behavior scales of hyperactivity and distractibility. The level of T4 was the stongest predictor of poorer cognitive attention, while TSH levels correlated directly with hyperactivity. (Rovet J, Alvarez M. Thyroid hormone and attention in school-age children with congenital hypothyroidism. <u>J Child Psychol Psychiat</u> July 1996;37:579-585). Reprints: Dr Joanne Rovet, Psychology Department, The Hospital for Sick Children, 555 University Ave, Toronto, Ontario, Canada M5G 1X8).

COMMENT. Higher levels of T4 and TSH, consistent with a resistance to thyroid hormone, are associated with poorer attention and less hyperactive behavior in children with congenital hypothyroidism. Children with CH should be closely monitored to maintain levels of T4 and TSH within the normal range and to avoid elevations of hormone that could impede attention. Thyroxine and thyrotropin have unique effects on specific aspects of attention and behavior.

The incidence of ADHD is 10 times higher in children with thyroid hormone resistance than in those with normal thyroid function. (Hauser P et al. <u>N Engl J Med</u> 1993;328:997). See <u>Progress in Pediatric Neurology II</u>, 1994, pp 177-8. Studies of thyroid function should be included more frequently in the clinical evaluation of children with ADHD. -Editor. *Ped Neur*

Briefs Sept 1996.

TOXIC FACTORS IN ADHD

COCAINE-INDUCED BEHAVIORAL CHANGES
Behavioral and hormonal responses in 30 preterm cocaine-exposed infants were compared with a cohort of 30 non-cocaine-exposed preterm infants at the Touch Research Institute, University of Miami School of Medicine, FL. Cocaine-exposed infants had smaller head circumference at birth, longer stays in the intensive care unit, a higher incidence of intraventricular hemorrhage, inferior performance on the Brazelton Neonatal Behavioral Assessment Scale (range of state, regulation of state, and depression clusters), decreased periods of quiet sleep, and increased levels of agitated behavior, including tremulousness, limb movements, and clenched fists. They also had higher urinary norepinephrine, dopamine, and cortisol levels and lower plasma insulin levels than controls. Epinephrine and glucose levels were unchanged. (Scafidi FA, Field TM et al. Cocaine-exposed preterm nenates show behavioral and hormonal differences. <u>Pediatrics</u> June 1996;97:851-855). (Reprints: Dr Tiffany M Field, Touch Research Institute, University of Miami School of Medicine, PO Box 016820, Miami, FL 33101).

COMMENT. Cocaine-exposed infants require careful follow-up for early diagnosis and therapy of neurobehavioral complications. A frequent history of prenatal cocaine exposure in foster children with attention deficit hyperactivity disorders is of interest in relation to the changes in catecholamine metabolism noted in the above study. For reference to neurological correlates of fetal cocaine exposure, see <u>Ped Neur Briefs</u> Feb 1996;10:9-10; and <u>Progress in Pediatric Neurology I and II</u> PNB Publishers, 1991 and 1994.

IN UTERO COCAINE EXPOSURE AND INFANT BEHAVIOR

The effects on neurobehavior in 20 infants with prenatal exposure to cocaine, alcohol, marijuana, and cigarettes, compared to 17 infants exposed to alcohol and/or marijuana and cigarettes without cocaine and 20 drug-free infants, were assessed using the Neonatal Intensive Care Unit Network Neurobehavioral Scale at Brown University School of Medicine, Women and Infants Hospital, Providence, RI. Cocaine-exposed infants showed increased tone and motor activity, more jerky movements, startles, tremors, back arching, and signs of central nervous system and visual stress than unexposed infants. Visual and auditory following responses, and birth weight and length of cocaine-exposed infants were also reduced. (Napiorkowski B, Lester BM et al. Effects of in utero substance exposure on infant neurobehavior. <u>Pediatrics</u> July 1996;98:71-75). (Reprints: Barry M Lester PhD, Women and Infant's Hospital, 101 Dudley St, Providence, RI 02905).

COMMENT. Meconium testing was used to confirm lack of illicit drug use in the unexposed group. Positive meconium or urine assays were found in 5 women who had denied prenatal drug use. Urine toxicology can detect cocaine within 1 to 4 days of last use. Cocaine-exposed infants had neurobehavioral changes especially involving increased tone and motor activity. Synergistic effects of cocaine with alcohol and marijuana could not be ruled out.

Dose-related effects of cocaine on 3-week neurobehavior were demonstrated in a study at Children's Hospital, Boston, MA. Comparing 38 heavily exposed infants, 73 lightly exposed, and 94 unexposed, after controlling for covariates, a significant dose effect was observed, heavily exposed infants showing poorer regulation of arousal and greater excitability at 3-week examination but not in the first few days of life. (Tronick EZ et al. Late dose-response effects of prenatal cocaine exposure on newborn neurobehavioral performance. <u>Pediatrics</u> July 1996;98:76-83). (Reprints:

Edward Z Tronick PhD, Children's Hospital, 300 Longwood Ave, Boston, MA 02115).

Since regulation of arousal and attention are important to learning, infants exposed to cocaine in utero may be expected to show decreased developmental scores and to have attention deficit disorders in childhood. (<u>Ped Neur Briefs</u> Feb 1996;10:9-10). -Editor. *Ped Neur Briefs* July 1996.

PRENATAL COCAINE AND INFANT BEHAVIOR

The Brazelton Neonatal Behavioral Assessment Scales (BNBAS) were administered to 23 infants exposed to cocaine in utero and 29 nonexposed infants recruited from the low-risk nursery, Wayne State University Hospital, Detroit. Cocaine exposure was determined by quantitative analysis of the infant's meconium stool. Exposed infants performed less well than controls on 6 of the 7 BNBAS clusters, particularly in tests for autonomic stability. A dose-response relationship was evident, with a negative effect of meconium cocaine concentration on motor, orientation, and regulation of state. (Delaney-Black V, Covington C, Ostrea E Jr et al. Prenatal cocaine and neonatal outcome: evaluation of dose-response relationship. <u>Pediatrics</u> Oct 1996;98:735-740). (Reprints: Virginia Delaney-Black MD, Children's Hospital of Michigan, 3901 Beaubien, Detroit, MI 48201).

COMMENT. Significant adverse behavioral effects may be demonstrated in neonates born to cocaine addicted mothers. Quantitative determination of cocaine exposure by meconium analysis is essential, since screening by history alone is found to be inadequate.

Three additional studies of the effects of prenatal cocaine on neurobehavior are summarized as follows. The Brazelton NBAScale, used at the Western Psychiatric Institute, University of Pittsburgh, showed impaired scores in motor maturity and tone, autonomic instability, and an increased number of abnormal reflexes on the 2nd day postpartum, but not at day 3. (Richardson GA et al. The effects of prenatal cocaine use on neonatal neurobehavioral status. <u>Neurotoxicol Teratol</u> Sept/Oct 1996;18:519-528). Heavy cocaine exposure early in pregnancy was related to faster responsiveness on an infant visual expectancy test but poorer recognition memory and information processing in 464 inner-city, black infants tested at 6, 12, and 13 months in the Psychology Department, Wayne State University, Detroit, MI. (Jacobson SW et al. New evidence for neurobehavioral effects of in utero cocaine exposure. <u>J Pediatr</u> Oct 1996;129:581-590). The motor development of 28 infants exposed to cocaine in utero compared to that of an unexposed group followed from birth through 15 months at Boston University, Department of Physical Therapy and Child Development Unit, Children's Hospital, Boston, showed impairments in performance at 4 and 7 months of age but not at 15 months. However, all infants, both exposed and unexposed, were motor impaired when compared to norms, a reflection of the effects of poverty and malnutrition in inner-city infants. (Fetters L, Tronick EZ. Neuromotor development of cocaine-exposed and control infants from birth through 15 months: poor and poorer performance. <u>Pediatrics</u> Nov 1996;98:938-943). The combination of cocaine exposure and poor nutrition is a cumulative risk factor for impaired infantile motor performance in minority subjects and potentially detrimental to later neurocognitive development. -Editor. *Ped Neur Briefs* Dec 1996.

PCB NEUROBEHAVIORAL TOXICITY

Developmental neurotoxicity of polychlorinated biphenyls (PCBs) in humans is reviewed from the Institute of Environmental studies, University of Illinois at Urbana-Champaign, Urbana, IL. (Schantz SL. <u>Neurotoxicol and Teratology</u> May/June 1996;18:217-227). Studies included those in Yusho, Japan; Yucheng, Taiwan; Michigan; North Carolina; Oswego, NY; New Bedford, MA; on Inuit people in the Arctic regions of Quebec; and in Faroe Islanders. Concurrent methylmercury poisoning may be an issue in interpretation of some studies.

Children born to mothers exposed to PCBs showed abnormalities in behavior and development, including higher activity levels, behavior problems, lower IQ scores, decreased birth weight and head circumference, lowered scores on the Brazelton Neonatal Battery, deficits in memory at 4 years, and delays in psychomotor development. Although the deficits in cognition were often small, the public health implications of low-level PCB exposure was compared to that of lead exposure. At a population level, a decrease of 4 points on the Bayley Scales is estimated to result in a 50% increase in the number of children with subnormal scores.

COMMENT. Subtle alterations in neuro-psychological functioning caused by exposure to these environmental toxins were proposed as explanations for some cases of ADHD, either by a direct effect on the brain in the prenatal period or secondary to effects on thyroid function. The potential impact of postnatal exposure to PCBs via breast milk was also reviewed. Other prenatal toxic factors that may underly cognitive, behavioral, and attentional deficits in childhood include alcohol and nicotine. -(see Chap. 14). -Editor. *Ped Neur Briefs* June 1996.

POLYCHLORINATED BIPHENYLS AND ATTENTION DEFICITS

The effects of in utero exposure to polychlorinated biphenyls (PCBs) on cognitive function in 212 children at 11 years of age were tested at Wayne State University, Detroit, MI. Prenatal exposure to PCBs from maternal ingestion of contaminated Lake Michigan fish was associated with significantly lower full-scale and verbal IQ scores. Concentrations of PCBs in maternal serum and milk at delivery, only slightly higher than in the general population, caused long-term intellectual impairment, especially affecting memory, attention, and reading comprehension. (Jacobson JL, Jacobson SW. Intellectual impairment in children exposed to polychlorinated

biphenyls in utero. <u>N Eng J Med</u> Sept 12 1996;335:783-9).
(Reprints: Dr Joseph L Jacobson, Department of Psychology,
Wayne State University, Detroit, MI 48202).

COMMENT. Deficits in short-term memory and
developmental delays, previously noted in infants and
at 4 years of age in children exposed to PCBs in utero,
have now been demonstrated in children tested at 11
years of age. PCBs may have a long-term adverse effect
on cognitive function, and prenatal exposure to these
environmental toxins should be included among
potential causes of attention deficit disorders in
children. -Editor. *Ped Neur Briefs* Oct 1996.

EPILEPSY AND HYPERKINETIC BEHAVIOR

A 4-year-old boy with benign partial epilepsy
and hyperkinetic behavior between seizures is
reported from Sapporo Medical University, Japan.
Hyperactivity was noted at age 3, and seizures began at
4 years 6 months. Attacks consisted of a terrified
expression, crouching, and rubbing his forehead on
the floor. They occurred in sleep and awake. An ictal
EEG in sleep showed theta rhythm, predominant over
the left hemisphere, followed by voltage depression,
but no spike and wave complexes. Both seizures and
hyperkinetic behavior responded to carbamazepine.
The epilepsy was characterized as benign partial
epilepsy with affective symptoms. (Wakai S et al.
Benign partial epilepsy with affective symptoms:
Hyperkinetic behavior during interictal periods.
<u>Epilepsia</u> July/Aug 1994;35:810-812). (Reprints: Dr S Wakai,
Dept Pediatrics, Sapporo Medical University, School of
Medicine, South 1 West 16, Chuo-ku, Sapporo, 060, Japan).

COMMENT. Behavioral and emotional disorder as a
form of epilepsy is a controversial topic, and the
response to antiepileptic drugs in treatment is not
proof of epilepsy. This patient tends to support the
concept of a specific epileptic syndrome, BPEAS, but the
EEG evidence could be more convincing.

The following study provides evidence against the concept of a so-called "masked epilepsy" in some hyperkinetic children. A comparison of the emotional and behavioral problems of 53 children, aged 6-12 years, with epileptiform EEG discharges and those of children without this EEG abnormality showed no significant differences, in a study at the Tokyo Medical and Dental University; the Nihon University; Asai Hospital, Chiba; and National Center for Neurology and Psychiatry, Kodaira, Japan. The authors conclude that the emotional and behavioral problems are coincidental and not directly related to the epileptiform discharges. (Okubo Y et al. Epileptiform EEG discharges in healthy children: Prevalence, emotional and behavioral correlates, and genetic influences. <u>Epilepsia</u> July/Aug 1994;35:832-841). -Editor. *Ped Neur Briefs* Nov 1994.

ATTENTION DISORDERS IN EPILEPSY

The relation of laterality of the epileptogenic focus to cognition and attention in 43 unmedicated children, mean age 10 years, with benign rolandic epilepsy of childhood was assessed at Clinica Neurologica Universita, Perugia, Italy. Children with right sided or bilateral paroxysmal foci scored worse on a figure cancellation task, whereas those with left-sided foci performed as well as controls. The task measures attentive processes and visuospatial orientation. (Piccirilli M et al. Attention problems in epilepsy: possible significance of the epileptogenic focus. <u>Epilepsia</u> Sept/Oct 1994;35:1091-1096). (Reprints: Dr M Piccirilli, Clinica Neurologica Universita, Via E Dal Pozzo, 06100 Perugia, Italy).

COMMENT. Attentional difficulties in children with benign rolandic epilepsy are related to right hemisphere dysfunction and impaired visuospatial processing. The data did not support an hypothesis of left spatial neglect. The laterality of the epileptic focus is linked to the type of cognitive deficit. Left hemisphere dysfunction affects language-related abilities. Attentional disorders in epileptic children can be explained by paroxysmal activity, and is independent of any effect of antiepileptic drugs. -Editor. *Ped Neur Briefs* Dec 1994.

ADVERSE FAMILY-ENVIRONMENT FACTORS AND ADHD

The influence of exposure to parental psychopathology and conflict on functioning and comorbidity in 140 children with ADHD and 120 normal controls was studied at the Pediatric Psychopharmacology Unit in Psychiatry, Massachusetts General Hospital and Harvard Medical School, Boston. Increased levels of environmental adversity were found among ADHD compared with control probands for all adversity variables and especially for parental conflict, diminished family cohesion, number of parents with psychiatric illness, and time exposed to maternal psychopathology (p<.01). Superior IQ protected ADHD subjects from negative influences of parental psychopathology. The risk of developing comorbidity (conduct disorder, depression, anxiety) in ADHD subjects was not influenced by environmental adversity. (Biederman J et al. Impact of adversity on functioning and comorbidity in children with attention-deficit hyperactivity disorder. <u>J Am Acad Child Adolesc Psychiatry</u> Nov 1995;34:1495-1503). (Reprints: Dr Biederman, Pediatric Psychopharmacology Unit (ACC 725), Massachusetts General Hospital, 15 Parkman Street, Boston, MA 02114).

COMMENT. Adverse family environments, including chronic family conflict, decreased family cohesion, and exposure to maternal psychopathology, are risk factors in children with ADHD. Early recognition of these environmental factors should lead to intervention and improved outcome.

The investigation of children with ADHD is multimodal and requires cooperation between various specialties involved. Parents will usually not accept from a neurologist the reality of their own behavior as a factor in the child's disorder. The expertise of a psychologist or psychiatrist is required when parental conflict is suspected. -Editor. *Ped Neur Briefs* Nov 1995.

Psychiatric and Developmental Disorders in Families of Children with ADHD were studied in the Department of Pediatrics, Wyler and La Rabida Children's Hospitals, University of Chicago. (Roizen NJ et al. Arch Pediatr Adolesc Med Feb 1996;150:203-208). Children with ADHD were more likely than control children (with Down syndrome) to have a parent affected by alcoholism, other drug abuse, depression, delinquency, learning disabilities, and/or ADHD. Anticipatory guidance and psychosocial intervention were recommended for families affected. The Editor, Dr DeAngelis, notes that children with a family history of psychiatric disorders should be screened for ADHD. -Editor. *Ped Neur Briefs* March 1996.

RISK FACTORS FOR ADHD PERSISTENCE INTO ADOLESCENCE

Predictors of persistence and the timing of remission of ADHD at a 4-year follow-up of 128 patients were studied prospectively using DSM-III-R criteria at the Massachusetts General Hospital, Boston. The diagnosis of ADHD had persisted in 109 (85%) and had remitted in 19 (15%). Of those no longer meeting the diagnostic criteria, 9 (47%) were late remitters (after age 12 years), and 10 (53%) were early remitters (by age 12 years). Risk factors for persistence included: 1) *genetic* familiality of ADHD, 2) *environmental* psychosocial adversity and exposure to parental conflict, and 3) comorbidity with conduct, mood, and anxiety disorders. (Biederman J et al. Predictors of persistence and remission of ADHD into adolescence: results from a four-year prospective follow-up study. J Am Acad Child Adolesc Psychiatry March 1996;35:343-351). (Reprints: Dr Biederman, Pediatric Psychopharmacology Unit, Massachusetts General Hospital, ACC 725, 15 Parkman Street, Boston, MA 02114).

COMMENT. The majority of children diagnosed with ADHD in childhood will continue to be affected after 12 years of age, into adolescence, and sometimes into adulthood. The frequently repeated prediction that a child will outgrow ADHD by 12 years of age is no longer tenable. These authors also found that the intensity of treatment of ADHD did not alter the incidence of persistence or remission.

The prognosis for ADHD seems to be bleaker than previously perceived. By using stimulant medication, special education, and counselling during early grade school years, the improvements in attentiveness and behavior are expected to result in better study habits and academic achievement. To assure continued success in high school and also, in college, ADHD appears to require persistent medical attention.

Treatment should also be directed more aggressively toward lessening the influence of environmental and familial adverse factors, which appear to be important in persistence of ADHD. Parents are often oblivious or in denial of their role in the etiology of a child's attention deficits and behavior problems. Family counselling, often neglected as part of the multimodal therapy for ADHD, should receive greater emphasis. -Editor. *Ped Neur Briefs* March 1996.

PERSISTENCE OF ADHD IN ADULTS AND RISK OF SUBSTANCE ABUSE

The association between attention deficit hyperactivity disorder (ADHD) and psychoactive substance use disorders in 120 adults with childhood-onset ADHD was evaluated with attention to comorbid mood, anxiety, and antisocial disorders in the Pediatric Psychopharmacology Unit, Psychiatric Service, Massachusetts General Hospital, Harvard Medical School, Boston. The lifetime risk of drug and drug plus alcohol use disorders in the ADHD adults was 52% compared to 27% of 268 control non-ADHD adults. The increased risk of drug and alcohol abuse or dependence related to ADHD was independent of psychiatric comorbidity. Antisocial disorders increased risk of drug abuse independent of ADHD. Mood and anxiety disorders were associated with increased drug abuse in both ADHD and control non-ADHD adults. (Biederman J et al. Psychoactive substance use disorders in adults with attention deficit hyperactivity disorder (ADHD): effects of ADHD and comorbidity. <u>Am J Psychiatry</u> Nov 1995;152:1652-1658). (Reprints: Dr Biederman, ACC 725, Massachusetts General Hospital, Boston, MA 02114).

COMMENT. Childhood onset ADHD persisting in adults without comorbidity carried a 40% risk of a lifetime diagnosis of substance use disorders. Drug abuse or dependence and drug plus alcohol abuse, but not alcohol abuse alone, were significantly increased in grown-up ADHD children compared to non-ADHD adult controls. Psychiatric comorbidity increased the risk of drug abuse. Marijuana was most commonly used (30 ADHD adults), cocaine in 10, and stimulants in 8.

There were no differences in the preferred drugs of abuse between ADHD adults and normal comparison subjects. These results contradict the commonly held view that ADHD patients may show a predilection for stimulant drug abuse. -Editor. *Ped Neur Briefs* Dec 1995.

ADHD in adults is reviewed from the New York State Psychiatric Institute (Shaffer D. <u>Am J Psychiatry</u> May 1994;151:633-638. Editorial).
• Placebo-controlled studies of methylphenidate in adults are infrequent and largely disappointing.
• Psychoactive substance use disorder is commonly associated with diagnoses of ADHD in adults and stimulant medication should be used with caution.
• Adult ADHD is often a self-diagnosed condition, and an excuse for job failure, divorce, and spousal abuse. -Editor. *Ped Neur Briefs* July 1994.

CO-MORBID DISORDERS, ADHD, AND DIFFERENTIAL DIAGNOSIS

DYSTHYMIA AND MAJOR DEPRESSIVE DISORDERS COMPARED

Clinical presentation, course, and outcome of childhood-onset dysthymic disorder (DD) in 55 school-age referrals were compared with a group of 60 youngsters whose first affective episode was major depressive disorder (MDD) in a prospective 3- to 12-year study at Psychiatric Departments of the University of Pittsburgh, Western Psychiatric Institute, University of California at San Diego, and Harvard Medical School. Dysthymic disorder was associated with earlier age at onset than MDD, similarly frequent symptoms of feeling unloved, friendless, irritability, anger, and self-deprecation, but relatively low rates of anhedonia (5% cf 70%), guilt (13% cf 30%), social withdrawal (8% cf 50%), impaired concentration (40% cf 67%), loss of appetite (5% cf 47%), insomnia (22% cf 62%), somatic complaints (36% cf 67%) and fatigue (22% cf 64%). Risk of affective disorders, including first-episode MDD (76%) and bipolar disorder (13%), was greater among dysthymic patients. After the first episode of MDD complicating DD, the clinical course of DD was similar to MDD in rates of recurrent major depression and bipolar disorder. In dysthymic children with subsequent MDD, the first episode of MDD is the "gateway" to recurrent affective illness. (Kovacs M et al. Childhood-onset dysthymic disorder. Clinical features and prospective naturalistic outcome. <u>Arch Gen Psychiatry</u> May 1994;51:365-374). (Reprints: Dr Kovacs, Western Psychiatric Institute and Clinic, 3811 O'Hara St, Pittsburgh, PA 15213).

COMMENT. Pediatric neurologists are frequently faced with the differentiation of organic and psychiatric causes for behavioral and mood disorders and somatic complaints. The recognition of early onset childhood dysthymic disorder should permit prompt referral to colleagues specialized in child psychology and psychiatry. Early diagnosis and treatment of dysthymia may prevent the occurrence of major depressive disorders.

The distinctions between major depression without dysthymia, dysthymia without major depression, and double depression in 62 child psychiatry inpatients were evaluated at the Department of Psychology, State University of New York at Stony Brook. Externalizing disorders (oppositional defiant and conduct disorders) were present more often in the dysthymic group compared to the major depression and double depression groups, whereas major depression and double depression groups revealed higher rates of depressive symptoms. In contrast to the Pittsburgh report, this study found social functioning to be least impaired in children with major depression. (Ferro T et al. Depressive disorders: distinctions in children. <u>J Am Acad Child Adolesc Psychiatry</u> June 1994;33:664-670).

The role of the Children's Depression Rating Scale-Revised in assessing depression in children with sickle-cell anemia was evaluated at the University of South Alabama Children's Medical Center, Mobile, AL. Excessive fatigue and physical complaints contributed to a high false-positive rate of depression on the standardized screening test, whereas the actual prevalence of depression in these children based on clinical interviews by a child psychiatrist was not increased. (Yang Y-M et al. Depression in children and adolescents with sickle-cell disease. <u>Arch Pediatr Adolesc Med</u> May 1994;148:457-460). -Editor. *Ped Neur Briefs* June 1994.

ADHD AND ADOLESCENT MANIA

An association between adolescent mania and ADHD is reported from the Department of Psychiatry, University of Cincinnati College of Medicine. (West SA et al. <u>Am J Psychiatry</u> Feb 1995;152:271-273). Of 14 adolescent bipolar patients who were admitted to hospital for the treatment of acute mania or hypomania, 8(57%) also met the DSM-III-R criteria for ADHD. Patients with ADHD had a higher mean total score on the Young Mania Rating Scale than patients with bipolar disorder alone. This finding may have important implications regarding pharmacological therapy. -Editor. *Ped Neur Briefs* March 1995.

OPPOSITIONAL DEFIANT DISORDER, CONDUCT, AND ADHD

The link between oppositional defiant disorder (ODD) and conduct disorder (CD) was evaluated in 140 children with attention-deficit hyperactivity disorder (ADHD) and 120 normal controls examined at baseline and 4 years later, in midadolescence, at the Pediatric Psychopharmacology Unit, Psychiatric Service, Massachusetts General Hospital, Boston, MA. Of ADHD children, 65% had comorbid ODD and 22% had CD at baseline. Of ODD children, 32% had comorbid CD. Children with CD also had ODD that preceded CD by several years. Children with both ODD and CD had more severe symptoms of ODD, more psychiatric disorders, more bipolar disorder, and more abnormal behavior scores compared to ADHD children without comorbidity. Risk of CD at 4-year follow-up was not increased in children with ODD without CD at baseline. Two subtypes of ODD associated with ADHD were evident: one prodromal to CD and one that is not. (Biederman J et al. Is childhood oppositional defiant disorder a precursor to adolescent conduct disorder? Findings from a four-year follow-up study of children with ADHD. <u>J Am Acad Child Adolesc Psychiatry</u> Sept 1996;35:1193-1204). (Reprints: Dr Biederman, Pediatric Psychopharmacology Unit (ACC 725), Massachusetts General Hospital, Fruit Street, Boston, MA 02114).

COMMENT. The majority of ODD children with ADHD do not have comorbid CD, whereas CD is almost always comorbid with ODD which precedes the onset of CD by several years. The majority of children with ADHD and CD had developed CD before age 12 years. Adolescent onset CD is rare. CD with ADHD is associated with higher frequency of substance abuse in adolescence, and higher levels of anxiety disorders and mood disorders. Two ODD subtypes, one prodromal to CD and one without, have different outcomes. -Editor. *Ped Neur Briefs* Sept 1996.

AUTISM, ADHD, AND TUBEROUS SCLEROSIS

In a population-based psychiatric study of 28 patients with tuberous sclerosis (TS) at the University of Goteborg, Sweden, 24 had autistic symptoms and 17 met all DSM-III-R criteria for autistic disorder (AD). Of the 17 with AD, 7 were severely mentally retarded, 7 had mild retardation, 3 were near average IQ, and 11 had ADHD. One girl of average IQ had Asperger syndrome. Only 3 were free of psychiatric/behavioral problems, all having average IQs. Of the 24 with autistic behavior, 14 had a history of infantile spasms. Infantile spasms were not specifically associated with later development of autistic behavior. TS predisposes to both autism and infantile spasms. Nine per cent of all children and 20% of females with autism may have TS. Autistic behavior in children < 5 years of age has a stronger correlation with TS than facial angiofibromas, a sign often not clearly defined until later childhood. (Gillberg IC et al. Autistic behavior and attention deficits in tuberous sclerosis: a population-based study. <u>Dev Med Child Neurol</u> Jan 1994;<u>36</u>:50-56). (Respond: Christopher Gillberg MD, Annedal Clinics, Child Neuropychiatry Clinic, University of Goteborg, S-413 45 Goteborg, Sweden).

COMMENT. An epidemiological study of TS in Western Sweden by the same authors showed a peak prevalence of 1 in 6800 in the 11 to 15 year-old age group, almost double that reported in earlier studies. In the whole cohort, 0-20 years, the prevalence was 1 in 12900. (Ahlsen G,Gillberg IC et al. Tuberous sclerosis in Western Sweden. <u>Arch Neurol</u> Jan 1994;<u>51</u>:76-81). -Editor. *Ped Neur Briefs* Feb 1994.

EARLY SIGNS OF AUTISM

A blinded comparison of parental and clinical observations of the behavior of 26 autistic children (23 boys and 3 girls) younger than age 48 months is reported from the Vanderbilt University School of Medicine, Nashville, TN, and The Children's Mercy Hospital, Kansas City. Five most prevalent behavioral characteristics both reported by parents and observed by clinicians were as follows: 1) abnormal social play (eg. nonparticipation in peekaboo and itsy bitsy spider games); 2) lack of awareness of others (eg. noninteraction); 3) impaired imitation (eg. wave goodbye, patty-cake); 4) deficient nonverbal communication (eg. absent social smile or eye contact); and 5) absent imaginative play (eg. pretend games). Autistic behaviors rarely endorsed by parents and clinicians included: abnormal comfort seeking, abnormal speech, distress over change, and insistence on sameness and routines. Parents were more likely than clinicians to report absence of imaginative play and presence of stereotyped movements. (Stone WL, Hoffman EL et al. Early recognition of autism. Parental reports vs clinical observation. <u>Arch Pediatr Adolesc Med</u> Feb 1994;<u>148</u>:174-179). (Reprints: Dr Stone, Child Development Center, Vanderbilt University Medical Center S, Room 426, 2100 Pierce Ave, Nashville, TN 37232).

COMMENT. Improved awareness of early signs of autism should help physicians recognize and refer patients for specialized intervention. Parents are better judges of a child's imaginative play and peer friendships, whereas physicians may be more objective about a child's social awareness, interactive play, imitation skills, and nonverbal communication.

Decreased plasma concentrations of the C4B complement protein are reported in a group of 42 autistic subjects examined at the Center for Persons with Disabilities and Department of Biology, Utah State University, Logan, UT. (Warren RP et al. <u>Arch Pediatr Adolesc Med</u> Feb 1994;<u>148</u>:180-183). -Editor. *Ped Neur Briefs* Feb 1994.

ABNORMAL EEG IN AUTISM: VALPROATE RESPONSE

Three children, ages 3, 4, and 5 years, with autism and epileptiform EEG discharges showed clinical improvement with valproic acid therapy at Mercy Hospital and Medical Center, Chicago, IL. None had a history of seizures. Within one month of VPA 125 mg tid treatment, language and social skills improved and the DSM-III-R criteria for autism no longer applied. Improvement had been maintained at follow-up 7 to 11 months later. (Plioplys AV. Autism: electro-encephalogram abnormalities and clinical improvement with valproic acid. <u>Arch Pediatr Adolesc Med</u> Feb 1994;<u>148</u>:220-222). (Reprints: Dr Plioplys, Division of Neurology, Mercy Hospital and Medical Center, Stevenson Expressway at King Drive, Chicago, IL 60616).

COMMENT. The author stresses the importance of sleep EEGs to uncover epileptiform discharges in young autistic patients without history of clinical seizures. Further trials of anticpileptic drugs in autistic children seem justified. -Editor. *Ped Neur Briefs* Feb 1994.

POSTERIOR FOSSA ABNORMALITIES IN INFANTILE AUTISM

Previously published cerebellar vermis measures of 78 autistic patients from 4 separate MRI studies have been reanalysed at the Neurosciences Department, School of Medicine, University of California at San Diego, La Jolla, CA. Abnormalities were in 2 groups: vermal hypoplasia in 80-90% and vermal hyperplasia in 8-16% patients. These subgroups also differed significantly from normal controls. Failure to recognize these variations in vermal structure among patients may have lead to disparate reports of cerebellar maldevelopment in infantile autism. (Courchesne E et al. The brain in infantile autism: Posterior fossa structures are abnormal. <u>Neurology</u> Feb 1994;<u>44</u>:214-223). (Reprints: Dr Eric

Courchesne, Neuropsychology Research Laboratory, Children's Hospital, 3020 Children's Way, San Diego, CA 92123).

COMMENT. Cerebellar pathology and hypoplasia have been reported in Rett and Down syndromes as well as autism. Attentional asynergia and dysfunction following cerebellar damage are linked to impaired social communication skills. Cerebellar mutism and personality changes have followed surgical removal of medulloblastoma.(Ped Neur Briefs Feb 1992;6:15-16). The finding of subtypes of neuroanatomic changes supports the belief that autism is a heterogeneous disorder. Editor. *Ped Neur Briefs* Feb 1994.

ASPERGER SYNDROME AND AUTISM COMPARED

The validity and neuropsychological characterization of Asperger syndrome (AS) was investigated by comparison with Higher-Functioning Autism (HFA) (ie autism associated with overall normal intelligence) in 73 potential subjects recruited from a consecutive case series seen at the Developmental Disabilities Clinic, Child Study Center, Yale University School of Medicine, New Haven, CT. A full scale IQ >70 and a diagnosis of AS or autism according to ICD-10 research criteria were required for inclusion. The sample selected included 21 with AS and 19 with HFA. The AS group had a higher Verbal IQ and lower Performance IQ in comparison with the HFA group. There was a significant interaction between clinical diagnosis and IQ type. A high degree of concordance between AS and the condition of Nonverbal Learning Disabilities (NLD) was observed when overlap between psychiatric diagnosis (ie AS/HFA) and neuro-psychological characterization (ie NLD assets and deficits) was examined. The NLD profile was an adequate neuropsychological model for individuals with AS but not for HFA. The AS and HFA groups differed significantly in 11 neuropsychological areas. (Klin A et al. Validity and neuropsychological characterization of Asperger syndrome: convergence with nonverbal learning disabilities syndrome. J Child Psychol Psychiat Oct 1995;36:1127-1140). (Reprints: Ami Klin, Child Study Center, Yale University School of Medicine, 230 South Frontage Road, New Haven CT 06520).

COMMENT. The neuropsychological profile obtained for children with Asperger syndrome (AS) coincided with that of the nonverbal learning disabilities syndrome (NLD) and differed from patients with higher-functioning autism. The defining criteria for NLD included assets in auditory perception and memory, vocabulary, and spelling, and deficits in motor skills, visual-motor integration, visual-spatial perception, visual memory, verbal content, reading comprehension, arithmetic, and social and emotional competence. The authors suggest that intervention strategies for AS should differ from those for autism, directly addressing specific neuropsychological deficits and building on neuropsychological assets, an approach found useful in individuals with nonverbal learning disabilities syndrome. -Editor. *Ped Neur Briefs* Dec 1995.

NONSPECIFIC BRAIN ANOMALIES IN AUTISM

Measurements of the cerebellar vermis in 125 normal individuals and 102 patients with a variety of neurogenetic abnormalities were compared, using quantitative MRI analysis in a study at the Universities of Nebraska, Omaha; Oklahoma, Norman; West Virginia, Morgantown; and Texas, San Antonio. The average size of cerebellar vermal lobules (CBL) VI and VII in patients with infantile autism was not significantly different from that in age-matched normal subjects. Relative CBL VI-VII hypoplasia occurred in patients with Rett syndrome and Sotos' syndrome, both having autistic behaviors, but the same was true for conditions without autistic behaviors. CBL VI-VII hypoplasia is not limited to disorders with autistic behavior and is not a specific neuroanatomical marker for autism. (Schaefer GB, Thompson JN Jr, Bodensteiner JB et al. Hypoplasia of the cerebellar vermis in neurogenetic syndromes. <u>Ann Neurol</u> March 1996;39:382-385). (Respond: Dr Schaefer, University of Nebraska Medical Center and Meyer Rehabilitation Institute, 600 S 42nd Street, Omaha, NE 68198).

COMMENT. Several neurogenetic disorders have relative CBL VI-VII hypoplasia, and cerebellar vermal hypoplasia is not specific for autism.

Temporal lobe morphology in childhood-onset schizophrenia was studied by MRI in 21 patients examined at the NIMH, the University of Maryland School of Medicine, Baltimore, and Northwestern University School of Medicine, Chicago. (Jacobsen LK et al. <u>Am J Psychiatry</u> March 1996;153:355-361). These schizophrenic patients had smaller cerebral volumes, but larger volume of the superior temporal gyrus. They lacked the normal (right-greater-than-left) hippocampal asymmetry. Early onset schizophrenia was not associated with a severe medial temporal lobe lesion in these patients. -Editor. *Ped Neur Briefs* May 1996.

LEAD INTOXICATION IN CHILDREN WITH AUTISM

The incidence of reexposure to lead poisoning in 17 children with pervasive developmental disorders (PDD), including autism, compared to a randomly selected group of 30 children without PDD who were treated for plumbism over the same six year period, was evaluated by a retrospective chart review at the lead treatment program, Children's Hospital, Harvard Medical School, Massachusetts Poison Control System, Boston, MA. Despite close monitoring, inspection and lead hazard reduction or alternative housing, 75% of children with PDD were reexposed to lead compared to 23% without PDD. Those with PDD were older at diagnosis (46 vs 30 months) and had a longer period of elevated lead (39 vs 14 months) during management. (Shannon M, Graef JW. Lead intoxication in children with pervasive developmental disorders. <u>Clin Toxicology</u> March 1996;34:177-181). (Respond: Dr Michael

Shannon, Children's Hospital, 300 Longwood Ave, Boston, MA 02115).

COMMENT. Children with developmental delays and PDD are at increased risk of lead poisoning beyond 3 years of age. Children with PDD and other behavior disorders should be tested for lead at regular intervals beyond 4 years of age. More importantly, primary preventive measures designed to abate lead from the environment before lead intoxication occurs may be the only successful method of management. -Editor. *Ped Neur Briefs* May 1996.

TREATMENT OF ADHD

MULTIMODAL TREATMENT APPROACH
The importance of a multimodal treatment approach to ADHD is emphasized by The National Institute of Mental Health's recently initiated 5-year, multisite study. Questions to be answered include the influence of comorbid conditions, gender, family history, home environment, age, nutritional status; and effects of various treatments (stimulants, behavior therapy, parent training, school-based intervention) on different functions (cognitive, academic, behavioral), for how long (short versus long term), to what extent, and why? (Richters JE et al. NIMH collaborative multisite multimodal treatment study of children with ADHD: I. Background and rationale. <u>J Am Acad Child Adolesc Psychiatry</u> August 1995;34:987-1000). -Editor. *Ped Neur Briefs* Aug 1995.

PHARMACOTHERAPY

Pharmacotherapy of ADHD is reviewed in a special article from the Massachusetts General Hospital. (Spencer T, Biederman J, Wilens T et al. <u>J Am Acad Child Adolesc Psychiatry</u> April 1996;35:409-432). The efficacy of stimulants in 70% of subjects has been documented in 155 controlled studies of 5,768 children, adolescents, and adults reported in the literature. Stimulants improve abnormal behaviors in ADHD, self-esteem, cognition, and social and family function. Response varied with age and comorbid conditions. The efficacy of tricyclic antidepressants in ADHD is also documented in more than 1000 subjects. Increased interest in comorbidity in ADHD has not been followed by related therapeutic advances. Data are limited on the response of medications in comorbid ADHD, and on the effects and safety of combined pharmacotherapy. -Editor. *Ped Neur Briefs* May 1996.

CNS STIMULANTS

METHYLPHENIDATE TREATMENT IN ADHD

METHYLPHENIDATE RESPONSE PREDICTION

Predictors of response to methylphenidate (MPH) among 47 children with ADHD and mental retardation (MR) were studied at the University of Pittsburgh School of Medicine, and the Western Psychiatric Institute and Clinic, Pittsburgh, PA. A double-blind, placebo-controlled evaluation of two doses of MPH (0.3 and 0.6 mg/kg), using Conners Scales, with data collected on weekday and Saturday laboratory classrooms, showed that: 1) higher parent ratings of impulsivity and activity level at baseline were associated with greater gains in weekday classroom dependent measures; 2) higher weekday teacher measures of activity level, impulsivity, inattention, and conduct problems at baseline were related to improvement on Saturday laboratory classroom dependent measures; and 3) male Caucasians of higher socioeconomic status were more likely to show clinical improvements than other subjects. Race and conduct problems had predictive utility specific to children with MR. (Handen BL et al. Prediction of response to methylphenidate among children with ADHD and mental retardation. <u>J Am Acad Child Adolesc Psychiatry</u> October 1994;33:1185-1193). (Reprints: Dr Handen, John

Merck Outpatient Program, Western Psychiatric Institute and Clinic, 3811 O'Hara St, Pittsburgh, PA 15213).

COMMENT. The higher the level of hyperactivity and associated inattention in children with ADHD and mental retardation (MR), the greater the beneficial response to methylphenidate. Similar findings have been reported previously in a study of 30 children of normal IQ with ADHD, using actometer measurements of motor activity and a neuropsychological test battery, and also in animals with hyperactivity induced by prefrontal cortical lesions. (Millichap JG. <u>Ann N Y Acad Sci</u> 1973;205:321; <u>Ped Neur Briefs</u> Oct 1987; June 1991).

Children with ADD without hyperactivity or moderate levels of abnormality on Conners Scales are less likely to benefit from stimulant medication than those with ADD and H. Baseline measures of behavior by Conners Scales in ADHD children with MR were more predictive of medication response than the measures obtained in the laboratory classroom. -Editor. *Ped Neur Briefs* Oct 1994.

METHYLPHENIDATE IN ADHD & EPILEPSY

The safety of methylphenidate (MPH), 0.3 mg/kg, in 9 boys and 8 girls, ages 6 to 16 years, with ADHD and epilepsy, studied in Jerusalem, Israel, was reported at the Annual Meeting of the Child Neurology Society, Oct 2-8, 1994, in San Francisco, CA. Of 17 patients treated with MPH for 1-month, following a placebo period of 1-month, 15 children who were seizure-free had no recurrence of seizures, while 2 with 1 to 2 seizures weekly before MPH had a moderate exacerbation of epilepsy. The EEGs showed no "major" changes. AED levels (CBZ and VA) were therapeutic during placebo and MPH periods. ADHD symptoms were benefited by MPH in 12 patients. (Gross-Tsur V et al. Methylphenidate for children with epilepsy and attention deficit hyperactivity disorder. <u>Ann Neurol</u> Sept 1994;36:501 [abstr]).

COMMENT. The authors recommend caution in the

use of methylphenidate in ADHD children with an active seizure disorder. The PDR states that: "In the presence of seizures, the drug (MPH) should be discontinued." Based on the present and previous reports there appears to be some justification for trials of MPH in selected patients with ADHD and epilepsy whose seizures are controlled with antiepileptic drugs.

Pemoline (Cylert) is generally considered to have less tendency to lower seizure threshold than MPH. Some recommend an EEG in all ADHD patients considered for stimulant medications; those with a history of seizures and/or epileptiform discharges in the EEG should receive concomitant AED therapy. Children with ADHD have a 7% incidence of epileptiform EEGs. (Ped Neur Briefs Oct 1989; Progress in Pediatric Neurology I, 1991, p 190). -Editor. *Ped Neur Briefs* Oct 1994.

STIMULANT MEDICATION IN TEENAGERS

Results of biennial surveys, 1975 - 1993, by school nurses of medication use for hyperactive/inattentive (HA/I) public elementary and secondary school students are reported from the Baltimore County Health Department and the Johns Hopkins University School of Medicine, Baltimore, MD. Over a 10 to 20 year period, the rate of medication use rose from 1.07 to 3.58% in elementary schools, 0.59 to 2.98% in middle schools, and 0.22 to 0.70% in high schools. The average rate increase per year was 15% (elementary), 28% (middle), and 31% (high school). One-third of all public school students on medication for HA/I in the 1990s were attending secondary schools. The female to male ratio of medicated students in secondary schools narrowed from 1:12 in 1980 to 1:6 in 1993. The majority (97%) of students had treatment initiated in the elementary school at 7 to 8 years of age. Methylphenidate was the medication prescribed in 90 to 95% of the total. (Safer DJ, Krager JM. The increased rate of stimulant treatment for hyperactive/inattentive students in secondary schools. Pediatrics Oct 1994;94:462-464). (Reprints: Daniel J Safer MD, ECMHC 9100

Franklin Square Drive, Rosedale, MD 21237).

COMMENT. Physician and parent concerns about possible substance abuse and adverse effects of stimulant medication prescribed for teenagers appear to be lessening. This survey demonstrates that the continuation of methylphenidate treatment into adolescence is favored with increasing frequency. Contrary to popular belief, children with ADHD do not generally outgrow their symptoms at 12 years of age. The increased rate of motor vehicle crashes among adolescent and young adult drivers with ADHD is one factor suggested as a reason for continued therapy. (see <u>Progress in Pediatric Neurology</u> Vols I and II, Millichap, Ed, PNB Publ, 1991 and 1994). -Editor. *Ped Neur Briefs* Oct 1994.

METHYLPHENIDATE AND SLEEP PATTERNS

The effects of methylphenidate (0.3-0.4 mg/kg) cf placebo on sleep in 10 children with ADHD are reported in a double-blind crossover study at the Bnai Zion Medical Center and the Technion-Israel Institute of Technology, Haifa, Israel. Sleep duration was significantly shorter during the drug period compared to placebo or baseline periods. The percent of quiet sleep was lower in the ADHD study group compared with controls in baseline measures, but not during methylphenidate treatment. (Tirosh E et al. Effects of methylphenidate on sleep in children with attention-deficit hyperactivity disorder. <u>AJDC</u> Dec 1993;<u>147</u>:1313-1315). (Reprints: Dr Tirosh, Hannah Khoushy Child Development Center, Bnai Zion Medical Center, POB 4940, Haifa, Israel).

COMMENT. Children with ADHD have significantly prolonged sleep duration and a trend toward a lower percentage of quiet sleep, possibly attributed to hypoarousal or fatigue. Normalization of sleep patterns and decreased sleep duration achieved by methylphenidate could result from increased arousal. Insomnia, frequently reported as a side effect of methylphenidate, requires closer study. -Editor. *Ped Neur Briefs* Jan 1994.

METHYLPHENIDATE WITHOUT SLEEP PROBLEMS

The effects of methylphenidate (MPH) administered at 4 PM on behavior and sleep in 12 child psychiatric inpatients with ADHD were evaluated in a double-blind, crossover study at the Division of Child and Adolescent Psychiatry, Long Island Jewish Medical Center, New Hyde Park, NY. Early morning and noon doses of MPH were continued through the study period. MPH in 10 and 15 mg doses administered at 4 PM for 12 consecutive days improved evening behavior without altering sleep latencies. The average time to sleep onset in treated and control groups was 49 minutes. Sleep adequacy was improved after 10 mg MPH doses compared to 15 mg MPH and placebo nights. The child seemed tired after waking more often after 15 mg MPH and placebo than on nights after 10 mg MPH. Ten of 12 patients lost an average of 1.2 kg weight, but dinner intake was not altered by the 4 PM dose of MPH. (Kent JD, Blader JC et al. Effects of late-afternoon methylphenidate administration on behavior and sleep in attention-deficit hyperactivity disorder. <u>Pediatrics</u> August 1995;96:320-325). (Reprints: Joseph C Blader PhD, Room SCH 416, Schneider Children's Hospital, Long Island Jewish Medical Center, New Hyde Park, NY 11042).

COMMENT. The authors recommend three daily doses of MPH in patients who show a beneficial response to two doses at school but who are hyperactive and disruptive at home in the evening. However, they caution that the study was performed at an inpatient setting, the analysis did not exclude possible adverse sleep effects in some individual patients, and the third dose did result in significant weight loss. The effects in outpatients may be different and insomnia and anorexia may require dosage modification. If well tolerated, a third dose of MPH may benefit homework compliance, bedtime habits, and family relations.

-Editor. *Ped Neur Briefs* Sept 1995.

MPH EFFECTS ON PEER RELATIONS

Perceptions of methylphenidate effects on peer interactions of ADHD children were studied by psychologists at the University of California, Los Angeles and Irvine. (Granger DA et al. <u>J Abnormal Child Psychol</u> 1993;<u>21</u>:535). Analyses of observations of videotapes by 96 undergraduates showed that medication increased social withdrawal and dysphoria/disengagement, suggesting negative interpersonal consequences of these unintended internalizing behavior changes, even when not cued by rating scales. A positive medication effect was obtained in the category of leader/planner, behaviors requiring social organization and foresight. -Editor. *Ped Neur Briefs* Jan 1994.

METHYLPHENIDATE RESPONSE PREDICTION

The dose-response, clinical effectiveness, and response prediction in 76 children with ADHD treated with methylphenidate (MPH) were evaluated by a double-blind, placebo-controlled, crossover study at the Department of Psychology, University of Hawaii, Honolulu. Four dose levels (5, 10, 15, and 20 mg) were employed. Effects on classroom functioning, (on-task attention, correct completion of assignments, and teacher ratings), were linear and dose related. Accuracy was enhanced at all dose levels, and task completion was significantly greater at doses above 5 mg. Academic improvement was associated with behavioral gains on teacher ratings. In children failing to respond to low dose MPH, attention changes were responsive to dose increments whereas academic and behavioral improvements failed to occur. A significant subset failed to gain academically from treatment with MPH. (Rapport MD et al. Attention deficit disorder and methylphenidate: Normalization rates, clinical effectiveness, and response prediction in 76 children. <u>J Am Acad Child Adolesc Psychiatry</u> July/Aug 1994;33:882-893). (Respond: Dr Rapport, Dept of

Psychology, University of Hawaii, 2430 Campus Rd, Gartley Hall, Honolulu, HI 96822).

COMMENT. Methylphenidate is again proven effective in the treatment of children with ADHD, and improvements in behavior, attention, and academic functioning may be expected in a large percentage. Response to MPH is related to the dose, especially in tasks requiring attention. In one subset, however, academic performance is unrelated to attentional and behavioral response to MPH. In another subset, MPH is ineffective in all domains of classroom functioning. A child's academic functioning is most important in assessing response to methylphenidate and the need for dose increments. -Editor. *Ped Neur Briefs* July 1994.

RESPONSE PREDICTION TO MPH IN ADHD

The pattern of individual responses to methylphenidate (10 mg) and factors that predict drug response in 46 children, 6-13 years old, with attention-deficit hyperactivity disorder (ADHD) were examined at the Department of Child and Adolescent Psychiatry, and the Rudolf Magnus Institute for Neurosciences, University of Utrecht, The Netherlands. Methylphenidate (MPH) normalized school behavior in one half the subjects, and behavior at home in one third. Behavior both at school and at home was normalized in 17%. Prediction of response to MPH was only successful when stringent, ie cross-situational, response definitions were used. Predictors were a high IQ, much inattentiveness, young age, low severity of disorder, and low rates of anxiety. Positive behavioral changes, measured by the Abbreviated Conners Rating Scales, after a single dose of MPH were predictive of cross-situational improvement after 4 weeks of MPH treatment. (Buitelaar JK et al. Prediction of clinical response to methylphenidate in children with attention-deficit hyperactivity disorder. <u>J Am Acad Child Adolesc Psychiatry</u> August 1995;34:1025-1032). (Reprints: Dr Buitelaar, Department of Child Psychiatry, PO Box 85500, 3508 GA Utrecht, The Netherlands).

COMMENT. The clinical judgment of severity of ADHD and improvement observed after a single dose of methylphenidate are useful predictors of a beneficial long-term response. -Editor. *Ped Neur Briefs* Aug 1995.

METHYLPHENIDATE AND FLEXIBLE THINKING IN ADHD

The acute effects of methylphenidate (MPH) in 3 dosages (0.3, 0.6, and 0.9 mg/kg) on the performance of 17 ADHD children in tests of cognitive flexibility were evaluated at the Departments of Psychology and Pediatrics, McGill University-Montreal Children's Hospital Research Institute, Canada. On five tasks designed to assess divergent and convergent thinking, problem solving, speed and accuracy of processing, perseveration, and ability to shift mental set, linear improvement across dosages was the usual pattern and deleterious effects on flexible thinking and other cognitive processes were minimal, either in the total ADHD group or in subgroups. On the Wisconsin Card-Sorting Test, nonperseverative errors decreased significantly with increasing dosage of MPH. Perseverative errors showed a similar pattern. On the Trailmaking Test, subjects completed task (Form A) more quickly on higher dosages of MPH than on placebo. Alternate Uses and Contingency Naming Tests also showed significant dosage effects and linear trends, refecting more valid responses or fewer errors. (Douglas VI et al. Do high doses of stimulants impair flexible thinking in attention-deficit hyperactivity disorder? <u>J Am Acad Child Adolesc Psychiatry</u> July 1995;34:877-885). (Reprints: Dr Virginia I Douglas, Department of Psychology, McGill University, 1205 Docteur Penfield Ave, Montreal, Quebec, Canada H3A 1B1).

COMMENT. Methylphenidate in acute doses caused no perseverative effects but rather, improved persistence in children with ADHD, and scores on tests measuring cognitive flexibility were increased. The authors recommend a dose range of MPH not exceeding

0.3 to 0.6 mg/kg in clinical practice. They find little advantage in higher doses and have concerns about side effects and possible impairment of cognitive functioning with multiple daily doses. -Editor. *Ped Neur Briefs* July 1995.

MPH IN ADHD WITH COMORBID ANXIETY

In a total of 40 ADHD children, 18 with comorbid anxiety and 22 without, who were treated with MPH in a placebo-controlled, crossover trial with MPH (0.3, 0.6, 0.9 mg/kg) at the Department of Psychiatry- Research Unit, Hospital for Sick Children, Toronto, the performance on a working memory cognitive task was enhanced in the ADHD group but not in children with comorbid anxiety. Both groups showed a lessening of motor activity. (Tannock R et al. Differential effects of methylphenidate on working memory in ADHD children with and without comorbid anxiety. <u>J Am Acad Child Adolesc Psychiatry</u> July 1995;34:886-896). -Editor. *Ped Neur Briefs* July 1995.

ROLE OF REWARD AND MOTIVATION IN MPH EFFECTS IN ADHD

The importance of rewards such as money and the role of motivation in explaining the effects of stimulant medication in children with ADHD were suggested by a study of 16 ADHD boys receiving MPH or placebo at the Department of Educational Psychology, University of Utah, Salt Lake City. ADHD subjects earned significantly more money on a button pressing test during drug treatment compared to placebo. Drug-related improvements in cognitive tasks may be a consequence of increased effort. (Wilkinson PC, Kircher JC et al. Effects of methylphenidate on reward strength in boys with attention-deficit hyperactivity disorder. <u>J Am Acad Child Adolesc Psychiatry</u> July 1995;34:897-901). -Editor. *Ped Neur Briefs* July 1995.

ADHD TREATMENT IN GREAT BRITAIN

Our British colleagues now recognize the

diagnosis of ADHD and have begun to treat with methylphenidate in a limited way. (Taylor E, Hemsley R. Treating hyperkinetic disorders in childhood. Treatment needs care but is worthwhile. <u>BMJ</u> 24 June 1995;310:1617-1618). At a meeting in England in the 1970s, Dr Ronald C Mac Keith of the Spastics Society once scolded me for my interest and research in the hyperkinetic child with MBD. It was his opinion that the entity was over emphasized in America and did not exist in the UK. (Millichap JG, Ed. Learning Disabilities and Related Disorders: Facts and Current Issues. Chicago, Year Book Medical Publishers, 1977). -Editor. *Ped Neur Briefs* July 1995.

METHYLPHENIDATE ABUSE

The clinical findings associated with IV methylphenidate/pentazocine abuse in emergency department visits are reported from the University of Missouri-Kansas City, MO. Twenty nine patients seen between 1987 and 1992 were treated 34 times. The mean age was 32 +/- 9 years. Central nervous system complications in 7 were anxicty/agitation (5%), seizures (9%), or loss of consciousness (6%). The typical symptom complex of chest pain, anxiety, muscle spasm, dizziness, and nausea was present in 58%. Treatment was mainly supportive and included oxygen and fluids. (Carter HS, Watson WA. IV pentazocine /methylphenidate abuse - the clinical toxicity of another Ts and Blues combination. <u>Clinical Toxicology</u> 1994;32:541-547). (Reprints: Dr William A Watson, Department of Emergency Medicine, Truman Medical Center, 2301 Holmes, Kansas City, MO 64108).

COMMENT. IV abuse of methylphenidate is unlikely in children with ADHD but the increased use of stimulant medication in teenagers (see <u>Ped Neur Briefs</u> October 1994) provides a possible source of concern. The combination of crushed Talwin® (pentazocine) tablets and Ritalin® (methylphenidate) is called "Ts and Blues" in Kansas City, MO, and has resulted in acute myelopathy in one reported case. The

CNS complications are reviewed by Caplan LR et al. (<u>Neurology</u> 1982;32:623). -Editor. *Ped Neur Briefs* Nov 1994.

METHYLPHENIDATE DOSING SCHEDULES

Efficacy and side effects of twice daily (bid) and three times daily (tid) methylphenidate (MPH) dosing schedules (mean dose, 8 mg, 0.3 mg/kg) in 25 boys with attention deficit hyperactivity disorder (ADHD) were compared in a 5-week, placebo-controlled, crossover evaluation at the Departments of Psychiatry and Pediatrics, University of Chicago. Three times daily dosing provided greater improvement than the bid schedule on Hyperactivity/Impulsivity Conners Parent and Teacher Rating scales. Compared to placebo, appetite and total sleep time were adversely affected by tid dosing but not bid schedules. The incidence of side effects with tid compared to bid dosing was not significantly different. No effect on weight was noted in this short time period. (Stein MA, Blondis TA, Schnitzler ER, Roizen NJ et al. Methylphenidate dosing: twice daily versus three times daily. <u>Pediatrics</u> Oct 1996;98:748-756). (Reprints: Dr Mark A Stein, Section of Child and Adolescent Psychiatry, 5841 S Maryland Ave, Chicago, IL 60637).

COMMENT. This short term study shows that more frequent, smaller dose, three times daily MPH treatment is often preferable to twice daily dosing schedules. The incidence of insomnia, usually regarded as a disadvantage of afternoon doses, is not increased, and teacher and parent ratings of MPH efficacy are benefited. Doses of MPH for ADHD should be selected for each individual child according to the time of occurrence of symptoms and not with regard to the pattern of possible side effects. An evening free from parent-child conflict and a home-work assignment satisfactorily completed may lead to improved self esteem and better classroom performance. Closer monitoring of MPH dosing schedules, using both parent and teacher abbreviated reports, should result in optimal treatment efficacy.

The benefits of a group treatment developmental approach, involving patients and their families, as a supplement to medication, are reported from the Department of Psychiatry and Behavioral Sciences, Stanford University School of Medicine, CA. (Lock J. Developmental considerations in the treatment of school-age boys with ADHD: an example of a group treatment approach. <u>J Am Acad Child Adolesc Psychiatry</u> Nov 1996;35:1557-1559). -Editor. *Ped Neur Briefs* Nov 1996.

PEMOLINE IN TREATMENT OF ADHD

The effects of pemoline (Cylert) in 28 children with attention deficit disorder (ADD), 23 with and 5 without hyperactivity, were evaluated for dose-response, timing of response after ingestion, and duration of effect, in a double-blind, placebo-controlled, crossover study at the Child Development Clinic of the Department of Neurology, Hospital for Sick Children, Toronto, Canada. Using doses of 18.75, 37.5, 75, and 112.5 mg of pemoline, q.a.m., each dose administered at 9 am for 1 week, performance was measured by number of math problems completed correctly, teacher-recorded on-task behavior and noncompliance, and Abbreviated Conners Teacher Rating Scale. Tests were completed immediately and beginning 2, 4, and 6 hours after drug ingestion. Beneficial effects of pemoline on classroom behavior and academic performance were linear, beginning 2 hours after ingestion and lasting at least 7 hours. Side effects during observation were minimal, and response was comparable to that reported in studies of methylphenidate. (Pelham WE Jr et al. Pemoline effects on children with ADHD: A time-response by dose-response analysis on classroom measures. <u>J Am Acad Child Adolesc Psychiatry</u> November 1995;34:1504-1513). (Reprints: Dr Pelham. Western Psychiatric Institute and Clinic, 3811 O'Hara Street, Pittsburgh, PA 15213).

COMMENT. The commonly held belief that

response to pemoline is gradual and sometimes delayed for 3 or 4 weeks was contradicted by the results of this study that demonstrate an acute beneficial effect, comparable to that of methylphenidate. The authors recommend that doses of pemoline higher than 18.75 or 37.5 mg may be needed for optimal benefit, and a prolonged response may be expected after a single morning dose.

The side-effect of insomnia, reported in 32% of patients in one previous long-term trial, could not be evaluated in the present study because parent and sleep evaluations were not included. In my own patients with a complaint of sleep disturbance during treatment with pemoline, the side-effect was reported soon after initiation of therapy, suggesting a more acute onset of response than that noted in the manufacturer's reports. The present study confirms the need to consider increments of dosage more rapidly than recommended in the PDR. -Editor. *Ped Neur Briefs* Nov 1995. (Abbott Laboratories have recently reported several deaths from liver failure in patients treated with Cylert. Pemoline is not recommended as a first line drug treatment for ADHD. -*Editor.*).

STIMULANT THERAPY FOR BENIGN CHOREA AND ADHD

A 6-year-old boy with benign familial chorea diagnosed at 1 year and ADHD evaluated and treated with methylphenidate (MPH) at 6 years is reported from the Department of Pediatrics, David Grant Medical Center, Travis Air Force Base, California. After MPH beginning with 2.5 mg BD and gradually increasing to 7.5 mg BD, his attention span, self-control, handwriting, and school performance were benefited as expected, but in addition, the chorea improved and his independent walking skills developed. On drug holidays, the chorea and gait problems regressed. (Friederich RL. Benign hereditary chorea improved on stimulant therapy. <u>Pediatr Neurol</u> May 1996;14:326-27). (Respond: Dr Friedrich, 60 MOS/SGOC, 101 Bodin Circle, Travis AFB, CA 94535).

COMMENT. The author suggests that chorea complicating ADHD should not contraindicate a cautious trial of stimulant medication. If methylphenidate improves a child's performance in school and lessens stressful situations, it may also result in a reduction in chorea and improved motor abilities. -Editor. *Ped Neur Briefs* Aug 1996.

USAGE OF CNS STIMULANTS BY PEDIATRIC NEUROLOGISTS

An overuse of methylphenidate (MPH) in the treatment of attention deficit disorders (ADHD) has been reported by the International Narcotics Control Board, and the potential for drug abuse has prompted media criticism and cause for concern among some parents and physicians. A questionnaire was mailed to 160 pediatric neurologists and clinic directors in the United States, and 53 (33%) located in 28 different States responded. A diagnosis of ADHD was made in <5 to 100% (mean 33%) of patients treated, and 10 to 96% (mean 51%) of ADHD patients received stimulant medications. The age groups of patients receiving MPH were 3 - 5 years (8.7%), 6 - 12 years (70.3%), 13 - 18 years (20.4%), and adults (0.6%). The drug of choice was MPH (90%). Pemoline and dextroamphetamine were equally favored as 2nd or 3rd choice stimulants. The mean average daily dose of MPH was 20 mg (range 10-40 mg); the mean maximum daily dose was 52 mg (range 25-85 mg). Drug holidays at weekends and school vacations were recommended by 65%. The duration of therapy with stimulants ranged from 1 to 5 years (mean 3.5 years). The adverse effects of MPH were as follows: personality changes in 7%, tics (5%), weight loss (4%), seizures (0.9%), and miscellaneous (2.3%), including insomnia (3), headache (2), increased activity (2), and parental anxiety (1). (Millichap JG. Usage of CNS stimulants for ADHD by pediatric neurologists. A questionnaire survey. <u>Ped Neur Briefs</u> Sept 1996;10:65).

COMMENT. An overuse of methylphenidate by

physicians treating attention deficit hyperactivity disorders in the United States was not supported by this questionnaire survey of pediatric neurologists. The side effects reported, especially personality changes, are usually dose related.

Contraindications or factors requiring extra caution in the use of stimulants for ADHD are as follows: 1) Tourette's syndrome or tics, 2) family history of tics, 3) history of seizures and/or EEG dysrhythmia, 4) history of drug abuse/dependence, 5) family history of drug abuse, 6) psychosis or anxiety/depression, 7) poor nutrition or short stature, 8) headaches, sleep disturbance, 9) liver dysfunction (pemoline), 10) treatment with other medications eg. clonidine, MAO inhibitors. -Editor. *Ped Neur Briefs* Sept 1996.

GROWTH AND WEIGHT DEFICITS IN ADHD

The hypothesis that stimulant medications may cause growth deficits in children with attention deficit hyperactivity disorder (ADHD) was reevaluated in 124 children and adolescents with ADHD and 109 controls at the Massachusetts General Hospital, Boston, MA. Small, significant deficits in height (average, 3 cm) were found in early but not late adolescent ADHD children, and height deficits were unrelated to weight deficits or stimulant treatment. In 10% of ADHD children cf 1% of controls, height deficits were more than 2 standard deviations (approx 14 cm in 15-yr-old males) below the average height of controls. The larger growth deficits occurred in patients with comorbid major depression but not in those with anxiety disorders. Neither recent nor past history of stimulant therapy significantly affected height measures in either early or late pubertal ADHD children. Pubertal development and weight measures of ADHD children were not different from controls. (Spencer TJ, Biederman J, Harding M, O'Donnell D, Faraone SV, Wilens TE. Growth deficits in ADHD children revisited: evidence for disorder-associated growth delays? <u>J Am Acad Child Adolesc Psychiatry</u> Nov 1996;35:1460-1469). (Reprints: Dr Spencer, Pediatric Psychopharmacology Unit (ACC 725), Massachusetts

General Hospital, Fruit Street, Boston, MA 02114).

COMMENT. ADHD may be associated with a temporary delay in the rate of growth in height in early adolescence that may be corrected by late adolescence. ADHD-associated height deficits are unrelated to stimulant-associated weight loss and may represent a manifestation of ADHD, mediated by a maturational delay. The dysmaturity hypothesis of ADHD, usually confined to neurobehavioral and attentional deficits, may be extended to physical deficits that can be outgrown. Small weight deficits in some ADHD children receiving stimulant therapy can usually be offset by adjusting the timing of medication and by food supplements if indicated.

In a Northwestern University, prospective study of the growth of 36 boys with ADHD, 5 to 10 years of age, who were treated with methylphenidate,
only 2 had a significantly decreased rate of annual growth, compared to normal growth patterns of children of the same age group. In 6 children under 8 years of age the growth rate was significantly increased. (Millichap JG. Growth of hyperactive children treated with methylphenidate: a possible growth stimulant effect. In: <u>Learning Disabilities and Related Disorders.</u> Chicago, Year Book Med Publ, 1977) (Millichap JG, Millichap MG. Growth of hyperactive children. <u>N Engl J Med</u> 1975;292:1300).

Predictors of weight loss in children with ADHD treated with stimulant medication were studied retrospectively at the Schneider Children's Hospital, New Hyde Park, New York. (Schertz M et al. <u>Pediatrics</u> Oct 1996;98:763-769). Using body mass index as a measure, pretreatment weight was a significant predictor of stimulant-related weight loss, heavier children losing more weight than thinner children. In overweight ADHD children, stimulant medication may provide a secondary benefit, improving self-esteem. -Editor. *Ped Neur Briefs* Nov 1996.

CARDIOVASCULAR EFFECTS OF TRICYCLIC ANTIDEPRESSANTS

Twenty-four pediatric studies, published from various centers between 1967 and 1996, involving 730 children and adolescents treated with imipramine, amitryptiline, desipramine, or nortryptiline, were surveyed for cardiovascular side effects at the Massachusetts General Hospital, Boston, MA. Treatment with tricyclic antidepressants (TCA) caused small increases in blood pressure and heart rate, and lengthening of PR, QRS, and QT conduction parameters on the ECG. Imipramine may be associated with lower rates of sinus tachycardia and intraventricular conduction lengthening than other TCAs, and desipramine may have the greatest tendency to cause QT prolongation. ECG abnormalities were related to the dose and relatively higher serum TCA levels. ECG monitoring is recommended with doses of TCAs of 2.5 mg/kg day (1 mg/kg day for nortryptyline), and doses more than 5 mg/kg day should be avoided. Lightheadedness or headaches signal the need for a check of vital signs, ECG, and TCA serum levels. Guidelines for monitoring ECG and vital signs in children receiving TCAs are suggested. (Wilens TE, Biederman J, Baldessarini RJ et al. Cardiovascular effects of therapeutic doses of tricyclic antidepressants in children and adolescents. <u>J Am Acad Child Adolesc Psychiatry</u> Nov 1996;35:1491-1501). (Reprints: Dr Wilens, ACC 725, Massachusetts General Hospital, Boston, MA 02114).

COMMENT. Tricyclic antidepressants are a second-line choice of medication for ADHD, sometimes favored in children with psychiatric comorbidity or enuresis. Although in general the cardiovascular effects are minor, tachycardia and shortness of breath, and occasional reports of idiosyncratic fatalities in TCA-treated children are a concern to some practitioners. Without frequent ECG monitoring, it is likely that these cardiovascular abnormalities and associated symptoms are often unrecognized. Children engaged in sporting activities especially should be closely examined for cardiac related side effects, and alternative treatments substituted.

Protriptyline for ADHD. Side effects were particularly prominent in a trial of protriptyline in 13 children with ADHD, and less than 50% showed a positive response. (Wilens TE, Biederman J, Abrantes AM, Spencer TJ. A naturalistic assessment of protriptyline for attention-deficit hyperactivity disorder. <u>J Am Acad Child Adolesc Psychiatry</u> Nov 1996;35:1485-1490). -Editor. *Ped Neur Briefs* Nov 1996.

CARBAMAZEPINE: A THERAPY FOR ADHD

The efficacy of carbamazepine (CBZ) in treatment of ADHD has been determined by meta-analysis of 10 reports from the international literature reviewed at Columbia University, St Luke's-Roosevelt Hospital Center, and New York University Medical Center. In 7 open studies involving a total of 189 patients with features of motor overactivity, impulsivity, and distractibility, 70% showed a marked improvement in target symptoms following treatment with CBZ for periods varying from 1 week to 8 years. Outcome was significantly correlated with duration of treatment; the longer the treatment the better the outcome. In 3 placebo-controlled, double-blind studies, 71% of 53 patients treated with CBZ were benefited whereas only 26% of 52 receiving placebo showed similar improvement in attentiveness and behavior. The difference was significant (p=.018). The most frequent side effects were sedation and skin rash occurring in 7.5% and 5.7% of CBZ-treated patients, respectively. (Silva RR et al. Carbamazepine use in children and adolescents with features of attention-deficit hyperactivity disorder: a meta-analysis. <u>J Am Acad Child Adolesc Psychiatry</u> March 1996;35:352-358). (Reprints: Dr Silva, St Luke's/Roosevelt Hospital Center, Division of Child and Adolescent Psychiatry, 411 W114th Street, Suite 3A, New York, NY 10025).

COMMENT. The authors conclude that carbamazepine may be an effective alternate treatment for ADHD. A response rate of 70% in both open and controlled studies is about the equivalent effectiveness of stimulant medication.

From a neurologist's perspective, the obvious questions would relate to the incidence of epilepsy and epileptiform EEG's in these patients selected for treatment with an anticonvulsant medication. Unfortunately, these data were not discussed and were tabulated for the entire sample and not the subsample with ADHD.

My own meta-analysis of these data show that abnormal EEGs occurred in 69% of 57 patients in the controlled studies and in 82% of 50 patients in the one open study providing EEG data. Seizures were mentioned in 4 of the studies, affecting 13 plus patients, but the total number of patients affected was not given. The frequency of abnormal EEGs in these patients is considerably higher than that usually reported for ADHD. It seems that CBZ might be indicated for the treatment of ADHD symptoms in some patients with abnormal EEGs and/or a history of seizures. On a negative note, see <u>Progress in Pediatric Neurology II</u>, 1994, pp188-190, for references to cognitive impairment and impulsivity caused by CBZ treatment of epilepsy. -Editor. *Ped Neur Briefs* March 1996.

CLONIDINE FOR SLEEP DISORDERS WITH ADHD

A retrospective analysis of 62 children and adolescents treated with clonidine for sleep disturbances associated with ADHD is reported from the outpatient Pediatric Psychopharmacology unit, Massachusetts General Hospital, Boston. Using the National Institute of Mental Health global assessment of sleep improvement, 85% of patients treated with nighttime clonidine (50-800 mcg, mean 157) for 35 months were much to very much improved. Concurrent pharmacotherapy and comorbidity showed no relation to response. Mild adverse effects in 31% included morning sedation and fatigue. (Prince JB, Wilens TE, Biederman J et al. Clonidine for sleep disturbances associated with attention-deficit hyperactivity disorder: a systematic chart review of 62 cases. <u>J An Acad Child Adolesc Psychiatry</u> May 1996;35:599-605). (Reprints: Dr Wilens, ACC 725, Massachusetts General Hospital, Boston, MA 02114).

COMMENT. Two thirds of the patients had medication-induced ADHD-associated sleep disturbance, mainly stimulants. The addition of clonidine in combination with stimulants such as methylphenidate in this study appeared to be safe and effective in correcting sleep disturbances. Fatalities have been reported using clonidine and methylphenidate together, and this combination therapy is being discouraged. The authors recommend further systematic assessment in large groups of children to clarify this issue. Clonidine is indicated in the treatment of ADHD, tic disorders, and comorbid ADHD and tic disorders. Somnolence, the most common side-effect of clonidine, often reduces its usefulness. -Editor. *Ped Neur Briefs* May 1996.

BUPROPION cf. METHYLPHENIDATE IN ADHD

The efficacy of bupropion and methylphenidate in the treatment of ADHD was compared in a double-blind, crossover study of 15 patients (7 to 17 years of age) at the University of Iowa, Iowa City. Methylphenidate titrated from 0.4 to 1.3 mg/kg per day (mean 0.7 mg/kg/d) and bupropion 1.4 to 5.7 mg/kg/d (mean 3.3 mg/kg/d) over a 6 week period were followed by a 2 week wash out period. Both drugs were effective in the treatment of ADHD, but rating scales trended in favor of methylphenidate. (Barrickman LL, Perry PJ et al. Bupropion versus methylphenidate in the treatment of attention-deficit hyperactivity disorder. <u>J Am Acad Child Adolesc Psychiatry</u> May 1995;34:649-657). (Reprints: Dr Perry, 2271 Quadrangle, University of Iowa, Iowa City, IA 52242).

COMMENT. Side effects were minor with both drugs in this study. Seizures may be induced or exacerbated by bupropion and methylphenidate, and appropriate precautions are recommended in patients with a history of seizures or an abnormal EEG. -Editor. *Ped Neur Briefs* June 1995.

BUSSELTON STUDY OF BEHAVIOR DISORDER PREVENTION

The long-term follow-up in 1993 of 209 adults, aged 27 to 29 years, who as children were enrolled in the Busselton Population six-year controlled study of prevention of children's behavior disorders is reported from Claremont, Western Australia. Ninety percent of the original cohort responded to a questionnaire detailing their present social situation and habits, educational achievements, and emotional well-being. In the initial Busselton study, 1964-1973, a 20- to 30-minute interview between physician and mother about the preschool child had reduced the incidence of behavioral disturbances at age 6 years. As adults, the study subjects had fewer neurotic symptoms and less depressive symptoms than controls, and more had a university degree. Study women were less obese and smoked less than controls. Behavior patterns noted at 6 years of age after preschool interventional counselling were reflected in the improvements recorded as adults when compared to controls. (Cullen KJ, Cullen AM. Long-term follow-up of the Busselton six-year controlled trial of prevention of children's behavior disorders. <u>J Pediatr</u> July 1996;129:136-9). (Reprints: Dr AM Cullen, 37 Riley Rd, Claremont 6010, Western Australia).

COMMENT. The interviewing and counselling of mothers of preschool children benefits the children's behavior at 6 years of age, and leads to increased emotional well-being and higher academic achievement in adult life. Women were benefited more than men. The decrease in eating problems among study children at 6 years of age were reflected in the lesser incidence of obesity, less anxiety and depressive symptoms, and reduced tendency to smoke in female study subjects. University degrees had been attained by 34% of experimental women compared to 24% of the male subjects and 15% of both male and female controls.

The adoption of a positive and gentle parental attitude toward modifying a child's behavior, as promoted in the Busselton study, should be encouraged early in a child's development. The obvious importance of services and expertise of child and family psychologists in Mental Health Programs should be emphasized in the management of ADHD. -Editor. *Ped Neur Briefs* Aug 1996.

CHAPTER **4**

LEARNING DISABILITIES

INTRODUCTION

The neural basis of dyslexia and other learning disabilities has been investigated using the MRI, EEG, PET, and magnetoencephalography. Different developmental pathways are suggested for specific learning disabilities and those with comorbid behavioral disorders.

Toxic, metabolic, endocrine, and other environmental factors are invoked in causation of neuropsychological delays and cognitive dysfunction. These include PCBs, methylmercury, lead, iodine deficiency diseases, and especially cranial irradiation. The adverse effects of HIV infection and congenital toxoplasmosis on cognitive function, speech and language, and motor development have been stressed.

Developmental disorders complicated by impaired intelligence and learning disabilities include hydrocephalus, and neurofibromatosis-1. Several studies have correlated the low IQ scores in neurofibromatosis-1 with UBOs on the MRI. The effects of epilepsy and antiepileptic drugs on learning have received continued and deserved attention.

Innovative treatments for language and learning impaired, including dyslexic children have included training with acoustically modified, synthetic, speech stimuli, and dietary supplements, notably the free fatty acid, docosahexaenoic acid (DHA). DHA is a key fatty acid in both the retina and brain, and low levels of DHA have previously been demonstrated in hyperactive children with learning disabilities.

J. Gordon Millichap, M.D.   Editor

DYSLEXIA

ARTICULATORY FEEDBACK DEFICIT IN DYSLEXIA

An efferent or "motor-articulatory feedback" hypothesis for developmental dyslexia-phonological type is proposed from the Departments of Neurology and Psychiatry, University of Florida College of Medicine, Gainesville, FL. Most children learn to read by the alphabetic system, requiring phonological awareness and conversion of letters (graphemes) into speech sounds (phonemes). Most dyslexics have deficient phonological awareness and difficulty converting graphemes into phonemes. The left inferior frontal lobe is important in phonological reading, as suggested by patients with acquired lesions and PET studies of normal subjects. Dyslexic children are unable to perceive the position and movement of the articulatory apparatus (mouth, lips, tongue) during speech, impairing phonological awareness and conversion of graphemes to phonemes. Deficits in motor-articulatory programming or feedback may be related to this lack of awareness of articulators. (Heilman KM et al. Developmental dyslexia: a motor-articulatory feedback hypothesis. <u>Ann Neurol</u> March 1996:39:407-412). (Respond: Dr Kenneth M Heilman, Box

100236, University of Florida, Gainesville, FL 32610).

COMMENT. Other current hypotheses for developmental dyslexia are 1) visual hypothesis, with dysfunction in the visual perception system, and 2) auditory hypothesis, with abnormalities in the rapid discrimination of low-contrast, complex sounds and associated speech and language disturbances.

A disconnection syndrome hypothesis for developmental dyslexia is proposed based on evidence from PET scanning studies conducted at the MRC Cognitive Development Unit, London, UK. (Paulesu E, Frith U et al. <u>Brain</u> Feb 1996;119:143-157). A rhyming and a short-term memory task with visually presented letters was used to study brain activity in 5 compensated adult developmental dyslexics. Brain regions normally activated in phonological processing were defective, and weak connections between anterior and posterior language areas are proposed. -Editor. *Ped Neur Briefs* April 1996.

MRI CHANGES IN DYSLEXIA: REAPPRAISAL

The convolutional surface area of the planum temporale, temporal lobe volume, and brain volume were compared by MRI in 17 dyslexic children (7 girls) and 14 controls (7 girls) at Yale University School of Medicine, New Haven. All measurements were significantly larger in boys. Age was directly correlated with brain region volumes. Analyses that controlled for age and overall brain size failed to confirm smaller left hemisphere structures previously reported in dyslexics. The authors suggest that differences in sex, age, handedness, and definition of dyslexia as well as methods of measurement of the planum temporale may explain apparent discrepancies in results of neuroimaging studies in dyslexic subjects. (Schultz RT et al. Brain morphology in normal and dyslexic children: The influence of sex and age. <u>Ann Neurol</u> June 1994;35:732-742). (Respond: Dr Shaywitz, Department of Pediatrics, PO Box 3333, New Haven, CT 06510).

COMMENT. This important study casts doubt on the significance of reports of differences in brain morphology in children with dyslexia and other learning disabilities. It should be noted in the Massachusetts General Hospital report of corpus callosal changes in ADHD children, a smaller splenium was unrelated to the age of the children. -Editor. *Ped Neur Briefs* July 1994.

DYSLEXIA AND SMALL CORPUS CALLOSUM

Corpus callosum morphology was studied by MRI in 16 children (mean age, 9.7 yrs) with developmental dyslexia and matched controls at the Center for Clinical and Developmental Neuropsychology, University of Georgia, Athens, and the Department of Neurology, Medical College of Georgia, Augusta, and the Athens Magnetic Imaging. The genu of the corpus callosum was significantly smaller in the dyslexic children. Familial left-handedness, and ADD with and without hyperactivity distinguished the dyslexic children from controls. (Hynd GW et al. Dyslexia and corpus callosum morphology. <u>Arch Neurol</u> January 1995;52:32-38). (Respond: Dr George W Hynd, Center for Clinical and Developmental Neuropsychology, 570 Aderhold Hall, The University of Georgia, Athens, GA 30602).

COMMENT. Studies of MRI morphology of the corpus callosum in monozygotic twins at Dartmouth Medical School Program in Cognitive Neuroscience showed wide variations in size and shape of the human corpus callosum. Measurements revealed greater similarity in twin pairs than in randomly paired controls. (<u>Ann Neurol</u> 1989;26:100). The anatomy of the corpus callosum appears to be under genetic control as well as being influenced by nongenetic factors. How much this natural variation in size of the corpus callosum influenced the results of the above study in dyslexia is debatable. (see <u>Progress in Pediatric Neurology I</u>, PNB Publ, 1991, pp 168-9). -Editor. *Ped Neur Briefs* Jan 1995.

BRAIN ACTIVITY DURING READING

PET was used to study the functional anatomy of reading in the intact brain of subjects examined at the Hammersmith Hospital, London, and other centers. The type of reading task and the exposure duration of the word stimuli were variables that influenced the patterns of brain activity. Three tasks were applied as follows: reading aloud, reading silently, and distinguishing words and pseudowords in a lexical decision task. Reading aloud and reading silently produced activity in the left posterior temporal lobe. Lexical decision involved the left inferior and middle frontal cortices and the supplementary motor area. Brain activity was greater for short exposure durations than for long durations. (Price CJ et al. Brain activity during reading. The effects of exposure duration and task. <u>Brain</u> Dec 1994;117:1255-1269). (Respond: Dr Cathy Price, MRC Cyclotron Unit, Hammersmith Hospital, Ducane Road, London W12 OHS, UK).

COMMENT. Small variations in experimental design may influence brain activity as measured by PET. The association of specific reading tasks with discrete anatomical areas must be interpreted with caution. The authors stress that the aim of their study was to determine reasons for inconsistencies in previous reports. -Editor. *Ped Neur Briefs* March 1995.

READING EPILEPSY

The electroclinical manifestations and natural history of reading epilepsy (RE) in 20 patients diagnosed between 1949 and 1989 are reported from the Mayo Clinic, Rochester, Minnesota. Age at onset ranged from 10 to 46 years (median 17 years). Juvenile myoclonic epilepsy occurred in 4, and a positive family history for epilepsy in 4, with RE in 1. Seizures were myoclonic, involving orofacial and jaw muscles, and the upper limbs also in 5. Generalized tonic-clonic seizures occurred at least once in 16. The EEG showed generalized spike or spike-and wave discharges in 15 cases and left hemisphere discharges in 5. RE was persistent into late adult life but not progressive; it responded to valproic acid. Higher cognitive processes acting as trigger mechanisms other than reading included calculation in 6, speaking under stress in 5, writing in 2, and playing chess in 1. (Radhakrishnan K, Silbert PL, Klass DW. Reading epilepsy. An appraisal of 20 patients diagnosed at the Mayo Clinic, Rochester, Minnesota, between 1949 and 1989, and delineation of the epileptic syndrome. <u>Brain</u> Feb 1995;118:75-89). (Respond: Donald W Klass MD, Section of Electroencephalography, Mayo Clinic, 200 First Street SW, Rochester, MN 55905).

COMMENT. The authors dedicate their article to Dr Reginald G Bickford on his 81st birthday and we add our congratulations! Bickford (1954) and Bickford, Klass et al (1956) first described the syndrome of reading epilepsy and stressed the importance of precipitating factors in the mechanism of seizures and EEG epileptiform discharges in general. Christie S (1988) found a combination of factors involved in the precipitation of reading epilepsy: saccadic eye movements, articulation, and difficulty of linguistic content. Bickford had alluded to the degree of difficulty of reading matter in his original article. (See <u>Progress in Pediatric Neurology</u> I, 1991, p45). -Editor. *Ped Neur Briefs* May 1995.

READING-INDUCED ABSENCE SEIZURES

A 12-year-old girl with a 2-year history of absence seizures induced by reading and diagnosed by video EEG is reported from The University of Texas Southwestern Medical Center, Dallas, and Riyadh Armed Forces Hospital, Saudi Arabia. The reading of complex material especially, either silently or aloud, produced staring episodes lasting several seconds and occasionally followed by headaches. Attacks were one to two a day at first and later increased to five to six daily. Two siblings had a history of febrile seizures. Routine EEG, including hyperventilation and photic stimulation, was normal. Video-EEG showed no spontaneous seizures in a 6-hour baseline period, but hyperventilation induced generalized 3-Hz spike-and-wave discharges and a clinical absence seizure. Reading in Arabic from the Koran for 30 seconds induced an absence seizure lasting 30 seconds. The reading challenge repeated several times at 10-minute intervals induced absences within 30 seconds. Valproate therapy given for 2 years controlled seizures, and she has been seizure-free for 9 months since stopping treatment. The EEG is normal, both during prolonged reading and hyperventilation. (Singh B et al. Reading-induced absence seizures. Neurology August 1995;45:1623-1624). (Reprints: Dr Balbir Singh, Department of Pediatric Neurology, University of Texas Southwestern Medical Center, 5323 Harry Hines Blvd, Dallas, TX 75235).

COMMENT. The electroclinical manifestations and natural history of reading epilepsy in 20 patients was recently reported from the Mayo Clinic (see Ped Neur Briefs May 1995). Seizures were myoclonic, involving orofacial and jaw muscles, and generalized tonic-clonic seizures occurred in 16. The reading epilepsy persisted into late adult life. It resonded to valproic acid. The reading-induced absence seizures in the present report appear to be unique and previously unreported. The precipitating stimuli for reading epilepsy are reviewed in Progress in Pediatric Neurology I, PNB Publ, 1991, pp 45-46. -Editor. *Ped Neur Briefs* Sept 1995.

CORTICAL MOTOR OUTPUT OF BRAILLE READING HAND

Focal transcranial magnetic stimulation (TMS) was used to map the motor cortical outputs to the right and left first dorsal interosseous (FDI) and right abductor digiti minimi (ADM) muscles of the reading hand in 6 blind proficient Braille readers studied at the National Institute of Neurological Disorders and Stroke, NIH, Bethesda, MD. All subjects had learned Braille before age 13, using the right index finger for character recognition and the left index for line keeping. Comparison of cortical output maps obtained on working days and off days showed that the maps for the FDI of the reading hand were significantly larger in the evening after the working shift than in the morning after having not worked for 2 days. The map shrunk following vacation days and enlarged following a return to work. On control days, the motor threshold for the muscles stayed constant, whereas on the work day, the motor thresholds for the right FDI were significantly lower in the evening study session after practice than in the morning test before practice. The results illustrate the rapid modulation in motor cortical outputs effected by Braille reading. (Pascual-Leone A, Hallett M et al. The role of reading activity on the modulation of motor cortical outputs to the reading hand in Braille readers. <u>Ann Neurol</u> December 1995;38:910-915). (Respond: Dr Pascual-Leone, Unidad de Neurobiologia, Departemente Fisiologia, Universidad Valencia, Avda Blasco Ibanez 17, Valencia 46010, Spain: or Dr Hallett, NINDS, NIH, Bldg 10, Rm 5N226, 10 Center DR MSC 1428, Bethesda, MD 20892).

COMMENT. The authors emphasize the critical importance of timing when looking for changes in neural networks associated with learning skills. Learning a new skill requires plastic changes and rapid modulation of intracortical connections that result in temporary enlargement of the cortical motor output. These neurophysiological changes are supported by PET scanning studies in the same laboratory, showing that Braille reading is associated with an increased activation of the sensorimotor and striate cortex contralateral to the reading hand. (Sadato N et al. 1995). -Editor. *Ped Neur Briefs* Jan 1996.

NEURAL BASIS OF DYSLEXIA

Whole-head magnetoencephalography (MEG) was employed to track noninvasively the cortical activation sequences during visual word recognition in 6 adult dyslexic and 8 control subjects examined at the Brain Research Unit, Helsinki University of Technology, Espoo; and the Departments of Psychology and Radiology, University of Helsinki, Helsinki, Finland. Significant differences between the two groups were found for the time window 0 to 200 msec after single word presentation in the left inferior temporo-occipital cortex, for 200 to 400 msec in the left temporal lobe, and for 0 to 400 msec in the left inferior frontal lobe. Considerable interindividual variability was shown for spatiotemporal activation patterns. Dyslexics failed to activate the left inferior temporo-occipital cortex within 200 msec after word presentation. The left temporal lobe, including Wernicke's area, a region associated with phonological aspects of language, was strongly involved in controls but not in dyslexics. Dyslexics activated, instead, the left inferior frontal lobe, involving Broca's area, whereas activation of the right motor/premotor cortex, present in controls, was absent in dyslexics. Perception of words as specific units was impaired in dyslexics. (Salmelin R et al. Impaired visual word processing in dyslexia revealed with magnetoencephalography. <u>Ann Neurol</u> Aug 1996;40:157-162). (Respond: Dr Salmelin, Low Temperature Laboratory, Helsinki University of Technology, Rakentajanaukio 2, 02150 Espoo, Finland).

COMMENT. An impaired perception of visual word processing of written words, resulting from dysfunction of auditory language areas in the left inferior temporoparietal area, appears to be a factor in the causation of dyslexia in some subjects. Early training in auditory language might help in the prevention of dyslexia.

Poeppel D and Rowley HA, Biomagnetic Imaging Laboratory, University of California, San Francisco, comment that the utility of magnetic source imaging (MSI) lies in the combination of MEG with the anatomic images supplied by MRI, providing anatomic location of activity at a given time-sampling point. MSI may be used clinically for presurgical mapping in evaluation of patients with epilepsy and determination of hemispheric dominance. The cost of MEG installations and MSI systems limits their practical use at present.

(Magnetic sorce imaging and the neural basis of dyslexia. <u>Ann Neurol</u> Aug 1996;40:137-138). -Editor. *Ped Neur Briefs* Sept 1996.

READING DISABILITY AND BEHAVIOR PROBLEMS

The early characteristics of groups of children, aged 7 to 8 years, identified with reading disability (RD) only, behavior problem (BP) only, RD and BP, and neither RD nor BP, were compared by temperament and behavior indices, gathered in 5 periods between infancy and 6 years of age, at the Department of Psychology, University of Melbourne, Australia. The RD children with and without BP were different from each other from early childhood. BPs of both the BP-only and the comorbid group distinguished them from the non-BP groups at an early age. In contrast, the RD-only children were similar to the normal comparison group up to school age, except for lower maternal education and more difficult temperament. The early detection of RD could not rely on behavioral measures. Children at risk for developing pure RD were predominantly girls, and low educational stimulation from low maternal education was the only risk factor. The gender composition of the two RD groups differed, the RD-BP boys showing the most problems. Boys with difficult temperament, poor mother-child relationship, lower educational stimulation and relative social disadvantage were at risk of early development of BPs and later diagnosis of RD. (Sanson A, Prior M, Smart D. Reading disabilities with and without behavior problems at 7-8 years: Prediction from longitudinal data from infancy to 6 years. <u>J Child Psychol Psychiat</u> July 1996;37:529-541). (Reprints: Ann Sanson, Department of Psychology, University of Melbourne, Parkville, Victoria, Australia 3052).

COMMENT. This study suggests different developmental pathways for pure RD children and those with comorbid BPs. Sex differences were also evident, boys showing more behavioral problems and more difficult temperament from 1-3 years, more hostile-aggressive and hyperactive behavior from 3-4 years, and lower school readiness and task orientation.

Twin-sibling differences in ADHD children with reading and speech problems were reported from the Prince of Wales Hospital, University of New South Wales, Australia (Levy F et al. <u>J Child Psychol Psychiat</u> July 1996;37:569-578). Male twins had the highest rate of ADHD, speech and reading problems. The reading deficit in male twins becomes more marked in adolescence while that in female twins decreases. Pre- and perinatal insults were not the explanation for an increased incidence of ADHD among twins. -Editor. *Ped Neur Briefs* Sept 1996.

FATTY ACID SUPPLEMENTS IN DYSLEXIA

The effect of docosahexaenoic acid (DHA) supplements (480 mg daily) on five adult dyslexics with poor dark adaptation was studied at the University of Surrey, Guildford, UK. Compared to controls, dyslexics were benefited and dark adaptation (scotopic vision) improvement was associated with improved reading ability in some. (Stordy BJ. Benefit of docosahexaenoic acid supplements to dark adaptation in dyslexics. <u>Lancet</u> Aug 5, 1995;346:385). (Respond: B Jacqueline Stordy, School of Biological Sciences, University of Surrey, Guildford GU2 5XH, UK).

COMMENT. The author admits that the benefits of treating dyslexics with docosahexaenoic acid (DHA) are anecdotal, and further controlled studies are indicated.

This study corroborates previous reports of low serum levels of docosahexaenoic and other essential fatty acids in hyperactive children with dyslexia and other learning disabilities. (see <u>Progress in Pediatric Neurology I</u>, Chicago, PNB Publ, 1991:p179).

TOXIC AND METABOLIC FACTORS IN LEARNING DISORDERS

PRENATAL PCB EXPOSURE AND IQ

The neuropsychological effects of in utero exposure to PCBs and their related compounds were evaluated in 27 'Yu-Cheng' ('oil disease') children (ages 7 to 12 years) at the Departments of Pediatrics and Psychiatry, National Cheng Kung University, Tainan, Taiwan. Full-scale IQ scores on the WISC-R were significantly lower than in the 27 controls. Mean P300 latencies of auditory event-related potentials were significantly longer and the amplitudes reduced. Pattern visual evoked potentials and somatosensory evoked potentials were unaffected. Apart from a slight increase in soft signs, the neurologic examinations of the exposed children were not different from controls. (Chen Y-J, Hsu C-C. Effects of prenatal exposure to PCBs on the neurological function of children: A neuropsychological and neurophysiological study. Dev Med & Child Neurol April 1994;36:312-320). (Respond: Dr Yung-Jung Chen, Dept of Pediatrics, Medical College, National Cheng Kung University, 138 Sheng-Li Road, Tainan 70428, Taiwan, R.O.C.).

COMMENT. PCBs affect cognitive function of children exposed in utero. Evoked potentials are useful in examining the neurotoxicity of environmental pollutants in the young child. The P300 wave latency is related to the solving of cognitive tasks and the amplitude of P300 reflects concentration abilities. A significantly greater difference in P300 latencies was found for exposed children with lower IQ scores compared to controls.

Delayed effects of PCBs on newborns whose mothers consumed contaminated Lake Michigan fish during pregnancy have been reported. Smaller head circumference and growth retardation persisted beyond infancy, and short-term memory and behavioral deficits occurred at later follow-up (see Ped

Neur Briefs Jan 1990, and March 1993). -Editor. *Ped Neur Briefs* May 1994.

NEUROLOGICAL LONG-TERM EFFECTS OF METHYLMERCURY POISONING

The clinical, neuropsychological, and radiological features of a family, and the toxicological and neuropathological findings of one family member, who were acutely and severely intoxicated with methylmercury are reported after a 22-year follow-up from the Albuquerque Veterans Affairs Medical Center, the University of New Mexico School of Medicine, and the Environmental Health Sciences Center, the University of Rochester School of Medicine, NY.

In 1969 a family in New Mexico had consumed pork containing methylmercury. Three children and a neonate developed severe neurological signs. At 22-year follow-up, the 2 oldest patients, ages 42 and 35 years, had cortical blindness, impaired stereognosis and graphesthesia, poor hand coordination, ataxia, choreoathetosis, dysarthria, and attentional deficits. MRIs showed loss of tissue in calcarine cortices, parietal lobes, and cerebellar folia. The 2 youngest were quadriplegic, blind, and mentally retarded and they died at ages 29 and 21 years. The brain of the patient poisoned at 8 years and dying at 29 showed cortical atrophy, neuronal loss and gliosis. Total mercury level in the occipital cortex was 1,974 ng/gm, 50 times that of a control; the Hg was mainly inorganic. Hair and systemic organs had Hg levels comparable to controls. (Davis LE et al. Methylmercury poisoning: Long-term clinical, radiological, toxicological, and pathological studies of an affected family. <u>Ann Neurol</u> June 1994;35:680-688). (Respond: Dr Davis, Chief, Neurology Service (127), Albuquerque VA Hospital, 2100 Ridgecrest Drive SE, Albuquerque, NM 87108).

COMMENT. Methylmercury crosses the blood-brain barrier easily while inorganic mercury does not. Biotransformation to inorganic Hg over time may account for the high level of inorganic Hg and absence of methyl Hg in the patient's brain at autopsy. The possible role of inorganic Hg in the brain damage is debatable; it is usually considered to be inert and nontoxic. See <u>Environmental Poisons in Food</u> , Chicago, PNB Publishers, 1993, for an account of the sources, metabolism, epidemiology, clinical manifestations, treatment, and prevention of mercury poisoning.

Accidental exposure to mercury vapor is a persisting hazard in nurseries with broken thermometers and in school science labs. The symptoms of mild exposure, *micromercurialism*, are subtle and difficult to diagnose without a high index of suspicion. Acrodynia, or Pink disease, is a relatively rare occurrence, but a diagnosis which should be familiar to the pediatric neurologist and pediatrician. -Editor. *Ped Neur Briefs* July 1994.

IODINE DEFICIENCY AND LEARNING DISABILITIES

The effect of prolonged iodine deficiency on learning and motivation to achieve was studied in 100 male children selected from both severely iodine-deficient (SID) and mildly iodine-deficient (MID) villages and reported from the Department of Psychology, Kashi Vidyapeeth, Varanasi, and Department of Endocrinology, Banjay Gandhi Post Graduate Institute of Medical Sciences, Lucknow, India. Mean urinary iodine excretion and serum thyroxine concentration were significantly lower, and serum TSH was significantly higher, in the SID group than in the MID group. SID compared to MID children were slower learners, having lower scores on maze and pictorial learning tasks, and the SID group scored significantly lower on the achievement motivation scale. The SID and MID groups were matched for age, socioeconomic status, and formal education. Cretins were excluded, and study subjects were required to read and write. (Tiwari BD, Godbole MM et al. Learning disabilities and poor motivation to achieve due to prolonged iodine deficiency. <u>Am J Clin Nutr</u> May 1996;63:782-6). (Reprints: MM Godpole, Associate Professor, Department of Medical

Endocrinology, Sanjay Gandhi Post Graduate Institute of Medical Sciences, Lucknow 226014, India).

COMMENT. Iodine deficiency results in slow learning ability and impaired motivation to achieve. In severely iodine-deficient (SID) children, the number of errors and time taken in maze learning were negatively correlated with urinary iodine excretion and thyroxine concentrations, and showed a positive correlation with thyroid stimulating hormone. In contrast, tests involving verbal learning and free-recall, a less demanding cognitive task than maze learning, did not distinguish between severely and mildly iodine-deficient children, but SID children were slower on serial testing, showing impairment of formation of new stimulus-response associations or engrams. Optimal iodine nutrition is important in the prevention of learning disabilities and failure to achieve academically. The following report supports a correlation between neonatal triiodothyronine levels and later cognition.

Low triiodothyronine concentration in preterm infants was correlated with a mean 6.6 point deficit in overall IQ scores (8.5 deficit on verbal scale) on the WISC scales at 8-year follow up in a study of 236 infants examined at the Infant and Child Nutrition Group, Medical Research Council Dunn Nutrition Unit, Cambridge, UK. (Lucas A, Morley R, Fewtrell MS. <u>BMJ</u> 4 May 1996;312:1132-3). Brook CGD, of Cobbold Laboratories, Middlesex Hospital, London, in a Commentary: Do preterm infants need thyroxine replacement? (<u>BMJ</u> 1996;312:1133) cautions that thyroxine therapy for hypothyroid mothers is unlikely to benefit premature babies, and triiodothyronine replacement in premature infants may be dangerous. Neonatologists generally withhold therapy pending a retest after the infant reaches term. An increased risk of developing cerebral palsy and cognitive deficits has been reported in premature infants with low thyroxine levels in the first week of life (<u>N Engl J Med</u> March 28

1996).

Iodine deficiency diseases (IDD), a major international public health problem especially affecting developing countries, may be prevented by the administration of iodinized salt. My colleague, Dr Charles Swisher, provided me with several references to the topic, pointing out that estimates have shown 200 million affected by IDD and 800 million people at risk worldwide for IDD, a total of "1 billion brains" at risk of maldevelopment or malfunction! The most serious complication of IDD is endemic cretinism, but milder forms of IDD may be associated with impaired cognitive function and learning disabilities in later childhood. For further reviews of IDD, see Delange F. <u>Thyroid</u> Spring 1994;4:107-128; Lamberg BA. <u>Ann Med</u> Oct 1991;23:367-372; Hetzel BS et al. <u>Neuropath & Applied Neurobiol</u> 1988;14:93-104; Maberly GF. <u>J Nutrition</u> Aug 1994;124(8 Suppl):1473-78S. Editor. *Ped Neur Briefs* June 1996.

INFECTIONS AND LEARNING DISORDERS

HIV DISEASE, CT AND IQ SCORES

Measures of cognitive function and social-emotional behavior were correlated with CT abnormalities in 87 children with symptomatic human immunodeficiency virus type 1 disease (HIV) at the Pediatric Branch, National Cancer Institute, and the NIND & S, Bethesda, MD; Children's National Medical Center, Washington, DC; and Medical Illness Counselling Center, Chevy Chase, MD. The mean age of the patients was 4.3 yrs. Vertically infected children were 2.3 +/- 0.3 years, and transfusion-infected children were 8.4 +/- 0.6 years of age.

The Full Scale IQ (FIQ) was a mean of 85.2 for the total group; 80 for vertically infected; and 95.5 for transfusion-infected patients. A significant correlation was found between FIQ and the overall CT severity rating. The correlation was stronger in (younger) vertically infected compared with older transfusion-infected children. Calcifications, observed only in vertically infected children (16 of 58), were associated with greater delays in neurocognitive development, independent of the degree of brain atrophy. (Brouwers P, DeCarli C et al. Correlation between computed tomographic brain scan abnormalities and neuropsychological function in children with symptomatic human immunodeficiency virus disease. <u>Arch Neurol</u> Jan 1995;52:39-44). (Reprints: Dr Brouwers, Pediatric Branch, National Cancer Institute, National Institutes of Health Clinical Center, Room 13N240, Bethesda, MD 20892).

COMMENT. CT scans are recommended as a baseline for patients at risk for CNS manifestations and cognitive deficits due to HIV. Even when mild, CT abnormalities were of clinical significance.

Effects of HIV on Language. The above authors have studied the effects of HIV disease on receptive and expressive language in 36 children with symptomatic HIV and the relation to CT scan brain abnormalities (Wolters PL, Brouwers P et al. <u>Pediatrics</u> Jan 1995;95:112-119). Expressive language was more impaired than receptive language. Greater severity of CT abnormalities was correlated with poorer receptive and expressive language functioning. The language impairments were associated with the direct effects of HIV-related CNS disease.

Effects of HIV on Speech. A speech motor control disorder developed after HIV infection in 6 right-handed patients. They had an ataxic dysarthria, associated with ataxic gait and intention tremors. The motor speech disorder was due to a cerebellar dysfunction. (Lopez OL et al. <u>Neurology</u> 1994;44:2187-2189). -Editor. *Ped Neur Briefs* Jan 1995.

EFFECTS OF HIV ON COGNITIVE AND MOTOR DEVELOPMENT OF INFANTS

The cognitive and motor development of 126 infants born to nondrug-using,HIV-seropositive

Haitian women, assessed at 3-month intervals from birth to 24 months, is reported from the University of Miami School of Medicine, FL. By 18 months of age, 28 were HIV-infected, and these infants were compared to 98 uninfected infants used as controls. The mean mental and motor scores on the Bayley Scales of Infant Development were significantly lower for infected compared to uninfected controls. Initial differences between the two groups, noted at 3 months, increased over time. Cognitive development was within normal levels in one third of infected infants, despite low mean scores for the group, and motor development was normal in one half. (Gay CL, Armstrong FD et al. The effects of HIV on cognitive and motor development in children born to HIV-seropositive women with no reported drug use: Birth to 24 months. Pediatrics Dec 1995;96:1078-1082). (Respond: Dr F Daniel Armstrong, Department of Pediatrics-R131, Box 016960, Miami, FL 33101).

COMMENT. Infants perinatally infected with HIV are at risk of cognitive and motor delays in the first two years of life. Visual-motor integration, processing speed, verbal memory, and other neuropsychological measures, not tested in infants and toddlers, may be uncovered at later follow-up. -Editor. *Ped Neur Briefs* May 1996.

HIV INFECTION AND NEURODEVELOPMENT

The mental and motor development of 24 children with vertically transmitted human immunodeficiency virus (HIV) infection in the first 30 months of life was compared to 27 HIV exposed but uninfected children at the Boston City Hospital and Boston University Medical Center, MA. Bayley Scales of Infant Development, assessed at 4-16 months and at 17-30 months of age, showed that motor development in the infected group was delayed compared to the uninfected seroreverter group in both age periods. Mental development was similar in the two groups at 4-17 months, but was delayed in the HIV infected children at 17-30 months of age. (Chase C et al. Early neurodevelopmental growth in children with vertically transmitted human immunodeficiency virus infection. <u>Arch Pediatr Adolesc Med</u> August 1995;149:850-855). (Reprints: Dr Chase, Department of Pediatrics, D4S, Boston City Hospital, 818 Harrison Ave, Boston, MA 02118).

COMMENT. Neurodevelopmental outcome in children with HIV infection is variable. Early delay in motor development and late infantile deceleration in mental development can be expected. -Editor. *Ped Neur Briefs* Aug 1995.

DEVELOPMENTAL AND NEUROLOGIC OUTCOME OF CONGENITAL TOXOPLASMOSIS

Neurologic, cognitive, and motor outcomes for 36 children with congenital toxoplasmosis treated with pyrimethamine and sulfadiazine for 1 year are reported from Michael Reese Hospital, Chicago, IL, and other Centers. Active infection, seizures, and motor abnormalities resolved in most during therapy. Of 29 infants evaluated at 1 year of age, 23 (79%) had a Mental Developmental Index of 102, and 6 had scores <50. Sibling controls had higher scores than patients, but sequential IQ testing showed no deterioration over time. Six of eight children with obstructive hydrocephalus relieved by shunts had normal neurologic and developmental outcomes. In contrast, of 10 with hydrocephalus ex vacuo from birth, eight had severe disabilities. Nine of 34 (26%) children had microcephaly. Of those presenting with chorioretinal lesions (69%), the majority had residual visual loss after therapy.

Risk factors for poor outcome included diabetes insipidus, hypoxia, hydrocephalus with high CSF protein, and delay in medical treatment. These results compared to previous reports for untreated children were thought to justify treatment of pregnant women with acute gestational Toxoplasma infection and young infants with congenital toxoplasmosis. (Roizen N, Swisher CN et al. Neurologic and developmental outcome in treated congenital toxoplasmosis. <u>Pediatrics</u> January 1995;95:11-20). (Reprints:Dr Rima McLeod, 114 Baumgarten, Department of Medicine, Michael Reese Hospital, 2929 South Ellis Ave, Chicago, IL 60616).

COMMENT. One third of the patients treated for congenital toxoplasmosis were severely impaired neurologically, and two thirds of those with normal developmental outcomes had retinal lesions and visual problems. The need for prevention and improved therapies was emphasized. -Editor. *Ped Neur Briefs* Jan 1995.

NEONATAL VIRAL MENINGITIS AND NEURODEVELOPMENT

The neurodevelopmental outcome of 16 young infants with viral meningitis diagnosed under 3 months of age and a control group of 13 infants was evaluated at the Children's Hospital Medical Center, and University of Concinnati, Ohio. Subtle but significant deficits were found in the meningitis group involving the receptive component of the Receptive-Expressive Emergent Language Scale (REEL), all subsections of the Preschool Language Scale (PLS), the Revised Peabody Picture Vocabulary Test (PPVT-R), and the verbal comprehension/language-processing section of the Stanford-Binet. These deficits were recognized by 3 years of age, but required specific quantitative testing by a psychologist or speech and language pathologist for their detection. (Baker RC et al. Neurodevelopmental outcome of infants with viral meningitis in the first three months of life. <u>Clin Pediatr</u> June 1996;35:295-301).
(Reprints: Raymond C Baker MD, OSB 4, Children's Hospital Medical Center, 3333 Burnet Avenue, Cincinnati, Ohio 45229).

COMMENT. Children with enteroviral meningitis in early infancy should be monitored for impairments of language development, particularly receptive language. Those with deficits should receive increased language stimulation in the home prior to enrollment in school. -Editor. *Ped Neur Briefs* July 1996.

CRANIAL IRRADIATION AND LEARNING DISORDERS

POST-IRRADIATION COGNITIVE AND CNS DISABILITIES

The neurological, neuropsychological, and educational outcome in 14 children who received a second course of cranial radiotherapy or total body irradiation for relapsing lymphoblastic leukemia is reported from the Neurosciences Unit and Department of Haematology, Institute of Child Health, University of London. Nine (64%) had postirradiation somnolence syndrome characterized by lethargy, irritability, nausea, and vomiting. All patients had mild neurological deficits, including hyperreflexia, incoordination, dyspraxia, and hand muscle weakness. All were growth hormone deficient. MRI showed ventricular enlargements. Verbal comprehension and tests of attention and memory were impaired, girls showing greater impairments than boys. Of 9 children still at school, only 2 performed at age appropriate levels in reading, spelling, and math, and social outcome was poor. (Christie D et al. Neuropsychological and neurological outcome after relapse of lymphoblastic leukaemia. <u>Arch Dis Child</u> April 1994;70:275-280). (Respond: Dr D Christie, Neurosciences Unit, The Wolfson Centre, Mecklenburgh Square, London WC1N 2AP, UK).

COMMENT. After survival of the rigors of two and three year protocols of chemotherapy for lymphoblastic leukemia, children who relapse after initial remission now have to face the prospect of postirradiation cognitive and neurological deficits. The morbidity asssociated with cranial radiotherapy has been recognized for some time, and the results of this study certainly favor the omission of presymptomatic irradiation and the use of intrathecal methotrexate in more current protocols. The justification for overzealous treatments of relapsing leukemia in children needs re-evaluation in light of the long term adverse effects and the overall quality of life. -Editor. *Ped Neur Briefs* June 1994.

COGNITIVE EFFECTS OF CRANIAL IRRADIATION

The effects of cranial irradiation on neuropsychological test performance, 9 months after diagnosis of acute lymphoblastic leukemia (ALL), were evaluated in 74 children aged 3 to 6 years included in the Children's Cancer Group cooperative treatment trials. Children who received cranial irradiation (18 Gy divided in 10 fractions) plus intrathecal methotrexate had significantly lower scores on the McCarthy Motor Scale and the Token Test of receptive language and auditory comprehension, when compared to children receiving intrathecal methotrexate alone. Performance of tests of general cognition, visual motor integration, and receptive language requiring verbal recognition and visual recognition (Peabody Picture Vocabulary Test-R) showed no differences among the treatment groups. (MacLean WE Jr et al, for the Children's Cancer Group. Neuropsychological effects of cranial irradiation in young children with acute lymphoblastic leukemia 9 months after diagnosis. <u>Arch Neurol</u> February 1995;52:156-160). (Reprints: Dr D Hammond, Children's Cancer Group, PO Box 60012, Arcadia, CA 91066).

COMMENT. Recent issues of Ped Neur Briefs have included two previous reports of the adverse effects of cranial irradiation in children treated for acute lymphoblastic leukemia.

In a study from the Institute of Child Health, University of London, children who received a second course of cranial radiotherapy for relapsing leukemia suffered from neurologic deficits, growth impairment, ventricular enlargement on MRI, and impairments of tests of verbal comprehension, attention, and memory. Girls were affected more than boys. (<u>Ped Neur Briefs</u> June 1994;8:47).

Hypoplasia of the cerebellar vermis and cognitive deficits involving visual-spatial-motor coordination and memory were reported at 9 year follow-up in 13 children who received 24 Gy cranial radiation and intrathecal methotrexate at the University of New Mexico and centers in Canada. (Ped Neur Briefs Nov 1994;8:82).

The late morbidity associated with cranial radiotherapy has been recognized for some time. The Children's Cancer Group study demonstrates that cognitive deficits may become evident as early as 9 months after treatment, even with more moderate levels of irradiation. Whole-brain radiotherapy for brain tumors may also result in significant IQ deficits in children treated before age 7. (Progress in Pediatric Neurology II, 1994, p199). -Editor. *Ped Neur Briefs* Feb 1995.

RADIOTHERAPY-INDUCED COGNITIVE SEQUELAE

Long-term neurological and neuropsychological outcome in 25 irradiated children <15-years of age and 25 treated with surgery alone for low-grade astrocytoma was evaluated by two neurosurgeons and two psychologists independently at the Royal Manchester Children's Hospital, UK. Neurological function was not different in the irradiated group compared to the non-irradiated patients. In all neuropsychological tests used to assess intelligence, word reading, memory, learning and information processing, the performance of children with cranial radiation therapy was worse than those treated by surgery alone, and significant changes occurred in tests of IQ and information processing. Special education was required more frequently in the irradiated group. Both supratentorial tumor radiotherapy and local field irradiation to the posterior fossa for cerebellar tumors produced significant cognitive impairments. (Chadderton RD et al. Radiotherapy in the treatment of low-grade astrocytomas. II. The physical and cognitive sequelae.

<u>Child's Nerv Syst</u> August 1995;11:443-448). (Respond: Mr CGH West, Department of Neurological Surgery, Royal Manchester Children's Hospital, Manchester M27 1HA, UK).

COMMENT. This study confirms previous reports of cognitive impairments following irradiation for supratentorial tumors in children. Additionally, even local field irradiation to the posterior fossa can result in learning and academic problems. Children receiving cranial radiation therapy, locally or to the whole brain, should be followed with neuropsychological testing for longer than 3 years to determine effects on IQ and the need for special education. -Editor. *Ped Neur Briefs* Sept 1995.

DEVELOPMENTAL DISORDERS AND COGNITIVE DEFICITS

INTELLIGENCE OUTCOME IN SHUNTED HYDROCEPHALUS

The intelligence outcome of 44 children, tested between 2 and 17 years, and having a shunted hydrocephalus without tumor and with normal ventricular size, was evaluated at the Departments of Child Neurology and Neurosurgery, Instituto Nazionale Neurologico, Milan, Italy. IQ scores ranged from normal to highly defective. Verbal IQs were always higher than performance IQs. Variables without effect on IQ were: 1) site of obstruction; 2) number of shunt revisions; and 3) history of seizures.

Verbal IQ was influenced negatively by antiepileptic therapy and motor deficits, and positively by an older age at time of shunting. Non-verbal, performance IQ was lower in patients with cerebral hemisphere malformations, those with more than one shunt, pre- and perinatal problems, and antiepileptic therapy. The side of shunt placement was significantly correlated with non-verbal IQ, insertion on the right ensuring a better outcome. Posterior fossa malformations were not correlated with IQ. (Riva D et al. Intelligence outcome in children with shunted hydrocephalus of different etiology. <u>Child's Nerv Syst</u> Jan 1994;<u>10</u>:70-73). (Respond: Dr Daria Riva, Dept of Child Neurology, Instituto Nazionale Neurologico "C Besta", Via Celoria, 11, I-20133 Milan, Italy).

COMMENT. Shunted hydrocephalic children have a preferential loss of non-verbal IQ. Verbal and Performance IQs are influenced by different factors. Verbal IQ is correlated mainly with antiepileptic therapy, while non-verbal IQ was dependent on several surgical and medical variables.

A study of long-term outcome of hydrocephalus at the Service de Neurochirurgie Pediatrique, Hopital Necker-Enfants Malades, Paris, France, showed that IQ was related more to etiology than to ventricular dilatation, and to time of treatment. IQs are higher in patients with meningomyeloceles than in those with brain parenchymal lesions, toxoplasmosis, hemorrhage, or meningitis. IQs were above 80 in 60% of those shunted before 2 months of age and in only 29% treated after 2 years. (Hirsch J-F. Consensus: long-term outcome in hydrocephalus. <u>Child's Nerv Syst</u> Jan 1994;<u>10</u>:64-69). -Editor. *Ped Neur Briefs* Feb 1994.

INTELLIGENCE AND MRI CHANGES IN NEUROFIBROMATOSIS

Brain MRI changes were studied in relation to intelligence in a group of 28 children, aged 4 to 16 years, with neurofibromatosis 1. The mean FS IQ on the Wechsler scales (WPPSI, WISC-R) was 89 (range 54-148), mean VS was 95 and PS 84. Eight children who had neurological disease (epilepsy, hydrocephalus, tumor, or post-irradiation) scored significantly lower on IQ tests than the 20 without neurological disease. Eighteen children with hyperintense T2 weighted foci had a mean FS IQ comparable with the 10 without spots. In the group without neurologic disease, the 10 showing hyperintense spots had a higher mean FS IQ than 10 without. There was no significant relation between the number or location of T2 weighted foci and FS IQ. (Legius E et al. Neurofibromatosis type 1 in childhood: correlation of MRI findings with intelligence. <u>J Neurol Neurosurg Psychiatry</u> December 1995;59:635-640). (Respond: Dr Eric Legius, Center for Human Genetics, University Hospital Gasthuisberg, Herestraat 49, 3000 Leuven, Belgium).

COMMENT. Previous studies have shown that the mean full scale IQ in children with neurofibromatosis 1 is shifted to the left, between 88 and 94. T2 weighted hyperintense foci in the brain MRI were not correlated with intelligence of children with neurofibromatosis 1 in the present study, and similar results have been reported from other centers. (see <u>Progress in Pediatric Neurology I</u>, PNB Publishers, 1991, pp376-77). However, the authors cite two recent reports showing a significant correlation between a lowered IQ and the presence of T2 weighted hyperintensities in the MRI of 52 affected children who had no major neurologic complication or frank retardation. Further studies are needed to define the significance of these hyperintense foci. -Editor. *Ped Neur Briefs* Jan 1996.

LOW IQ AND MRI IN NEUROFIBROMATOSIS

The relationship between cognitive impairment and unidentified bright objects (UBOs) on the MRI in children with neurofibromatosis 1 (NF-1) was studied at the Kennedy Krieger Institute, and the Johns Hopkins University, Baltimore, MD. The data set included WISC-R-derived FSIQ for 20 pairs of children (NF-1 and unaffected sibling of NF-1); a "lesion count" for number of locations in which UBOs were seen; and the ratio of total volume of UBOs divided by total brain tissue volume. The number of locations occupied by UBOs accounted for IQ lowering in children with NF-1, whereas the total UBO volume was not associated with a discrepancy of IQ of NF-1 patients compared to their unaffected siblings (D-SIQ). The child's age, familiality, or summed UBO volume did not strengthen the regression model based on number of UBO locations.

The mean discrepancy (D-SIQ) for the NF-1 affected children was 13 points. The mean number of UBO-occupied locations was 3, with basal ganglia the most frequent site. (Denckla MB et al. Relationship between T2-weighted hyperintensities (Unidentified Bright Objects) and lower IQs in children with neurofibromatosis-1. <u>Am J Med Genet</u> 1996;67:98-102). (Reprints: Martha Bridge Denckla MD, The Kennedy Krieger Institute, 707 North Broadway, Suite 501, Baltimore, MD 21205).

COMMENT. In this study, the number of locations occupied by UBOs correlated with the lowering of IQ in children with neurofibromatosis-1. Previous studies have provided conflicting findings, some showing significant correlations between a lowered IQ and the presence of UBOs, and others failing to demonstrate a significant relation between intelligence and the number or location of T2 weighted foci in the brain. (see <u>Ped Neur Briefs</u> Jan 1996;10:3-4).

IQ correlated with UBOs in thalamus. A most recent paper from the University of Texas MD Anderson Cancer Center, and the UTMS, Houston, TX, reports that hyperintensities located in the cerebral hemispheres, basal ganglia, brainstem, or cerebellum show no correlation with neuropsychological functioning, whereas hyperintensities in the thalamus were significantly correlated with a lowered IQ. Mean scores for IQ, memory, motor, distractibility, and attention performance in children with UBOs in the thalamus were significantly lower than scores for those with UBOs located elsewhere. The presence or absence of UBOs and the number of UBOs were not significantly correlated with IQ. (Moore BD et al. Neuropsychological significance of areas of high signal intensity on brain MRIs of children with neurofibromatosis. <u>Neurology</u> June 1996;46:1660-1668). (Reprints: Dr Bartlett D Moore III, Division of Pediatrics (Box 87), UTMD Anderson Cancer Center, 1515 Holcombe Blvd, Houston, TX 77030). Location, location, location is the crucial factor!

Somatic mosaicism in neurofibromatosis is reported from the University of Florida, Gainesville, FL, and may possibly explain the discrepancies in patient selection and results of the above studies. (Colman SD et al. <u>Am J Hum Genet</u> March 1996;58:484-490). -Editor. *Ped Neur Briefs* July 1996.

MRI, BRAIN DEVELOPMENT AND IQ

Volumetric analysis of brain images obtained from MRI was used to study cerebral development in 85 normal children and adolescents, 5 to 17 years of age, at the Kennedy Krieger Institute, Johns Hopkins University, Baltimore; and Thomas Jefferson School of Medicine, Philadelphia, USA. Boys' brains were 10% larger than girls, and increased cortical grey matter contributed primarily to the larger brain volume. Age related changes included loss of cortical and subcortical grey volume and gain in white matter volume. Cerebral asymmetries were similar in both sexes: cortical and subcortical grey matter was prominent on the right side and CSF on the left. Total cerebral volume, particularly prefrontal grey matter, correlated with IQ. Subcortical grey matter volume showed a lesser but significant correlation with IQ variance. (Reiss AL, Abrams MT, Singer HS, Ross JL, Denckla MB. Brain development, gender and IQ in children. A volumetric imaging study. <u>Brain</u> Oct 1996;119:1763-1774). (Respond: Dr Allan L Reiss, Kennedy Krieger Institute, 707 North Broadway, Baltimore, MD 21205).

COMMENT. The finding that larger than normal brain volume is not always associated with superior cognitive function should allay fears that the investigators had any sexist bias in reporting boys' brains to be 10% larger than girls. Examples cited include children with neurofibromatosis-1 and the fragile X syndrome, both characterized by macrocephaly and below average IQ. -Editor. *Ped Neur Briefs* Dec 1996.

EPILEPSY AND LEARNING DISABILITIES

EPILEPSY AND COGNITIVE PERFORMANCE

Changes in left temporal interictal epileptiform activity during and after the performance of cognitive tasks are reported in an 18-year-old male with intractable complex partial seizures evaluated at the Radcliffe Infirmary, Oxford, UK. Epileptiform discharges were suppressed or enhanced depending on the nature and timing of the tasks. A posterior temporal spike focus occurred only during rest periods that followed verbal tasks. The mean left mid-to-anterior temporal spike count was halved during verbal tasks compared to the count during visuo-spatial tasks. A relatively low rate of right-sided temporal discharges was unchanged during or after the performance of tasks. (Boniface SJ et al. Changes in focal interictal epileptiform activity during and after the performance of verbal and visuospatial tasks in a patient with intractable partial seizures. <u>J Neurol Neurosurg Psychiatry</u> Feb 1994;<u>57</u>:227-228). (Respond: Dr SJ Boniface, Dept of Clinical Neurophysiology, Radcliffe Infirmary, Woodstock Road, Oxford OX2 6HE, UK).

COMMENT. Activation or suppression of EEG focal spike discharges in relation to psychological testing may have a role in the medical treatment of certain children with reading and other learning disabilities as well as the assessment of patients before and after surgery for epilepsy. -Editor. *Ped Neur Briefs* April 1994.

ANTIEPILEPTIC DRUGS AND LEARNING

PHENYTOIN AND COGNITIVE-MOTOR PERFORMANCE

Cognitive-motor function in 51 children with

seizures well controlled with phenytoin (PHT) monotherapy was assessed in relation to drug concentration, seizure type, and time of medication at the Departments of Psychiatry and Pharmacology, Auckland University School of Medicine, Australia. Age ranged from 4 to 14 years, and performance was significantly better in older patients. Diagnosis (partial vs generalized epilepsy), PHT concentration levels, and change from trough to peak concentration days had little effect. Fluctuations in PHT as great as 50% had no or minimal effects on performance of tests in low therapeutic doses. (Aman MG, Werry JS et al. Effects of phenytoin on cognitive-motor performance in children as a function of drug concentration, seizure type, and time of medication. <u>Epilepsia</u> Jan/Feb 1994;<u>35</u>:172-180). (Reprints: Dr MG Aman, Nisonger Center, Ohio State University, 1581 Dodd Dr, Columbus, OH 43210).

COMMENT. Maintenance phenytoin monotherapy, at relatively low therapeutic levels, had negligible or no effects on cognitive motor function in a group of children with well controlled seizures. Performance swings resulting from drug absorption and elimination were absent or minimal in this carefully monitored study. The importance of frequent determinations of phenytoin levels during evaluations of neuropsychological function in children is evident from the following report.

In a special article on the "role of therapeutic drug monitoring in pediatric anticonvulsant drug dosing," Walson PD at Children's Hospital, Columbus, OH refers to a rapid phenytoin clearance and a first order (linear) rather than saturated kinetics observed in some children found to have unusually low serum drug levels despite doses as high as 18 mg/kg/day. (<u>Brain & Dev</u> 1994;<u>16</u>:23). The effects of rate and extent of absorption on the interpretation of phenytoin concentrations and cognitive function are often unappreciated.

Various factors can modify phenytoin absorption

in children, including the dose and stool frequency. Doses well tolerated in healthy children may become toxic if the patient is constipated. High dose phenytoin loading can affect glucose homeostasis, with possible changes in cognition. The hyperglycemic effect of phenytoin was first demonstrated in the Division of Neurology and Neurochemistry Laboratories at Children's Memorial Hospital, Chicago (Belton NR, Etheridge JE Jr, and Millichap JG. Effects of convulsions and anticonvulsants on blood sugar in rabbits. <u>Epilepsia</u> 1965;<u>6</u>:234). -Editor. *Ped Neur Briefs* April 1994.

COGNITIVE EFFECTS OF PHT AND CBZ AFTER BRAIN TRAUMA

The effects of prophylactic anticonvulsant use of phenytoin (PHT) and carbamazepine (CBZ) on the cognitive and emotional status of a total of 80 brain trauma patients are compared and reported from the Division of Neurosurgery and Department of Neurology, St Louis University School of Medicine and School of Public Health. The median ages of the two groups were 40 (PHT patients) and 36 (CBZ) years. Both phenytoin and carbamazepine had some negative effects on performance measured by neuropsychological tests. Effects generally were small in magnitude and were evident on tasks with motor and speed components. Earlier hypotheses that phenytoin had a more marked effect on higher-level cognitive skills than did carbamazepine were not confirmed. CBZ had a slightly greater negative effect than PHT on verbal fluency, verbal and visual memory, and complex attentional tasks. Patients receiving PHT were possibly more anxious compared to CBZ-treated patients. (Smith KR Jr et al. Neurobehavioral effects of phenytoin and carbamazepine in patients recovering from brain trauma: A comparative study. <u>Arch Neurol</u> July 1994;51:653-660).(Reprints: Dr Smith, Division of Neurosurgery, St Louis University, Box 15250, 3635 Vista at Grand, St Louis, MO 63110).

COMMENT. The neurobehavioral effects of

phenytoin and carbamazepine were small and of limited functional significance. Most of the patients had no clinically detectable deficits while receiving either drug. Substantial variability was noted in drug serum concentrations at test sessions in individual patients, and between drug levels and test scores from subject to subject. Individual differences among patients and possible idiosyncratic responses to drugs are factors to be considered in the use or choice and evaluation of AEDs in brain trauma patients.

A previous randomized, double-blind study has shown that phenytoin prevents posttraumatic seizures only during the first week after severe head injury. (Temkin NR et al. <u>N Engl J Med</u> 1990;323:497). Some authorities have concluded that prophylactic drugs should be withheld, or administered only in a single loading dose, after severe head injury, minimizing the risk of idiosyncratic side-effects, especially exfoliative dermatitis. (<u>Progress in Pediatric Neurology</u>. Millichap JG, Ed, Chicago, PNB Publishers, 1991, pp 54-56). -Editor. *Ped Neur Briefs* Aug 1994.

CARBAMAZEPINE EFFECTS ON AUDITORY EVOKED POTENTIALS AND COGNITION

The effects of carbamazepine (CBZ) on cognitive function were evaluated by using measurements of auditory event-related potentials (ERPs) and P300 latencies in 23 patients, aged 7 to 16 years, with benign childhood epilepsy and centrotemporal spikes (BCECT), at the Department of Pediatrics, Toyama Medical and Pharmaceutical University, Toyama, Japan. As the epilepsy was controlled at the initiation of therapy, and with increasing age, the P300 latency was at first shortened. During the course of therapy with CBZ, P300 latency was prolonged, and the age-corrected P300 latency showed a significant correlation with the serum CBZ level. The dose of CBZ ranged from 10-23 mg/kg/day (mean 15.8). The latency became shorter when CBZ was discontinued. (Naganuma Y et al. Auditory event-related potentials in benign childhood epilepsy with centrotemporal spike: The effects of carbamazepine. <u>Clin Electroencephalogr</u> Jan 1994;<u>25</u>:8-12). (Reprints: Yoshihiro Naganuma MD, Department of Pediatrics, Toyama Medical and Pharmaceutical University, 2630 Sugitani, Toyama 930-01, Japan).

COMMENT. The major positive component of auditory event-related potentials, at a latency of 300 msec (P300) for rare tones (2000 Hz), has been correlated with cognitive function. Abnormalities in ERPs in patients with epilepsy, and particularly prolongation of P300 latency, have been ascribed to the effects of the seizures and to antiepileptic drug therapy.

Various epileptic syndromes have shown different degrees of abnormality in the ERPs. In this study, after a transient beneficial response, the cumulative effect of carbamazepine was associated with a chronic impairment of cognitive function, as measured by changes in auditory event-related potentials.

Studies of the effects of carbamazepine on auditory brainstem responses (ABR) in 21 epileptic patients examined at the Institute of Clinical and Experimental Neurology, Thilisi, Republic of Georgia, demonstrated prolongation of ABR peak latencies and interpeak intervals. In addition, CBZ was associated with increases in peak latencies of middle-latency responses and slow cortical potentials. CBZ has suppressive influences on central auditory structures and the acoustic nerve. (Japaridze G et al. <u>Epilepsia</u> Nov/Dec 1993;<u>34</u>:1105-1109). -Editor. *Ped Neur Briefs* Jan 1994.

COGNITIVE FUNCTION AND VALPROATE MONOTHERAPY

A test battery to assess neuropsychological and behavioral changes associated with anticonvulsant, particularly valproate, therapy in children is proposed from the Departments of Pediatrics (Neurology), and Clinical Health and Psychology, University of Florida, Gainesville, FL. This includes 1) intellectual functioning (WISC-III, WPPSI-R), 2) verbal memory, sentence recall, story recall, and verbal learning (Wide Range Assessment of Memory and Learning-WRAML, 3) nonverbal memory, picture memory and visual learning-WRAML, 4) attention, digit span, continuous performance task-Paced Auditory Serial Addition Task-PASAT, 5) motor speed-finger tapping test, verbal fluency-Controlled Oral Word Association, and 6) problem behaviors- Child Behavior Check List. These tests were found to be sensitive to AED-induced cognitive changes, and some tests are repeatable to allow for frequent monitoring. (Legarda SB et al. Altered cognitive functioning in children with idiopathic epilepsy receiving valproate monotherapy. <u>J Child Neurol</u> July 1996;11:321-330). (Respond: Dr Stella B Legarda, Division of Neurology, Department of Pediatrics, University of Florida College of Medicine, PO Box 100296, JHM Health Center, Gainesville, FL 32610).

COMMENT. The authors comment that the cognitive effects of valproate reported in normal adult volunteers and adults with epilepsy cannot reliably be applied to children. There is a relative paucity of well-controlled studies assessing memory and attentional differences in pediatric epilepsy patients treated with valproate monotherapy. Reports that cognitively impaired children on valproate therapy improve with L-acetylcarnitine supplements requires further study.

In one study involving children with epilepsy previously untreated, significant positive correlations were found between serum levels of valproate and the sum of 5 memory tests at 1 month and at 6 months after starting valproate monotherapy. Phenytoin had no adverse effects, whereas carbamazepine serum levels showed a negative correlation with memory and reading scores. (Forsythe I et al. <u>Dev Med Child Neurol</u> 1991;33:524). For reviews of Cognitive Effects of Antiepileptic Drugs, see <u>Progress in Pediatric Neurology II,</u> Chicago, PNB Publ, 1994. -Editor. *Ped Neur Briefs* Sept 1996.

CARBAMAZEPINE VS VALPROATE AND COGNITIVE FUNCTION

Effects of carbamazepine vs valproate on cognitive functioning in patients with previously unmedicated epilepsy were evaluated in a prospective, randomized, double-blind Veterans Affairs multicenter study. Patients with seizures showed deficits relative to a normal control group prior to AED therapy. No significant decline from baseline levels of neuropsychological performance was detected over 6- or 12-month treatment intervals for either drug. Patients with high serum VPA levels (mean, 94 mcg/mL) performed less well than controls on measures of concentration and memory. Subtle compromises of cognitive functioning following treatment with VPA or CBZ were suggested by absence of practice effects. (Prevey ML, Delaney RC, Cramer JA et al. Effect of valproate on cognitive functioning. Comparison with carbamazepine. <u>Arch Neurol</u> Oct 1996;53:1008-1016). (Reprints: Mary L Prevey PhD, Neurology 127, VA Medical Center, West Haven, CT 06516).

COMMENT. Carbamazepine and valproate monotherapies may have subtle effects on cognitive functioning.

COGNITIVE AND SPEECH DEFICITS WITH OPSOCLONUS-MYOCLONUS

Thirteen patients, aged 1.7 to 16 years, with opsoclonus-myoclonus syndrome were evaluated for neuropsychological, psychosocial and adaptive function at the Children's National Medical Center, George Washington University, Washington, DC. IQs of six older children ranged from 50 to 72 on the Wechsler scales. One infant had a Mental Index of 71 on the Bayley, and a 46-month-old child tested at the 20-month level. Severe problems related to motor output, involving ambulation, fine motor coordination and speech, while some age-appropriate cognitive skills were retained. Verbal and visual reasoning approached the borderline to normal range. On the Achenbach Child Behavior Checklist, mild to moderately severe behavioral irritability and emotional lability were reported in 8 of 12 non-medicated children. On Vineland Adaptive Behavior Scales, severe adaptive limitations were noted; self-care was significantly delayed in areas related to feeding, dressing and toileting. Motor problems contributed to low scores in daily living and communication scales. One child, aged 8 years examined while treated with ACTH, tested in the normal range. (Papero PH, Pranzatelli MR et al. Neurobehavioral and psychosocial functioning of children with opsoclonus-myoclonus syndrome. <u>Dev Med Child Neurol</u> 1995;37:915-932). (Respond: Dr Patricia H Papero, Department of Psychiatry, Children's National Medical Center, 111 Michigan Ave NW, Washington DC 20010).

COMMENT. In 27 patients with opsoclonus-myoclonus syndrome reported previously from the same center (Pranzatelli et al. 1995, see <u>Ped Neur Briefs</u> March 1995;9:19), the etiology was paraneoplastic in 46% and infectious in the remainder. Hammer, Larsen, and Stack, at Children's Memorial Hospital, Chicago, have reported on the developmental outcome of 11 children with opsoclonus-myoclonus syndrome, the majority having an associated neuroblastoma. (See <u>Ped Neur Briefs</u> August 1995;9:61). Delayed development with motor incoordination and speech delay occurred in 8 patients and 3 had behavioral problems. Development was normal in 2 of 3 patients without neuroblastoma and in only 1 of 8 whose opsoclonus was associated with neuroblastoma. While the majority of patients in this study had significant developmental delay, others have reported a 50% incidence of intellectual deficit. The poor outcome might possibly be related to etiology, but symptoms of ataxia and opsoclonus were not improved by removal of a neuroblastoma. -Editor. *Ped Neur Briefs* Jan 1996.

SYNTHETIC SPEECH USED TO TREAT LANGUAGE DELAY

Deficits in recognition and processing of rapidly successive phonetic elements of speech in language-learning impaired (LLI) children, aged 5 to 10 years, treated at Rutgers University, Newark, NJ, and University of California, San Francisco, were improved by listening to acoustically modified synthetic speech and by daily training with computer "games" designed to modify temporal processing and phoneme perception. A two-stage acoustic speech processing algorithm was developed:1) prolonging the duration of the speech signal by 50%, and 2) enhancing by 20dB the fast (3-30 Hz) consonant speech elements relative to the slowly modulated vowels. After 1 month of daily training with this acoustically modified speech presented as listening exercises on audiotapes, test scores significantly improved by approximately 2 years, with each of seven LLI children achieving normal levels of speech discrimination and language comprehension. In a second study involving 22 LLI children divided into two matched groups, both groups received the same training exercises used in the initial study but only one group was presented with temporally adaptive computer games and acoustically modified speech exercises. Significantly larger improvements in speech discrimination and language comprehension were achieved by the LLI children receiving the acoustically modified speech training as compared with improvements recorded for subjects receiving natural speech training. (Tallal P, Merzenich MM et al. Language comprehension in language-learning impaired children improved with acoustically modified speech. <u>Science</u> Jan 5, 1996;271:81-84).

(Respond: Dr Paula Tallal, Center for Molecular and Behavioral Neuroscience, Rutgers University, Newark, NJ 07102).

COMMENT. Remarkable and significant improvements in receptive speech and language comprehension were demonstrated in language-learning impaired (LLI) children who received training with acoustically modified speech stimuli. Brief, rapidly changing components of speech were temporally prolonged and emphasized, and coupled with adaptive training exercises.

LLI children have been found to have a temporal processing deficit, expressed by limited identification of brief phonetic elements of speech and impaired sequencing of short-duration acoustic stimuli presented in rapid succession. When presented in slower forms and rates, the stimuli are correctly perceived and receptive language is improved.

Temporal processing deficits of 11 LLI children studied at the Center for Integrative Neurosciences and Coleman Laboratory, University of California, San Francisco, were corrected by adaptive training exercises and computer games designed to modify temporal processing skills. (Merzenich MM, Tallal P et al. Temporal processing deficits of language-learning impaired children ameliorated by training. <u>Science</u> Jan 5, 1996;271:77-81). -Editor. *Ped Neur Briefs* Jan 1996.

KLUVER-BUCY SYNDROME FOLLOWING HEAT STROKE

A 12-year-old girl who developed a typical Kluver-Bucy syndrome (KBS) following heat stroke is reported from the University of Minnesota and Gillette Children's Hospital, Minneapolis, MN. The child collapsed and had a 20 min generalized seizure at the end of a 2 mile race run in 40-44 C ambient temperature. Cardiopulmonary resuscitation was necessary during a brief apnea. After iced normal saline infused during transport to the ER her rectal temperature was 102.7 F. Twelve days later she had bowel and bladder incontinence, her affect was flat, she examined objects orally and attempted to eat them, she had no language and could not imitate sounds or words, she could not identify objects, she did not recognize family members, she had marked motor restlessness. After 4 weeks, she was extremely distractible and had limited visual attention. She was unable to dress herself. She was absorbed with her body. Hypersexuality was demonstrated by moving and dancing suggestively, masturbating, and rubbing against objects. She attempted to sit on the lap of adults and to kiss adults of both sexes. Several weeks later, she developed aggressive behaviors. At discharge, she required constant supervision and was dependent on others for all daily needs. MRI at 11 months after heat stroke showed mild, diffuse atrophy. Fourteen months after onset, she did not respond consistently to language, did not communicate verbally, and was dependent on others. (Pitt DC, Kriel RL et al. Kluver-Bucy syndrome following heat stroke in a 12-year-old girl. <u>Pediatr Neurol</u> July/August 1995;13:73-76). (Respond: Dr Kriel, Hennepin County Medical Center #867-B, 701 Park Avenue South, Minneapolis, MN 55415).

COMMENT. The features of Kluver-Bucy syndrome include visual agnosia, hypermetamorphosis (distortion of objects), hypersexuality, language disorder and aphasia, hyperorality, placidity, flat affect, and memory dysfunction. The authors concluded that a metabolic/anoxic encephalopathy associated with heat stroke was the cause of the KBS in this child. In 12 additional reports cited from the literature, anoxic encephalopathy was the most commonly identified cause.

This article is especially appropriate during this exceptionally hot summer. Young athletes should be warned of possible serious consequences of exercise and heat stroke. -Editor. *Ped Neur Briefs* Aug 1995.

PERCEPTUAL-MOTOR DEFICITS AND CONGENITAL MUSCULAR DYSTROPHY

Fine motor and perceptual-motor abilities in 22 children with congenital muscular dystrophy, with and without MRI changes, were evaluated at the Hammersmith Hospital, London, UK. Perceptual-motor difficulties and minor neurological soft signs were present in those with diffuse MRI changes but not in those with normal MRI. (Mercuri E et al. Minor neurological and perceptuo-motor deficits in children with congenital muscular dystrophy: Correlation with brain MRI changes. <u>Neuropediatrics</u> June 1995;26:156-162). -Editor. *Ped Neur Briefs* Aug 1995.

CEREBELLAR MUTISM

Of a series of 15 children operated for cerebellar tumor at University Hospital Rotterdam-Dijkzigt, The Netherlands, 5 developed "cerebellar mutism" and subsequent dysarthria after surgery, and 2 had mild speech problems. Of 8 without speech problems, 7 had astrocytomas, with involvement of a cerebellar hemisphere. Of the 5 with mutism, 4 had medulloblastomas, and all had tumors that lined the fourth ventricle. Mutism was delayed for 1 to 2 days after surgery. Alternating movements of the tongue were impaired but no paresis of bulbar muscles was evident in mute patients. The duration of mutism varied from 3 to 8 weeks. Speech was regained suddenly and unexpectedly, and the severe dysarthria that followed lasted for 1 to 5 weeks. Recovery was associated with normalization of tongue movements. Factors predictive of mutism were 1) tumor filling and adherence to the floor of the fourth ventricle; 2) shunting for hydrocephalus prior to surgery; and 3) postsurgical edema of the pontine tegmentum. (van Dongen HR et al. The syndrome of 'cerebellar' mutism and subsequent dysarthria. <u>Neurology</u> Nov 1994;44:2040-2046). (Reprints: Dr HR van Dongen, Department of Neurology, University Hospital Rotterdam-Dijkzigt, dr Molewaterplein 40,3015 GD Rotterdam, The Netherlands).

COMMENT. The authors cite 36 cases of cerebellar mutism from the literature. An additional 2 cases are reported in <u>Progress in Pediatric Neurology Vol. II</u>, Chicago, PNB Publishers, 1994, pp219-220. The complication was correlated with the amount of the posterior vermis resected. One tumor was a medulloblastoma and the other an astrocytoma. Speech was regained after 2 months.

A case of mutism followed by dysarthria and agrammatic speech is reported in an adult after a right cerebellar infarction. (Silveri MC et al. The cerebellum contributes to linguistic production: a case of agrammatic speech following a right cerebellar lesion. <u>Neurology</u> Nov 1994;44:2047-2050). -Editor. *Ped Neur Briefs* Dec 1994.

NEUROLOGICAL ASSESSMENT OF DEVELOPMENTAL DELAY

The etiologic or diagnostic yield of the neurologic examination in 60 children referred to a pediatric neurologist for evaluation of global developmental delay was determined at the Montreal Children's Hospital-McGill University, Quebec, Canada. Examination at a mean age of 3.58 years revealed mild delay in development in 25, moderate delay in in 23, and severe delay in 12. EEG, MRI, metabolic screens, fragile X test and karyotype established an etiologic diagnosis in 38 (63%), including cerebral dysgenesis (17%), HIE (10%), chromosomal anomalies (10%), toxins (8%), and metabolic disorders (5%). (Majnemer A, Shevell MI. Diagnostic yield of the neurologic assessment of the developmentally delayed child. <u>J Pediatr</u> August 1995;127:193-199). (Reprints: Annette Majnemer PhD, Montreal Children's Hospital, 2300 Tupper St, Room A-509, Montreal, Quebec II3II 1P3, Canada).

COMMENT. Optimal management of children with developmental delay should include a neurologic examination and selected laboratory tests. An etiologic diagnosis provides physician and family with important information regarding risks of recurrence and choice of therapeutic intervention. -Editor. *Ped Neur Briefs* Sept 1995.

EARLY SCREENING FOR LEARNING DISABILITIES

The value of child health surveillance (CHS) practices in early detection of mild to moderate learning difficulties (LD) was investigated at the North and West Belfast Community Paediatric Unit, Belfast, N

Ireland. The prevalence of learning difficulties in this deprived inner city area was 16%. Only 6% of children with LD were identified by the CHS in the preschool period. Perinatal variables associated with LD were lower social class, prematurity, male sex, and birth to an unmarried mother. Risk factors used in the CHS which proved to be insensitive included speech delay, poor parenting, behavior problems, enuresis, poor visual acuity, and otitis media with effusion. (Corrigan N, Stewart M et al. Predictive value of preschool surveillance in detecting learning difficulties. <u>Arch Dis Child</u> 1996;74:517-521). (Respond: Dr N Corrigan, Altnagelvin Area Hospital, Londonderry, N Ireland).

COMMENT. Child Health Surveillance (CHS) by health visitors, at birth, 6 weeks, 6, 12, and 18 months, 2,3, and 4 years, failed to detect the majority of children with mild learning difficulties and missed 38% of the moderately learning disabled. Retrospective analysis of the child health record failed to identify a model to predict children with later LD. The failure of CHS in this setting was attributed to a combination of poor test sensitivity and the overlap of LD with variants of developmental norms. Nursery school and preschool surveillance, and increased parental and professional awareness could provide more accurate early detection of LD children. -Editor. *Ped Neur Briefs* Aug 1996.

LEARNING DISABILITIES AND TOURETTE'S SYNDROME

A retrospective study of 138 children with Tourette's syndrome examined the contribution of neurobehavioral concomitant symptoms to academic difficulties in the Department of Neurology, and Division of Biostatistics, University of Rochester Medical Center, Rochester, NY. A diagnosis of specific learning disorder (LD) was made in 30 (22%). Among 108 without a diagnosis of LD, 36 (33%) had school problems that included grade retention in 16 (15%) and/or special education placement in 41 (38%). The association of ADHD with TS was a significant predictor of school problems. (Abwender DA et al. School problems in Tourette's syndrome. <u>Arch Neurol</u> June 1996;53:509-511). (Respond: Dr Como, Department of Neurology, Box 673, University of Rochester Medical Center, 601 Elmwood Ave, Rochester, NY 14642).

COMMENT. Even when children with specific learning disabilities are excluded, TS is associated with academic problems in one third. Tics themselves were not the reason for the school problems, but rather the associated comorbid ADHD. These findings confirm those of the Johns Hopkins group of investigators, who found that children with TS + ADHD were at higher risk for a specific learning disability than those with TS alone (32% v 0%). (Schuerholz LJ et al. <u>Neurology</u> 1996;46:958-965).

For those readers interested in history, Lajonchere C et al, from Washington University, St Louis, MO, have published an English-language translation of an 1884 article by Gilles de la Tourette that led to his description of the Tourette syndrome published in 1885. (<u>Arch Neurol</u> June 1996;53:567-574). -Editor. *Ped Neur Briefs* Sept 1996.

INTRAVENTRICULAR HEMORRHAGE AND COGNITION

The effects of premature birth-related subependymal and mild intraventricular hemorrhage (S/IVH) on specific cognitive abilities in 2-year-old children were investigated at the Perinatology Center, New York Hospital, and Cornell and New York University Medical Colleges. Of 82 children included in the study, 27 had premature births complicated by Grade I or II hemorrhages, 28 prematurely born children had normal neonatal ultrasound, and 27 were born at term without complications. The premature group with S/IVH at birth performed significantly less well than children without hemorrhage on a measure of memory for location and on ability to change response set. Both groups of prematurely born children performed less well than full term children on systematic search for an object when the order of hiding was reversed. All groups performed equally on a visual attention task and on the global Bayley mental ability scores. (Ross G, Boatright S, Auld PAM, Nass R. Specific cognitive abilities in 2-year-old children with subependymal and mild intraventricular hemorrhage. <u>Brain Cogn</u> Oct 1996;32:1-13). (Reprints: Dr Gail Ross, Perinatology Center, New York Hospital, 525 East 68th Street, New York, NY 10021).

COMMENT. Prior testing of these prematures at age 10 months had shown that S/IVH affected global mental ability and habituation to visual patterns, and prematurity was associated with poorer memory for location. When reevaluated at 2 years, the premature groups with or without hemorrhage did not differ on the visual attention task, but prematures with S/IVH did poorly on the memory for location task and ability to change response set. Memory for location is a function of the caudate nucleus and thalamus and frontal cortex, areas affected by subependymal and intraventricular hemorrhage of prematurity. Fronto-striatal structural changes in the MRI have been demonstrated in patients with ADHD. (Denckla MB. In: Progress in Pediatric Neurology II, Chicago, PNB Publ, 1994:173-176). At a later age, the incidence of ADHD in the S/IVH affected children will be of interest.

Indomethacin prophylaxis against IVH in very low birth weight infants did not result in adverse cognitive or motor outcomes at 36 months, in a study at Yale University School of Medicine. (Ment LR et al. <u>Pediatrics</u> Oct 1996;98:714-718). The authors suggest that the early administration of intravenous low-dose indomethacin to neonates weighing 1250 g or less is beneficial and does not cause neurodevelopmental delay. However, Dr Henrietta Bada, University of Tennessee, Memphis, advises caution, and slow infusion, because of reported acute cerebral effects. (Commentary. Routine indomethacin prophylaxis: has the time come? <u>Pediatrics</u> Oct 1996;98:784-785). -Editor. *Ped Neur Briefs* Nov 1996.

MATERNAL DIABETES AND INFANT INTELLIGENCE

The intellectual development of 33 children born to 33 diabetic Japanese mothers (ODM) was compared to that of 34 control offspring of non-diabetics delivered at Kurume University Hospital, Fukuoka, Japan, between 1987 and 1989. Intelligence scores on the Tanaka-Binet test were significantly lower in the ODMs at 3 years of age than in controls. Maternal age and infant IQ were inversely correlated in ODMs but not in controls. (Yamashita Y, Kawano Y, Kuriya N et al. Intellectual development of offspring of diabetic mothers. <u>Acta Paediatr</u> Oct 1996;85:1192-1196). (Respond: Dr Y Yamashita, Department of Paediatrics and Child Health, Kurume University School of Medicine, 67 Asahi-machi Kurume-city, Fukuoka 830, Japan).

COMMENT. Infants of diabetic mothers may be at risk for impaired intellectual development, and especially infants born to older mothers. The difference in IQ between offspring of diabetics and non-diabetics was not associated with maternal toxemia or postnatal hyperbilirubinemia or hypoglycemia. A longer period of follow-up was considered important in determining the final cognitive outcome of these children.

Severe hypoglycemia and cognitive impairment in diabetes is reviewed and the link is considered not proven in a report from the Department of Psychology, University of Edinburgh, and Department of Diabetes, Royal Infirmary of Edinburgh. (Deary IJ, Frier BM. <u>BMJ</u> 28 Sept 1996;313:767-768). Among young adults with insulin dependent diabetes, recurrent episodes of severe hypoglycemia over a 5 to 15 year period have either a mild or negligible effect on cerebral function, except for a few subjects who are unusually vulnerable and suffer permanent brain damage. While strict glycemic control delays onset of retinopathy, nephropathy, and neuropathy, it is associated with a threefold increase in severe hypoglycemia. -Editor. *Ped Neur Briefs* Nov 1996.

CHAPTER **5**

TOURETTE SYNDROME AND OTHER MOVEMENT DISORDERS

INTRODUCTION

Advances in our understanding of Tourette's syndrome have included MRI studies of corpus callosum morphology, genetic factors, and treatment. The side effects of medications are particularly troublesome, and new methods of therapy would be welcome.

Co-morbid illness such as ADHD and bipolar disorders often complicate therapy, and drug combinations are sometimes contraindicated because of the risk of serious toxicity. For example, methylphenidate and clonidine or desipramine, prescribed together in cases of ADHD complicated by tics, have been linked to sudden unexplained fatalities in rare cases. These drug combinations are discouraged and best avoided if possible. Careful monitoring, especially of the cardiovascular system, is advised during treatment.

The relation of hemolytic streptococcal infection to Tourette's syndrome and co-morbid ADHD and obsessive-compulsive disorder is of interest, particularly in view of the observed acute, fluctuating enlargement of the basal ganglia on MRI. Further studies of the possible autoimmune basis for these diseases and immunological methods of treatment are indicated.   *J. Gordon Millichap, M.D.*, Editor.

GENETICS OF TOURETTE'S SYNDROME

Bilineal transmission (from maternal and paternal sides) of Tourette's syndrome, especially in families in which the proband's symptoms were most severe, was a frequent finding (approx 1/3) in a study at the University of Rochester School of Medicine, NY, and University College London Medical School, London, UK. (Kurlan R et al. <u>Neurology</u> Dec 1994;44:2336-2342). -Editor. *Ped Neur Briefs* Jan 1995.

FAMILY AND SOCIAL ASPECTS OF TOURETTE'S SYNDROME

Results of a prospective, longitudinal study of 21 children recruited at age 2 1/2 to 3 1/2 years without tics but with a first-degree relative with Tourette syndrome (TS) are reported from the Department of Psychology and Child Study Center, Yale University, New Haven, CT. All subjects were evaluated annually and for 2 to 4 years. Among these high risk children, 24% had developed TS, 9% chronic tics, and 9% transient tics. Obsessive-compulsive symptoms occurred in 19%, and obsessive-compulsive disorder in 5%. Other diagnoses included attention deficit disorder, speech problems, and anxiety disorder in 24%. Children in this sample demonstrated an increased risk for tic disorders as well as other psychiatric disorders. Family functioning, independent of parental psychopathology, was associated with attention-deficit and anxiety disorders, decreased adaptive and increased maladaptive behaviors, and lower self-esteem but not tics or learning disorders. (Carter AS et al. A prospective longitudinal study of Gilles de la Tourette's syndrome. <u>J Am Acad Child Adolesc Psychiatry</u> March/April 1994;<u>33</u>:377-385). (Reprints: Dr David L Pauls, Child Study Center, Yale University School of Medicine, 230 S Frontage Road, New Haven, CT 06510).

COMMENT. An autosomal dominant mode of transmission for TS is suggested by the rates of tic disorders observed. Stressors in family functioning play a role in comorbid disorders such as anxiety and attentional difficulties. The authors advise family, cognitive-behavioral, and interpersonal therapies to address the social-emotional difficulties that often accompany TS.

Clonazepam was a useful adjunctive treatment for tics in children with comorbid ADHD studied at the Children's Hospital, Boston (Steingard RJ et al. <u>J Am Acad Child Adolesc Psychiatry</u> March/April 1994;<u>33</u>:394). -Editor. *Ped Neur Briefs* Feb 1994.

TOURETTE'S SYNDROME AND STIMULUS-INDUCED TICS

Three patients with Tourette's syndrome (TS) and tic-related behaviors induced by external and internal stimuli are reported from the Department of Psychiatry, University College Medical School, Middlesex Hospital, London. All young adults whose tics began in childhood had developed a variety of obsessive compulsive disorders, sensory tics, reflex motor tics, or exaggerated startle responses, in response to internal (tightness in the chest) and external (people coughing or spitting) stimuli. The term "impulsions" has been used to describe these stimulus-induced behaviors which overlap with reflex tics and sensory tics. (Eapen V, Moriarty J, Robertson MM. Stimulus induced behaviours in Tourette's syndrome. <u>J Neurol Neurosurg Psychiatry</u> July 1994;57:853-855). (Respond: Dr Robertson,

Department of Psychiatry, Middlesex Hospital, Mortimer Street, London W1N 8AA, England).

COMMENT. The authors use the term "reflex tic" to describe those tics occurring in response to external stimuli (someone coughing), and "sensory tic" for those induced by sensations (tingling) felt in the soma or an internal stimulus (oneself coughing). The overlap between these various induced behaviors makes their separation difficult. -Editor. *Ped Neur Briefs* Aug 1994.

TIC DISORDERS AND TOURETTE'S SYNDROME

The relationship between Tourette's syndrome (TS) and chronic tic disorder was evaluated in 71 unselected children referred for psycho-pharmacological treatment at the Massachusetts General Hospital, Boston. Children with TS (32) and chronic tics (39) differed from controls in rates of comorbid psychiatric disorders including ADHD, obsessive-compulsive disorder, mood disorders (depression, bipolarity), antisocial disorders (conduct and oppositional defiant disorder), and anxiety disorders.

Both TS and chronic tic groups also suffered from cognitive impairments, lowered academic achievement (WRAT arithmetic), arithmetic learning disabilities, and school dysfunction. TS patients differed from tic disorder patients in the significantly higher rates of obsessive-compulsive disorder, oppositional defiant disorder, and simple phobia. TS and chronic tic disorder are related disease entities, with TS being a more severe form of tic disorder. (Spencer T, Biederman J et al. The relationship between tic disorders and Tourette's syndrome revisited. <u>J Am Acad Child Adolesc Psychiatry</u> September 1995;34:1133-1139). (Reprints: Dr Spencer, Psychopharmacology Unit (ACC-725), Massachusetts General Hospital, Fruit Street, Boston, MA 02114).

COMMENT. These findings are consistent with genetic studies showing that the TS gene is variably expressed as TS, transient tic disorders, or chronic tics. Comorbidity with ADHD, occurring in 50% of TS patients, is reported to cause more disability than the motor tics. The comorbidity with anxiety and mood disorders including mania affects the course, treatment, and outcome of tic disorders. -Editor. *Ped Neur Briefs* Sept 1995.

COMORBID TOURETTE'S AND BIPOLAR DISORDERS

Of 205 patients with Tourette's disorder in the North Dakota Longitudinal Tourette Syndrome Surveillance Project, 15 had comorbid bipolar disorder. The ratio of males to females was 5.2:1. The estimated risk of developing bipolar disorder among the study group of children and adolescents with Tourette's disorder was more than four times higher than the level expected by chance, significant at the 0.05 level. Males were at greater risk than females, and adults had comorbid developmental disorders as well. Shared common neural pathways, especially basal ganglia structures, and genetic factors may explain the comorbidity. (Kerbeshian J et al. Comorbid Tourette's disorder and bipolar disorder: an etiologic perspective. <u>Am J Psychiatry</u> November 1995;152:1646-1651). (Reprints: Mr Larry Burd, Medical Center Rehabilitation Hospital, 1300 South Columbia Rd, Grand Forks, ND 58202).

COMMENT. The authors have previously published case-reports of patients with comorbid Tourette's disorder and bipolar disorder, some with early histories of attention deficit hyperactivity disorder. The frequency and intensity of motor and vocal tics were positively correlated with manic symptoms and inversely with depressive symptoms. Noradrenergic, dopaminergic, and serotonergic mechanisms have been invoked in all three disorders. -Editor. *Ped Neur Briefs* Dec 1995.

GUANFACINE IN COMORBID ADHD & TOURETTE'S SYNDROME

An open-label study of guanfacine (1.5 mg/d), an a-adrenergic agonist, in 10 children with TS + ADHD, aged 8 to 16 years, was reported from the Yale University School of Medicine, New Haven, CT, and Johns Hopkins Medical Institutions, Baltimore, MD. At 4 to 20 weeks follow-up, significant decreases were observed in commission errors and omission errors on Continuous Performance Tests, and the severity of motor and phonic tics was also decreased. Side effects occurred in all patients and included transient fatigue, headaches, insomnia, and sedation. (Chappell PB, Riddle MA et al. Guanfacine treatment of comorbid attention-deficit hyperactivity disorder and Tourette's syndrome: preliminary clinical experience. <u>J Am Acad Child Adolesc Psychiatry</u> September 1995;34:1140-1146). (Reprints: Dr Chappell, Pfizer, Building 200, Eastern Point Road, Grozon, CT 06340).

COMMENT. The authors recommend guanfacine as a safe alternative to stimulants in the treatment of ADHD complicated by Tourette's syndrome. Guanfacine may be beneficial without having the hypotensive or sedative effects of clonidine *Ped Neur Briefs* Sept 1995;9:66.

Risperidone, a neuroleptic with both serotonin- and dopamine-blocking properties, reduced tic frequency and intensity in seven children and adolescents with Tourette's syndrome and chronic motor tic disorders. Weight gain was the most frequent side effect. (Lombroso PJ et al. Risperidone treatment of children and adolescents with chronic tic disorders: a preliminary report. <u>J Am Acad Child Adolesc Psychiatry</u> September 1995;34:1147-1152). -Editor. *Ped Neur Briefs* Sept 1995.

CLOMIPRAMINE FOR COMPULSIVE TICS

Reduction of adventitious movements and

compulsions during clomipramine treatment (25 mg - 200 mg daily at bedtime) in five prepubertal, autistic, retarded boys is reported from the Division of Child and Adolescent Psychiatry, Bellevue Hospital and New York University Medical Center, New York. Ratings were conducted before, after 2 and 4 weeks treatment, and every 4 weeks. All three classes of movements responded to medication: general dyskinesia, akathisia, and tics. Medications were administered in a nonblind trial in clinical emergencies to extremely disturbed patients with severe environmental and familial stresses. (Brasic JR et al. Clomipramine ameliorates adventitious movements and compulsions in prepubertal boys with autistic disorder and severe mental retardation. <u>Neurology</u> July 1994;44:1309-1312). (Reprints: Dr James R Brasic, Department of Psychiatry, New York University School of Medicine, 550 First Avenue, New York, NY 10016).

COMMENT. Medicated autistic patients frequently have akathisia and tics. The differentiation of various adventitious movements in a heterogeneous group of patients is difficult, and specificity of response to treatment is limited. -Editor. *Ped Neur Briefs* Aug 1994.

TREATMENT OF ADHD IN TOURETTE'S SYNDROME

A double-blind, placebo-controlled study of clonidine (.05 mg 4xd) and desipramine (25 mg 4xd) treatment of attention-deficit hyperactivity disorder (ADHD) behaviors in 34 children with TS + ADHD is reported from the Departments of Neurology and Pediatrics, Johns Hopkins University School of Medicine, Baltimore, MD. Desipramine was superior to clonidine in improving measures of ADHD, including parent-completed global linear analogue rating scale, hyperactivity subscale of the child behavior checklist (CBCL), and teacher CBCL subscales for nervous/overactive, anxious, and unpopular items. More than two thirds of families requested continuation of desipramine at the completion of the study. Neither drug made tics worse. (Singer HS, Denckla MB et al. The treatment of attention-deficit hyperactivity disorder in Tourette's syndrome: A double-blind placebo-controlled study with clonidine and desipramine. <u>Pediatrics</u> January 1995;95:74-81). (Reprints: Dr Harvey S Singer, Department of Neurology, Harvey 811, Johns Hopkins Hospital, 600 North Wolfe Street, Baltimore, MD 21287).

COMMENT. Desipramine is a more effective medication than clonidine for the treatment of ADHD in children with Tourette's syndrome. The authors hesitate to recommend the general use of desipramine. A review of the literature uncovered at least four sudden, unexplained deaths in children receiving desipramine. Careful monitoring, especially of the cardiovascular system, is advised.

Behavioral improvements found with tricyclic antidepressants and the positive effects of stimulant medication on cognitive tasks have prompted combined drug therapy of ADHD. Side effects occurred more frequently when a combination of desipramine and methylphenidate was employed compared to either medication used alone. (see <u>Progress in Pediatric Neurology II</u>, PNB Publ, 1994, pp210-211). -Editor. *Ped Neur Briefs* Jan 1995.

DEPRENYL IN TOURETTE'S SYNDROME AND ADHD

The efficacy of deprenyl, a monoamine oxidase inhibitor, was evaluated in the treatment of ADHD in 24 children and adolescents with comorbid Tourette's syndrome (TS) enrolled at the University of Rochester and Baylor College of Medicine. A double-blind placebo-controlled crossover design included two 8-week treatment periods separated by a 6-week washout period. A beneficial effect of deprenyl on tics was noted, but improvement of ADHD symptoms was limited to the first treatment period. (Feigin A et al. A controlled trial of deprenyl in children with Tourette's syndrome and attention deficit hyperactivity disorder. <u>Neurology</u> April 1996;46:965-968). (Reprints: Dr A Feigin,

North Shore University Hospital, 444 Community Drive, Suite 206, Manhasset, NY 11030).

COMMENT. Deprenyl is metabolized to amphetamine and methamphetamine. By inhibiting breakdown of dopamine and increasing synaptic dopamine levels, deprenyl might be expected to worsen tics. These authors report a controlling effect on tics, possibly due to an influence on dopamine receptors. The failure to demonstrate a significant beneficial effect on ADHD could be explained by the crossover study design and patient dropout. -Editor. *Ped Neur Briefs* May 1996.

ACUTE BASAL GANGLIA ENLARGEMENT WITH OBSESSIVE-COMPULSIVE DISORDER, TICS, AND STREP INFECTION

A 12-year-old boy with an acute exacerbation of obsessive-compulsive disorder (OCD) symptoms and tics following a Group A B-hemolytic streptococcal (GABHS) throat infection is reported from the National Institute of Mental Health, Bethesda, MD. Family history included Sydenham's chorea in a maternal grandfather, OCD in the mother and paternal aunt, and Tourette's syndrome in his 16-year-old brother. The boy had excessive throat-clearing, hyperactivity, and choreiform movements. Antistreptolysin O and DNAse B titers were elevated and a throat culture was positive for GABHS. Serial MRI scans performed to assess basal ganglia morphology in relation to symptom severity before and during plasmapheresis showed an initial caudate measure greater than two standard deviations above the mean for healthy boys. Within 1 day of the first plasmapheresis, the caudate volume decreased 24%, the putamen 12%, and the globus pallidus 28%. These fluctuations in the size of the basal ganglia correlated with the severity of symptoms of OCD which showed amelioration after plasmapheresis and a course of amoxicillin. The acute enlargement of the basal ganglia was most pronounced when the throat culture was positive for GAGHS. Less dramatic changes in size accompanied subsequent exacerbations of OCD, which occurred with negative throat cultures. (Giedd JN, Rapoport JL et al. Case study: Acute basal ganglia enlargement and obsessive-compulsive symptoms in an adolescent boy. <u>J Am Acad Child Adolesc Psychiatry</u> July 1996;35:913-915). (Reprints: Dr Giedd, NIMH, Child Psychiatry Branch, Building 10, Room 6N240, 10 Center Drive MSC 1600, Bethesda, MD 20892).

COMMENT. A link between obsessive-compulsive disorder and basal ganglia dysfunction is supported by this case-study. The swelling of the basal ganglia was thought to represent an inflammatory reaction with edema secondary to a cross-reaction of antibodies against the invading bacteria.

An association between B-hemolytic streptococcal infection and Tourette's syndrome in children with ADHD was previously correlated with serum antibodies against human caudate nucleus sections and elevated antistreptolysin titers in a study at Brown University, RI. (Kiessling LS et al. see <u>Progress in Pediatric Neurology II</u>, PNB Publ, 1994, pp236-7). Immunological treatments for autoimmune neuropsychiatric disorders associated with streptococcal infections, including ADHD and co-morbid symptoms, deserve further study. -Editor. *Ped Neur Briefs* Aug 1996.

CORPUS CALLOSUM SIZE IN TOURETTE'S SYNDROME

The size of the corpus callosum (CC) in Tourette's syndrome (TS) and ADHD was determined by analysis of MRI data in 77 children and adolescents, aged 6 to 16 years, including 27 controls, at the Kennedy Krieger Institute, Johns Hopkins University School of Medicine, Baltimore, MD. TS patients had significant increases in 4 of 5 subregions (splenium, isthmus/posterior body, mid-body, and rostral body), the total area, and the perimeter of the CC. ADHD was associated with a significant decrease in the rostral body size. Inspection of subgroup means demonstrated a statistical independence of the effects of ADHD versus effects of TS on CC size. The larger CC in TS was independent of age, handedness, intracranial area, and the association of ADHD. (Baumgardner TL, Singer HS, Denckla MB et al. Corpus callosum morphology in children with Tourette syndrome and attention deficit hyperactivity disorder. Neurology Aug 1996;47:477-482). (Reprints: Dr Thomas L Baumgardner, Behavioral Neurogenetics and Neuroimaging Research Center, Kennedy Krieger Institute, 707 N Broadway, Suite 509, Baltimore, MD 21205 or Dr HS Singer, Department of Neurology, Harvey 811, Johns Hopkins Hospital, 600 N Wolfe St, Baltimore, MD 21287).

COMMENT. The authors comment that TS and ADHD may result from distinct neurodevelopmental processes, and the three syndrome groups, comprising TS only, ADHD, and TS + ADHD, may represent different degrees of expression of the same gene. In addition to genetic transmission, environmental influences include prenatal factors, anabolic steroids, and antineural antibodies induced by streptococcal infection. (Singer HS, in Progress in Pediatric Neurology II, 1994, pp 227-231). -Editor. *Ped Neur Briefs* Sept 1996.

LEARNING DISABILITIES AND TOURETTE'S SYNDROME

A retrospective study of 138 children with Tourette's syndrome examined the contribution of neurobehavioral concomitant symptoms to academic difficulties in the Department of Neurology, and Division of Biostatistics, University of Rochester Medical Center, Rochester, NY. A diagnosis of specific learning disorder (LD) was made in 30 (22%). Among 108 without a diagnosis of LD, 36 (33%) had school problems that included grade retention in 16 (15%) and/or special education placement in 41 (38%). The association of ADHD with TS was a significant predictor of school problems. (Abwender DA et al. School problems in Tourette's syndrome. Arch Neurol June 1996;53:509-511). (Respond: Dr Como, Department of

Neurology, Box 673, University of Rochester Medical Center, 601 Elmwood Ave, Rochester, NY 14642).

COMMENT. Even when children with specific learning disabilities are excluded, TS is associated with academic problems in one third. Tics themselves were not the reason for the school problems, but rather the associated comorbid ADHD. These findings confirm those of the Johns Hopkins group of investigators, who found that children with TS + ADHD were at higher risk for a specific learning disability than those with TS alone (32% v 0%). (Schuerholz LJ et al. <u>Neurology</u> 1996;46:958-965).

For those readers interested in history, Lajonchere C et al, from Washington University, St Louis, MO, have published an English-language translation of an 1884 article by Gilles de la Tourette that led to his description of the Tourette syndrome published in 1885. (<u>Arch Neurol</u> June 1996;53:567-574). -Editor. *Ped Neur Briefs* Sept 1996.

HEMIFACIAL SPASMS AND CEREBELLAR ANGLE TUMORS

Two children, aged 3 years, with hemisomatic spasms caused by tumors in the ipsilateral cerebellopontine angle are reported from the Division of Pediatric Neurology and Department of Neurology, University of Texas Southwestern Medical Center, Dallas, TX. Patient 1 had persistent hemifacial spasms with onset soon after birth; some were complicated by flexion of the arm and extension of the leg. An initial diagnosis of partial seizures was not confirmed by video-EEG monitor, and anticonvulsants were of no benefit. CT and ultrasound were normal, but MRI revealed a C-P angle tumor. Following partial resection of a low-grade ganglioneuroma, the spasms were less severe. Patient 2 developed left sided jerks at 2 years of age, turning of the head to the right, and flexion of left elbow and hip, without loss of consciousness. Movements were worse while speaking or watching television. The EEG was normal and carbamazepine without benefit. MRI uncovered a left sided angle tumor, and spasms ceased after partial resection of a ganglioneuroma. (Al-Shahwan SA, Roach ES et al. Hemisomatic spasms in children. <u>Neurology</u> July 1994;44:1332-1333). (Reprints: Dr ES Roach, Department of Neurology, University of Texas Southwestern Medical Center, 5323 Harry Hines Blvd, Dallas, TX 75235).

COMMENT. The absence of impaired consciousness, normal EEG, and lack of response to antiepileptic drugs should help to distinguish hemifacial or hemisomatic spasms from partial epilepsy and lead to confirmation of a posterior fossa tumor by MRI. -Editor. *Ped Neur Briefs* Aug 1994.

HEREDITARY ESSENTIAL TREMOR

Twenty index patients with hereditary essential tremor, and 93 first degree and 38 more distant relatives were studied at the Institute of Neurology, Queen Square, London, and Oldchurch Hospital, Romford, UK. Tremor presented in the arms. It was symmetrical in 75% and first noted in the dominant hand in 25%. In index patients, tremor spread to affect the legs, head, voice, tongue, face, and rarely the jaw. Affected relatives had tremor of the upper limbs, and spread occurred in a minority. The median age of onset for index patients was 15 yrs (range 5 - 52). The age at onset for both index and secondary cases was bimodal, peaking in the second and fifth and sixth decades. Of 14 relatives under 15 years old, 4 were described as tremulous and 2 had definite tremor, beginning as early as 2 years of age. Disability occurred in the majority but none before 15 years of age. Hunger, emotion, fatigue, and heat exacerbated tremor and disability, whereas alcohol was of benefit in 50%. Classical migraine was associated in 25% cases. Dystonia, included in some previous studies, was not encountered. Inheritance was autosomal dominant and penetrance was complete by age 65. (Bain PG, Marsden CD et al. A study of hereditary essential tremor. <u>Brain</u> 1994;117:805-824). (Respond: Dr PG Bain, MRC Human

Movement and Balance Unit, Institute of Neurology, Queen Square, London WC1N 3BG, UK).

COMMENT. The diagnosis should be considered in older children described as tremulous or having a mild symmetrical postural tremor of the upper limbs. Genetic counselling is pertinent in a parent with tremor and a currently unaffected child. The authors' data show that at birth, the risk of ever developing essential tremor is 46%, and the risk of being affected by 20 years is 30%. In an unaffected child of 15 years of age, the risk of tremor by 20 years is 8%, and by 40 years, 20%. -Editor. *Ped Neur Briefs* Nov 1994.

MANGANESE SUPPLEMENTS AND DYSTONIA

A 7 month old girl who developed dystonic movements of the arms after a 3 month period of parental nutrition for jejunal atresia and bowel resection is reported from Great Ormond Street Hospital, London, UK. Development and head growth stopped at 12 months. Liver function tests showed cholestatic liver disease, a complication of parenteral nutrition. MRI showed basal ganglia changes in T1 weighted images compatible with trace metal deposition. A high blood manganese of 1740 nmol/L (ref. 73-210 nmol/L) was diagnosed at 17 months. She died 1 month later with neurological deterioration. A subsequent investigation of 53 children who had been on parenteral nutrition for more than 6 weeks showed that all those with cholestatic liver disease (35/53), and consequent impairment of biliary excretion of manganese, had whole blood manganese levels of >360 nmol/L. The parenteral supplement in the UK contained 55 times more manganese than that recommended by the American Society for Clinical Nutrition. This product has now been replaced with one containing 1 mcg/kg manganese, in line with the American guidelines. (Reynolds AP, Kiely E, Meadows N. Manganese in long term paediatric parental nutrition. <u>Arch Dis Child</u> Dec 1994;71:527-528). (Respond: Dr Reynolds, Department of Chemical Pathology, Great Ormond Street Hospital, Great

Ormond St, London WC1N 3JH, UK).

COMMENT. Blood manganese should be monitored in patients on parenteral nutrition, especially those who develop cholestatic liver disease. MRI is recommended if blood manganese is >360 nmol/L and/or if patient develops dystonia.

Manganese poisoning with dystonia in an 8 year old girl with Alagille's syndrome (hepatic duct hypoplasia, chronic cholestasis, facial dysmorphism, vertebral malformations, retarded development, and cardiac murmur) responded to treatment with ursodeoxycholic acid (see <u>Progress in Pediatric Neurology II</u>, Chicago, PNB Publ, 1994, pp438-9). Toxicity from dietary sources of manganese appears to require a prolonged period of exposure before neurologic symptoms develop. -Editor. *Ped Neur Briefs* Jan 1995.

MRI IN KERNICTERUS

The magnetic resonance images (MRI) of three children with athetotic cerebral palsy and severe neonatal jaundice were examined in the Department of Pediatric Neurology, Ohzora-no-iye Hospital and Seirei-Mikatahara General Hospital, Shizuoka, Japan. High intensity areas in the posteromedial border of the globus pallidus on T2-weighted images were found bilaterally in all 3 children. No abnormalities were demonstrated on T1-weighted imaging. (Yokochi K. Magnetic resonance imaging in children with kernicterus. <u>Acta Paediatr</u> August 1995;84:937-9). (Respond: Dr K Yokochi, Ohzora-no-iye Hospital, 7448 Nakagawa, Hosoe, Inasa, Shizuoka 431-13, Japan).

COMMENT. Kernicteric encephalopathy is a rare neonatal disorder since the introduction of phototherapy. Autopsy findings have revealed bilirubin staining of the globus pallidus, subthalamic nucleus, hippocampus, and dentate and olivary nuclei. The posteromedial border of the globus pallidus is the most sensitive region to kernicterus in MR imaging.

Perinatal hypoxic-ischemic encephalopathy is distinguished by involvement of the putamen and thalamus on pathological and MR studies. The author lists other diseases with MR lesions in the globus pallidus including Leigh syndrome, Hallervorden-Spatz disease, hemolytic uremic syndrome (associated with E coli 0157:H7 and *Shigella dysenteriae* food poisoning), carbon monoxide intoxication, hepatic encephalopathy, and neurofibromatosis. See <u>Progress in Pediatric Neurology II</u> (PNB Publishers, 1994, pp242-3) for a previous article by the same author and commentary on MRI in 22 athetotic cerebral palsied children. The value of the MRI in the timing of basal ganglia pathology has been alluded to in other reports of dyskinetic and dystonic cerebral palsy (*ibidem.* pp243-4). Of 219 dyskinetic CP cases seen between 1955 and 1986 in the Cheyne CP Centre, Chelsea, London, 25% had been diagnosed with kernicterus. -Editor. *Ped Neur Briefs* Oct 1995.

MRI CHANGES IN SYDENHAM'S CHOREA

Cerebral MRIs of 24 children with Sydenham's chorea and 48 matched controls were compared at the National Institutes of Health, Bethesda, MD. The caudate, putamen, and globus pallidus in the chorea group were all significantly greater in volume, whereas the total hemispheres, prefrontal, midfrontal, or thalamus areas were not increased. (Giedd JN et al. Sydenham's chorea: Magnetic resonance imaging of the basal ganglia. <u>Neurology</u> Dec 1995;45:2199-2202). (Reprints: Dr Jay N Giedd, National Institutes of Health, NIMH, Child Psychiatry Branch, 9000 Rockville Pike, Building 10, Room 6N240, Bethesda, MD 20892).

COMMENT. A cross-reactive antibody-mediated inflammation of the basal ganglia is suggested as the pathophysiology of Sydenham's chorea. The authors admit that volumetric MRI is of limited diagnostic value because of large variability and overlap in basal ganglia size between chorea and control subjects. **Chorea   in   an   infant   with**

holoprosencephaly is reported from the College of Physicians and Surgeons, New York. (Louis ED et al. <u>Pediatr Neurol</u> 1995;13:355-357). MRI showed small, fused frontal lobes with hypoplastic caudate nuclei. This example of chorea associated with a congenital structural anomaly and undersized basal ganglia contrasts with the inflammatory hyperplasia of the caudate in Sydenham's chorea. -Editor. *Ped Neur Briefs* March 1996.

CLASSIFICATION OF PAROXYSMAL DYSKINESIAS

Forty six patients, ages ranging 1 to 77 years, with paroxysmal dyskinesias and classified according to precipitating factors and duration of attacks were reported from the Movement Disorder Clinic, Department of Neurology, Baylor College of Medicine, Houston, TX. Paroxysmal kinesigenic dyskinesia (PKD), occurring abruptly after a sudden movement, affected 13 patients; paroxysmal nonkinesigenic dyskinesia (PNKD) occurred spontaneously in 26; exertion-induced attacks (PED) affected 5; and episodes were precipitated only by sleep (PHD) in 1. The etiology was idiopathic in 22 and secondary to psychogenic illness in 9, to stroke in 4, trauma (3), encephalitis (2), multiple sclerosis (2), kernicterus (1), and migraine (1). Short duration (<5 min) and long-lasting attacks (>5 min) were about equal in incidence. None had loss of consciousness or other evidence of seizures and EEGs were normal in 34 tested. MRI was normal in 25 tested. Nine of 10 (90%) patients with PKD improved with medications, mainly carbamazepine, phenytoin, or clonazepam, compared to only 7 of 19 (37%) with PNKD. (Demirkiran M, Jankovic J. Paroxysmal dyskinesias: clinical features and classification. <u>Ann Neurol</u> October 1995;38:571-579).

(Respond: Dr Jankovic, Department of Neurology, Baylor College of Medicine, 6550 Fannin, Suite 1801, Houston, TX 77030).

COMMENT. In contrast to the original (Mount and Reback, 1940) and other previous reports which empasized genetic and familial factors in etiology, the majority of the patients in the above series had sporadic and secondary paroxysmal dyskinesias. Menkes JH, in his <u>Textbook of Child Neurology</u> (Lea & Febiger, 1985), provides an excellent account of the various types of paroxysmal dyskinesia, classified according to 1) movement pattern - choreiform, athetoid, dystonic, or tonic; 2) familial or acquired; 3) kinesigenic or nonkinesigenic; 4) acquired etiology - perinatal asphyxia, reflex epilepsy, metabolic disorders (eg. idiopathic hyperparathyroidism), and multiple sclerosis.

The specificity of response of the kinesigenic dyskinesias to anticonvulsant drugs, especially phenytoin, has been documented previously. Rare cases of hypnogenic dyskinesia, responding to lorazepam, and one patient with paroxysmal diplopia due to superior oblique myokymia following head injury, responding to carbamazepine, are described in the present series. An overlap between paroxysmal dyskinesia and epilepsy, migraine, and paroxysmal ataxia is discussed. The possible relation between migraine and paroxysmal dyskinesia mentioned in this report has not previously been noted. -Editor. *Ped Neur Briefs* Nov 1995.

HEREDITARY MYOKYMIA AND PAROXYSMAL ATAXIA

A family with autosomal dominant hereditary myokymia and paroxysmal ataxia, linked to chromosome 12p, is described from University Hospital Groningen, The Netherlands. The proband, a 20 year old woman, had an onset of attacks of 'swinging legs', dizziness, involuntary jerky limb movements, dysarthria, and gait ataxia beginning at 6 years of age. Attacks up to four times daily and lasting 10 seconds to 5 min occurred at rest, during exercise, or when startled, standing up, or running. Myokymia of the hands and semirhythmical movements of fingers were noted on examination, and EMG showed myokymic discharges. An attack provoked by knee bends consisted of rhythmic involuntary shaking of limbs, and tremor and dysmetria on finger-to-nose test. Acetazolamide prevented attacks, but treatment was limited by paraesthesiae and development of tolerance. A 22 year old brother was also affected from 6 years of age, and the myokymia and ataxia were complicated by paroxysmal kinesigenic dystonia at 15 years, after a mild head injury. Another family member also had attacks of paroxysmal choreoathetosis. Carbamazepine controlled the attacks of dystonia and choreoathetosis but not the ataxia. Data on 6 affected family members are tabulated. (Lubbers WJ, Brunt ERP, et al. Hereditary myokymia and paroxysmal ataxia linked to chromosome 12 is responsive to acetazolamide. <u>J Neurol Neurosurg Psychiatry</u> October 1995;59:400-405). (Respond: Dr ERP Brunt, Department of Neurology, University Hospital Groningen, PO Box 30.001, 9700 RB Groningen, The Netherlands).

COMMENT. Provisional diagnoses of basilar migraine and epilepsy had been made initially in two of three children with familial paroxysmal ataxia reported in the UK (Hawkes CH, 1992). The EEG was normal and the MRI showed atrophy of the superior cerebellar vermis. All responded to acetazolamide. (see <u>Progress in Pediatric Neurology II</u>, PNB Publ, 1994, p149-150). MRI findings were not reported in the above series. An overlap and relation between paroxysmal types of ataxia, myokymia, choreoathetosis and dystonia is strengthened by this report, although different responses to acetazolamide and carbamazepine may suggest separate etiologies. -Editor. *Ped Neur Briefs* Nov 1995.

STIMULANT THERAPY FOR BENIGN CHOREA AND ADHD

A 6-year-old boy with benign familial chorea diagnosed at 1 year and ADHD evaluated and treated with methylphenidate (MPH) at 6 years is reported from the Department of Pediatrics, David Grant Medical Center, Travis Air Force Base, California. After MPH beginning with 2.5 mg BD and gradually increasing to 7.5 mg BD, his attention span, self-control, handwriting, and school performance were benefited as expected, but in addition, the chorea improved and his independent walking skills developed. On drug holidays, the chorea and gait problems regressed. (Friederich RL. Benign hereditary chorea improved on stimulant therapy. <u>Pediatr Neurol</u> May 1996;14:326-27). (Respond: Dr Friedrich, 60 MOS/SGOC, 101 Bodin Circle, Travis AFB, CA 94535).

COMMENT. The author suggests that chorea complicating ADHD should not contraindicate a cautious trial of stimulant medication. If methylphenidate improves a child's performance in school and lessens stressful situations, it may also result in a reduction in chorea and improved motor abilities. -Editor. *Ped Neur Briefs* Aug 1996.

OPSOCLONUS-MYOCLONUS SYNDROME

OUTCOME OF OPSOCLONUS WITH NEUROBLASTOMA

The neurologic and developmental outcomes in 10 children with opsoclonus-myoclonus ("dancing eyes syndrome") and neuroblastoma were reviewed by examination of records at Northwestern University Medical School and Children's Memorial Hospital, and the University of Illinois Hospital, Chicago. Ages ranged from 8 months to 30 months. Opsoclonus and ataxia had been present from 6 days to 1 year before diagnosis of neuroblastoma. All had localized disease and 50% had extraabdominal tumors. All are alive and without recurrence of tumor 8 months to 111 months after resection. All had opsoclonus-myoclonus or ataxia for at least 5 months after surgery, but eventually responded to ACTH therapy. Two were symptom-free 12 months after surgery, and 3 remitted after 36 months. Nine relapsed and had chronic deficits, including cognitive and motor delays, reading and language deficits, and behavioral abnormalities. Factors precipitating recurrences of opsoclonus-myoclonus or ataxia included discontinuance or reduction of ACTH, febrile illness, and immunizations. (Koh PS, Raffensperger JG et al. Long-term outcome in children with opsoclonus-myoclonus and ataxia and coincident neuroblastoma. <u>J Pediatr</u> Nov 1994;125:712-716). (Reprints: John G Raffensperger MD, Pediatric Surgery, Children's Memorial Hospital, 2300 Children's Plaza, Chicago, IL 60614).

COMMENT. All children with neuroblastoma and opsoclonus-myoclonus and ataxia had an excellent surgical outcome and their eye movement disorder eventually responded to ACTH. The majority have long-term learning and behavioral problems, requiring special remedial education and behavioral intervention. Immunizations should be delayed or withheld when possible to avoid relapse of opsoclonus and ataxia. -Editor. *Ped Neur Briefs* Dec 1994.

OPSOCLONUS-MYOCLONUS OUTCOME

The developmental outcome of 11 patients with opsoclonus-myoclonus, 8 having occult neuroblastoma, is reported from the Division of Pediatric Neurology, Children's Memorial Hospital, Chicago. Nine were treated with ACTH and 3 received prednisone. Symptoms recurred in 9 when ACTH was withdrawn. The response to predisone was minimal. Symptoms were not improved by removal of a neuroblastoma. The median age at presentation was 17 months. Follow-up ranged from 12 to 115 months. Delayed development with motor incoordination and speech delay occurred in 8 children and 3 had behavioral problems. IQs ranged from 56 to 75 in 7 children and one had a borderline IQ. Development was normal in 2 of 3 patients without neuroblastoma and in only 1 of 8 whose opsoclonus-myoclonus was associated with neuroblastoma. (Hammer MS, Larsen MB, Stack CV. Outcome of children with opsoclonus-myoclonus regardless of etiology. <u>Pediatr Neurol</u> July 1995;13:21-24). (Respond: Dr Hammer, Division of Pediatric Neurology, Children's Memorial Hospital, 2300 Children's Plaza, #51, Chicago, IL 60614).

COMMENT. Other terms for this syndrome include myoclonic encephalopathy of infancy (MEI), dancing eyes syndrome, and infantile polymyoclonia. The majority of children with opsoclonus-myoclonus in this study were found to have significant developmental delay. Others report that about 50% are left with intellectual deficits. (Boltshauser E et al. <u>Helv Pediatr Acta</u> 1979;34:119).

The criteria for diagnosis were 1) marked motor incapacity from myoclonic jerking and/or cerebellar ataxia, 2) opsoclonus, 3) acute or subacute onset, and 4) absence of central nervous system infection. All 3 children with MEI without neuroblastoma had a viral illness 1-2 weeks before symptoms began. The pathogenesis is multiple and is usually viral in origin, notably poliovirus, Coxsackie virus B3, and St Louis encephalitis virus. An autoimmune mechanism and DDT intoxication have also been invoked. (Menkes JH. <u>Textbook of Child Neurology</u>. 3rd ed. Philadelphia, Lea & Febiger, 1985). In treatment, some advocate ACTH for the acute stage followed by predisone for several months. (see <u>Progress in Pediatric Neurology</u> I, 1991, Chicago, PNB Publishers, p 486). -Editor. *Ped Neur Briefs* Aug 1995.

COGNITIVE AND SPEECH DEFICITS WITH OPSOCLONUS-MYOCLONUS

Thirteen patients, aged 1.7 to 16 years, with opsoclonus-myoclonus syndrome were evaluated for neuropsychological, psychosocial and adaptive function at the Children's National Medical Center, George Washington University, Washington, DC. IQs of six older children ranged from 50 to 72 on the Wechsler scales. One infant had a Mental Index of 71 on the Bayley, and a 46-month-old child tested at the 20-month level. Severe problems related to motor output, involving ambulation, fine motor coordination and speech, while some age-appropriate cognitive skills were retained. Verbal and visual reasoning approached the borderline to normal range. On the Achenbach

Child Behavior Checklist, mild to moderately severe behavioral irritability and emotional lability were reported in 8 of 12 non-medicated children. On Vineland Adaptive Behavior Scales, severe adaptive limitations were noted; self-care was significantly delayed in areas related to feeding, dressing and toileting. Motor problems contributed to low scores in daily living and communication scales. One child, aged 8 years examined while treated with ACTH, tested in the normal range. (Papero PH, Pranzatelli MR et al. Neurobehavioral and psychosocial functioning of children with opsoclonus-myoclonus syndrome. <u>Dev Med Child Neurol</u> 1995;37:915-932). (Respond: Dr Patricia H Papero, Department of Psychiatry, Children's National Medical Center, 111 Michigan Ave NW, Washington DC 20010).

COMMENT. In 27 patients with opsoclonus-myoclonus syndrome reported previously from the same center (Pranzatelli et al. 1995, see <u>Ped Neur Briefs</u> March 1995;9:19), the etiology was paraneoplastic in 46% and infectious in the remainder. Hammer, Larsen, and Stack, at Children's Memorial Hospital, Chicago, have reported on the developmental outcome of 11 children with opsoclonus-myoclonus syndrome, the majority having an associated neuroblastoma. (See <u>Ped Neur Briefs</u> August 1995;9:61). Delayed development with motor incoordination and speech delay occurred in 8 patients and 3 had behavioral problems. Development was normal in 2 of 3 patients without neuroblastoma and in only 1 of 8 whose opsoclonus was associated with neuroblastoma. While the majority of patients in this study had significant developmental delay, others have reported a 50% incidence of intellectual deficit. The poor outcome might possibly be related to etiology, but symptoms of ataxia and opsoclonus were not improved by removal of a neuroblastoma. -Editor. *Ped Neur Briefs* Jan 1996.

DANCING EYE SYNDROME SEQUELAE
A persisting disability was found at long-term follow-up in 88% of 54 patients with dancing eye

syndrome (DES) reported from the Hospital for Sick Children, Great Ormond Street, London. The disability was severe in 30 (62%), 34 (69%) had a motor disability, 29 (59%) had learning disabilities, and 23 (47%) had a combined motor and learning disability. Neurologic sequelae were independent of the severity of symptoms of the illness and age at onset. A malignancy was diagnosed in only 4: neuroblastoma in 3 and acute lymphoblastic leukemia in 1. An intercurrent illness, usually respiratory, preceded onset of DES in one half the cases. Presenting symptoms included ataxia, abnormal head and limb movements, and opsoclonus. Emotional outbursts of temper and affection were later features. A favorable initial response to corticotrophin or predisolone, observed in all patients, was not predictive of a good neurological prognosis. (Pohl KRE, Pritchard J, Wilson J. Neurological sequelae of the dancing eye syndrome. <u>Eur J Pediatr</u> March 1996;155:237-234). (Respond: Dr KRE Pohl, Newcomen Centre, Guys Hospital, St Thomas's Street, London SE1 9RT, UK).

COMMENT. Dancing eye syndrome (opsoclonus-myoclonus, infantile myoclonic encephalopathy) presents in infancy or early childhood (93% under 3 years) and neurologic sequelae may persist into adult life. Speech deficits, described as occasional in the above series, were more prominent in patient series reported from the Children's Memorial Hospital, Chicago, and the Children's National Medical Center, Washington, DC. (see <u>Ped Neur Briefs</u> Jan 1996;10:2). -Editor. *Ped Neur Briefs* March 1996.

CHAPTER **6**

NEUROMUSCULAR DISORDERS

INTRODUCTION

Deficiency of brain synaptic dystrophin in Duchenne muscular dystrophy (DMD) is one of the interesting reports among several important advances in neuromuscular disorders. Although a relationship between dystrophin deficiency in the synapse and cognitive function in DMD is undetermined, this possiblility requires further study. Cognitive dysfunction and psychiatric symptoms may be the major presenting features of Becker's and other muscular dystrophies. An elevated serum creatine kinase is a valuable screening test for boys with unexplained learning and behavior disorders, including ADHD.

Among MD patients having normal dystrophin, a primary adhalin deficiency is reported in three childhood-onset cases, including one Becker's MD and a limb-girdle type. The dystrophin-associated glycoprotein, adhalin, requires histochemical analysis in MD patients with normal dystrophin. Congenital muscular dystrophy syndromes are distinguished by muscle biopsy staining for alkaline and acid phosphatase, merosin, and dystrophin. The genetics of Fukuyama MD and facioscapulo-humeral dystrophy (FSHD) are further defined. Deletion size is correlated with disease severity in FSHD.

Since the initial clinical description of congenital mysathenia gravis more than 30 years ago, studies of the kinetics of the acetylcholine receptor (AChR) and ultrastructure of the endplate have uncovered a number of different syndromes. Recent additions to this complex problem include a deficiency and short open-time of the receptor, and a syndrome without endplate AChR deficiency, in which a defective neuromuscular transmission is explained by abnormal interaction of acetylcholine with its receptor. A dual center, large study of juvenile myasthenia gravis emphasizes race, sex, and puberty as influencing onset, severity, and outcome. Another study compares congenital and juvenile cases, clinical features, course, presence of AChR antibody, and response to treatment.

Factors responsible for neuropathies in childhood include infection, inflammatory demyelination, trauma, including obstetric palsies, and pyridoxine excess. *Campylobacter jejuni* infection is linked to Guillain-Barre and Chinese paralytic syndromes. Carpal tunnel syndrome may occur in children. Megadoses of pyridoxine may cause a sensory neuropathy when treatment or ingestion is protracted. Obstetric brachial plexus palsy continues to pose a problem and controversy, in mechanism, treatment, outcome, and in litigation. Caution is required in the interpretation of fibrillation potentials in the neonate EMG. Further studies are needed to determine more accurately the temporal relationship of injury to onset of denervation potentials in newborns. EMG findings alone cannot be used to assign cause of brachial plexus injury.   *J. Gordon Millichap, M.D.,* Editor.

GENETICS OF FUKUYAMA MUSCULAR DYSTROPHY

The Fukuyama congenital muscular dystrophy (FCMD) chromosome analysis has been further defined at the University of Tokyo; Department of Pediatrics, Tokyo Women's Medical College; Kobe General Hospital; Aichi Welfare Center, Kasugai; and Nagoya City University Medical School, Japan. The FCMD locus was first mapped to chromosome 9q31-33 by genetic linkage analysis, and further defined with additional markers and families between loci D9S127 and CA246, a region that includes the mfd 220 locus. The close proximity of mfd220 to FCMD is supported by tight linkage disequilibrium. (Toda T et al. Refined mapping of a gene responsible for Fukuyama-type congenital muscular dystrophy: Evidence for strong linkage disequilibrium. <u>Am J Hum Genet</u> November 1994;55:946-950). (Reprints: Dr Tatsushi Toda, Department of Human Genetics, School of International Health, University of Tokyo, 7-3-1 Hongo, Bunkyo-ku, Tokyo 113, Japan).

COMMENT. Fukuyama-type congenital muscular dystrophy is an autosomal recessive disorder of muscle complicated by CNS anomalies and neuronal migration defects. It is the second most common form of childhood muscular dystrophy in Japan, and 1 in 100 persons is a carrier. Weakness of facial and limb muscles and generalized hypotonia are evident before 9 months, and most patients never walk. Severe mental and speech retardation occur simultaneously, and survival beyond 20 years is rare. The biochemical and cytogenetic defects are unknown. -Editor. *Ped Neur Briefs* Nov 1994.

MUSCULAR FATIGUE IN DUCHENNE DYSTROPHY

The fatigability of the anterior tibial muscle in 11 boys with Duchenne muscular dystrophy (DMD) was compared to that of controls at the California Pacific Medical Center and the University of California, San

Francisco. The force generation of dystrophic muscle and compound muscle action potential amplitude were lower and relaxation time of tetanus was longer in patients than in controls at rest. During exercise, maximum voluntary contraction was better sustained, suggesting less central fatigue in DMD patients than in controls. (Sharma KR, Mynhier MA, Miller RG. Muscular fatigue in Duchenne muscular dystrophy. <u>Neurology</u> February 1995;45:306-310). (Reprints: Dr Khema R Sharma, University of Miami, Dept of Neurology, 1501 NW 9th Ave, Miami, FL 33136).

COMMENT. The intramuscular fatigability and recovery following sustained maximum voluntary contraction was similar in dystrophic muscles and controls, but patients with DMD had less central fatigue, possibly explained by longer training sessions and greater familiarity with the exercise. -Editor. *Ped Neur Briefs* Feb 1995.

PERCEPTUAL-MOTOR DEFICITS AND CONGENITAL MUSCULAR DYSTROPHY

Fine motor and perceptuo-motor abilities in 22 children with congenital muscular dystrophy, with and without MRI changes, were evaluated at the Hammersmith Hospital, London, UK. Perceptuo-motor difficulties and minor neurological soft signs were present in those with diffuse MRI changes but not in those with normal MRI. (Mercuri E et al. Minor neurological and perceptuo-motor deficits in children with congenital muscular dystrophy: Correlation with brain MRI changes. <u>Neuropediatrics</u> June 1995;26:156-162). -Editor. *Ped Neur Briefs* Aug 1995.

BRAIN DYSTROPHIN IN DUCHENNE MUSCULAR DYSTROPHY

To define the potential pathogenic role of dystrophin deficiency in the cognitive impairment characteristic of Duchenne muscular dystrophy (DMD), the protein in brain cortical synapses of an 8-year-old patient examined at autopsy and an age-matched control subject dying of myelogenous leukemia was analysed in the Department of Neuroscience and Cell Biology, Rutgers-The State University of New Jersey, Piscataway, NJ. Western blot analysis of protein in total homogenate, synaptic membrane, and the highly purified postsynaptic density (PSD) disc beneath the postsynaptic membrane, showed 427-kd dystrophin normally expressed in the PSD of the control tissue but was undetectable in the PSD from the DMD cerebral cortex. (Kim T-W, Wu K, Black IB. Deficiency of brain synaptic dystrophin in human Duchenne muscular dystrophy. <u>Ann Neurol</u> September 1995;38:446-449). (Respond: Dr Kim, Laboratory of Genetics and Aging, Department of Neurology, Massachusetts General Hospital East, 13th Street, Charlestown, MA 02129).

COMMENT. Human brain dystrophin is normally present in the cortical synapse but is absent in the brain of a child dying with Duchenne muscular dystrophy. Dystrophin deficiency in DMD may be a factor in both muscle and brain synaptic dysfunction. The patient examined in this report had no obvious cognitive impairment but a subclinical deficit was not excluded. The possible relationship between the dystrophin deficiency in the synapse and cognitive function was undetermined. That brain cortical dysfunction needs further study in patients with DMD is indicated by this report and by occasional observation of Babinski and other abnormal central nervous system signs. -Editor. *Ped Neur Briefs* Oct 1995.

ADHALIN DEFICIENCY AND MUSCULAR DYSTROPHY

Muscle biopsy specimens from 30 muscular dystrophy patients were examined for a deficiency of adhalin, the 50-kd dystrophin-associated protein, at the University of Pittsburgh School of Medicine, PA. Of 3 patients with neonatal-onset congenital MD, 11 with childhood-onset MD, and 16 with early adult-onset MD (limb-girdle MD), only one, a 16-year-old African-

American girl with childhood-onset MD, had adhalin gene mutations. All patients had autosomal recessive inheritance patterns, and all had serum CK levels higher than 1000 IU/liter. (Ljunggren A et al. Primary adhalin deficiency as a cause of muscular dystrophy in patients with normal dystrophin. <u>Ann Neurol</u> September 1995;38:367-372). (Respond: Dr Eric P Hoffman, BST W1211, University of Pittsburgh School of Medicine, Pittsburgh, PA 15261).

COMMENT. Primary adhalin deficiency in patients with muscular dystrophy with normal dystrophin is a relatively rare occurrence. It is not restricted to French families in which it was first reported. The phenotype is consistent with childhood-onset muscular dystrophy.

Approximately 60% of MD patients show absence or deficiency of dystrophin. Of the remaining 40% with normal dystrophin, most have the genetically heterogeneous severe childhood form of autosomal recessive MD, or limb-girdle dystrophy, and 1 in 30 may have a primary adhalin deficiency. -Editor. *Ped Neur Briefs* Oct 1995.

ADHALIN DEFICIENCY IN MUSCULAR DYSTROPHY

A 13-year-old boy previously diagnosed with Becker's muscular dystrophy and dilated cardiomyopathy was studied at the University of Wisconsin, Madison, and the University of Iowa College of Medicine, Iowa City, and was found to have a deficiency of the dystrophin-associated glycoprotein, adhalin. He was asymptomatic until 9 years of age, when proximal weakness developed. He had flexion contractures at the ankles, hypertrophy of calf muscles, and Gower's sign. The serum creatine kinase level was 11,560 U/L. Both his sister and mother had normal CK. There was no consanguinity. Analysis of dystrophin from the biceps by Western blot was normal. Congestive heart failure required heart transplantation. Immunostaining in both skeletal and cardiac muscle showed normal dystrophin, whereas adhalin was reduced in skeletal muscle and absent in cardiac muscle. (Fadic R, Lotz BP et al. Brief report: Deficiency of a dystrophin-associated glycoprotein (adhalin) in a patient with muscular dystrophy and cardiomyopathy. <u>N Engl J Med</u> Feb 8, 1996;334:362-365). (Reprints: Dr Lotz, Department of Neurology, University of Wisconsin Hospital and Clinics, 600 Highland Ave, Madison, WI 53792).

COMMENT. Adhalin deficiency is an autosomal recessive disorder and is indistinguishable from the dystrinopathies by clinical presentation and muscle pathology. The authors propose that constituents of the dystrophin-glycoprotein complex (adhalin) and merosin should be analysed histochemically in all patients with histological findings suggestive of a dystrophinopathy and with normal muscle dystrophin. The dystrophin-associated glycoprotein was named "adhalin" from the Arabic *adhal* (muscle). It has been linked in North African populations to a gene in chromosome 13q, but the deficiency is genetically heterogeneous. The adhalin gene has been mapped to chromosome 17q. See <u>Ped Neur Briefs</u> Oct 1995, pp73-74, for reference to a further case report of primary adhalin deficiency in a 16-year-old African-American girl with childhood-onset limb-girdle muscular dystrophy. -Editor. *Ped Neur Briefs* Feb 1996.

DIAGNOSIS OF CONGENITAL MUSCULAR DYSTROPHY

Patterns of alkaline and acid phosphatases were compared with the distribution of merosin and dystrophin staining in muscle biopsies from 20 children with congenital muscular dystrophy (CMD) examined at the Department of Neurology, Washington University School of Medicine, St Louis, MO. A ratio of AcP:AlkP staining was calculated for each biopsy. In 9 patients with CMD with normal dystrophin, the AcP:AlkP ratio was low, whereas in 3 patients with CMD and reduced dystrophin and in 7 with Duchenne muscular dystrophy, the ratio was up to 15 times higher. Low AcP:AlkP ratios were correlated with absence of AcP-positive cells. Merosin staining was absent in 5 of 17 CMD patients, none of whom could walk, whereas all 12 with merosin-positive stains walked. (Connolly AM, Pestronk A, et al. Congenital muscular dystrophy syndromes distinguished by alkaline and acid phosphatase, merosin, and dystrophin staining. <u>Neurology</u> March 1996;46:810-814). (Respond: Dr Alan Pestronk, Department of Neurology, Box 8111, Washington University School of Medicine, 660 S Euclid Ave, St Louis, MO 63110).

COMMENT. Biopsies showing few acid phosphatase-positive cells in association with numerous alkaline phosphatase staining muscle fibers are specific for congenital muscular dystrophy syndromes and histopathological support for the diagnosis. A finding of reduced merosin in muscle is predictive of severe weakness and disability.

Classical (Occidental) Merosin-positive form of CMD was milder and more slowly progressive than the merosin-negative form and Fukuyama type in a clinical and pathological study of 50 patients examined at the National Institute of Neuroscience, National Center of Neurology and Psychiatry, Kodaira, Tokyo, Japan. (Kobayashi O et al. Congenital muscular dystrophy: Clinical and pathological study of 50 patients with the classical (Occidental) merosin-positive form. <u>Neurology</u> March 1996;46:815-818).

Cognitive dysfunction in Becker's muscular dystrophy was the major presenting feature in 4 patients reported from the Children's Hospital, Boston, the Texas Children's Hospital, Houston, and other centers. (North KN, Miller G et al. <u>Neurology</u> March 1996;46:461-465). Psychiatric disturbance was also a feature in the absence of muscle weakness. An elevated serum creatine kinase may provide a valuable screening test in boys with unexplained cognitive or psychiatric disturbance. One patient had received various drugs used for ADHD before diagnosis was determined. -Editor. *Ped Neur Briefs* April 1996.

GENETICS OF FACIOSCAPULOHUMERAL DYSTROPHY

The relationship of phenotype to genotype in a clinically and genetically well defined population of 157 affected patients and 62 kindreds with facioscapulohumeral muscular dystrophy (FSHD) was examined at the University of Rochester School of Medicine, NY, and Ohio State University, Columbus, OH. Using isometric myometry scores to quantify disease severity, a significant correlation between disease severity and the size of the 4q35-associated deletion was evident, and the offspring were more severely affected than their parents. This generation effect and presence of anticipation in FSHD suggests a possible underlying dynamic mutation and an unstable repeat element within the region of the 4q35 deletion. (Tawil R et al. Evidence for anticipation and association of deletion size with severity in facioscapulohumeral muscular dystrophy. <u>Ann Neurol</u> June 1996;39:744-748). (Respond: Dr Tawil, University of Rochester, Department of Neurology, Box 673, 601 Elmwood Avenue, Rochester, NY 14642).

COMMENT. These findings have important significance in the genetic counselling of patients with FSHD. No differences in severity of disease were noted between paternally and maternally inherited FSHD, but a reduction in reproductive fitness in male compared to female patients was an unexpected finding.

FSHD with chromosome 9p deletion is reported in a 31-year-old man who also had congenital anomalies and mental retardation studied at Oita Medical University, Hasama-machi Oita 879-55, Japan. (Ueyama H et al. <u>Neurology</u> Feb 1996;46:566-569). A translocation between chromosome 4q and 9p was not detected. The FSHD was probably not attributable to the 9p deletion syndrome, which consists of the following: mental retardation, trigonocephaly, arched eyebrows, micrognathia, wide-spaced nipples, kyphosis, and inguinal hernias. -Editor. *Ped Neur Briefs* Aug 1996.

MYASTHENIA GRAVIS

CONGENITAL MYASTHENIC SYNDROMES

A new syndrome associated with a deficiency of acethylcholine receptor (AChR) and a short open-time of the AChR channel in a 5 year-old girl with myasthenic symptoms since birth is reported from the Neuromuscular Research Laboratory, Mayo Clinic, Rochester, MN. She required ventilatory support for the first 24 days after birth, nasogastric feeding for 6 months, and was hypotonic and weak. She had fluctuating ptosis, head control was delayed until 5 months, she walked unsteadily at 16 months, and had slurred speech when tired, and difficulty in chewing and closing her mouth. Her parents were healthy and mother was not myasthenic. On examination at 5 years, her head was dolichocephalic, the palate was high-arched, and teeth maloccluded. Myasthenic signs included ptosis, weakness of facial, laryngeal, and masticatory muscles, truncal and limb muscle weakness, and hypoactive deep tendon reflexes. Symptoms responded to pyridostigmine, 5 mg/kg/daily, and prednisone, 1 mg/kg, on alternate days. Tests for anti-AChR antibodies were negative. EMG studies with facial nerve stimulation evoked a 25% decremental response, and an intercostal muscle specimen for morphological and electrophysiological studies showed decreased numbers of endplate-specific I-BGT binding sites and attenuated immunostaining of endplates by anti-AChR antibodies. The neonatal onset, negative tests for anti-AChR antibodies, abnormal AChR kinetics, and other findings distinguished this case from autoimmune myasthenia gravis. (Engel AG et al. Congenital myasthenic syndromes: I. Deficiency and short open-time of the acetylcholine receptor. <u>Muscle & Nerve</u> Dec 1993;<u>16</u>:1284-1292). (Reprints: AG Engel MD, Department of Neurology, Mayo Clinic, Rochester, MN 55905).

COMMENT. Congenital myasthenia gravis is

distinguished from the *neonatal transient* form by absence of the disease in the mother, less severe generalized muscle weakness, and a relatively poor response to anticholinesterase treatment. Ptosis relieved by sleep is the most common presenting sign, and ophthalmoplegia and weakness of facial and masticatory muscles occur frequently during childhood and adult life. A family history of myasthenia in brothers, sisters, and cousins has been described. (Millichap JG, Dodge PR. Diagnosis and treatment of myasthenia gravis in infancy, childhood, and adolescence; a study of 51 patients. <u>Neurology</u> 1960;<u>10</u>:1007).

Since this clinical description more than 30 years ago, and the later discovery of the autoimmune origin of myasthenia gravis, the absence of antibodies against the acethylcholine receptor further delineated the congenital syndrome. Subsequently, Engel and his colleagues have identified and characterized a number of different congenital myasthenic syndromes, including endplate acethylcholine and AChR deficiencies, a slow-channel syndrome, and defects in resynthesis of ACh and kinetics of AChR. The investigation of congenital myasthenic syndromes is complex and requires studies of the kinetics of AChR, and ultrastructure of the endplate.

A further syndrome without endplate AChR deficiency, in which the defect of neuromuscular transmission is attributed to an abnormal interaction of acethylcholine with its receptor, is reported from the Mayo Clinic (Uchitel O, Engel AG et al. <u>Muscle & Nerve</u> Dec 1993;<u>16</u>:1293). -Editor. *Ped Neur Briefs* Jan 1994.

JUVENILE MYASTHENIA AND PUBERTY

The influence of race, sex, and puberty on incidence, severity, and outcome of juvenile myasthenia gravis beginning before age 20 years was evaluated in 115 patients seen at the University of Virginia, Duke University, and University of North Carolina at Chapel Hill. White patients with prepubertal disease onset had an equal sex ratio, and female predominance increased during and after puberty. Males had less severe disease than females. Black patients showed a constant F:M ratio of 2:1 in all pubertal-onset groups. Spontaneous remissions only occurred in white patients with prepubertal onset; and persistent symptoms for more than 10 years were least frequent in this group. Early thymectomy in white patients was followed by more remissions and milder symptoms than late thymectomy. Black patients had infrequent remissions, and similar disease severity after early or late thymectomy. (Andrews PI et al. Race, sex, and puberty influence onset, severity, and outcome in juvenile myasthenia gravis. <u>Neurology</u> July 1994;44:1208-1214). (Reprints: Dr P Ian Andrews, Division of Pediatric Neurology, Box 3533, Duke University Medical Center, Durham, NC 27710).

COMMENT. This study documents the importance of race, sex, and puberty on the incidence, severity, response to thymectomy, and outcome in juvenile myasthenia gravis. Thymectomy was most effective in white patients when performed within 1 year of peripubertal disease onset. See <u>Progress in Pediatric Neurology II</u>, Chicago, PNB Publ, August 1994, for further reports of juvenile myasthenia gravis from the University of Iowa, a multicenter study in Italy, and from the Mass General Hospital, Boston. -Editor. *Ped Neur Briefs* Aug 1994.

CONGENITAL AND JUVENILE MYASTHENIA GRAVIS

The clinical features, course, and presence of acetylcholine receptor antibody (AChRAb) were reviewed in 25 congenital (CMG) and 30 juvenile (JMG) cases of myasthenia gravis seen at Hacettepe University, Department of Paediatric Neurology, Ankara, Turkey. The age range of onset showed overlap: birth to 4 years for CMG, and 1.5 to 15 years for JMG. Parental consanguinity was present in 15 (60%) of CMG and only 3 (30%) of JMG patients. Motor development was delayed in 9 (36%) CMG infants and in

3 (10%) JMG patients. Initial symptoms were ocular in equal frequency for CMG (44%) and JMG (53%). After 1 year follow-up, only 4 (16%) CMG patients had ocular only involvement, 19 (76%) having progressed to ocular and bulbar or generalized weakness. Symptoms were limited to ocular muscles in 47% of JMG patients after 1 year. Unlike CMG, JMG patients showed spontaneous remissions in 20% and myasthenic crises in 33%. Good response to anticholinesterase drugs was more frequent in JMG than CMG (63 versus 41%). AChRAbs were present in 9 (34%) of JMG patients, all were girls with a later disease onset (>11 yrs) than antibody-negative cases. Pure ocular forms of MG were more often seronegative. None of the antibody-positive cases were in remission. The response to treatment was not significantly different between seropositive and negative cases. (Anlar B et al. Myasthenia gravis in childhood. <u>Acta Paediatr</u> July 1996;85:838-842). (Respond: Dr B Anlar, Hacettepe University, Department of Paediatric Neurology, Ankara 06100, Turkey).

COMMENT. In this series of childhood onset myasthenic patients, the proportion of congenital cases was much larger than previously reported. Facial muscle involvement and malformation often described in congenital cases was not alluded to in the above report. (see <u>Progress in Pediatric Neurology I and II</u>, PNB Publ, 1991 & 1994). Family and developmental histories, severity and distribution of weakness, and response to therapy are supportive criteria for the differentiation of congenital and juvenile cases. -Editor. *Ped Neur Briefs* Aug 1996.

CONGENITAL AND OTHER MYOPATHIES

CONGENITAL NEMALINE MYOPATHY

A female neonate with a rapidly fatal course of nemaline myopathy is reported from the University of Siena, Italy. Positive pressure ventilation was required and postasphyxia suspected. Despite improved cardiorespiratory function, severe hypotonia, muscle weakness and areflexia persisted. At 2 months, fractures of both femurs and left humerus were noted, and a myopathy was considered in diagnosis. Muscle biopsy of quadriceps showed rod-shaped nemaline bodies. The infant died at 4 months of pneumonia. Nemaline bodies were found in diaphragm, intercostal, psoas, and quadriceps muscles. The heart was also involved. The parents were healthy and their muscle biopsies normal. (Buonocore G et al. A new case of severe congenital nemaline myopathy. <u>Acta Paediatr</u> Dec 1993;<u>82</u>:1082-4). (Respond: Dr G Buonocore, Division of Neonatology, University of Siena, via P Mascagni, 46 53100 Siena, Italy).

COMMENT. Persistence of severe hypotonia in a neonate, together with dependence on assisted ventilation, should prompt investigation of a possible myopathy.

Intranuclear rods were present in muscle fibers of one infant with a rapid, fatal course of nemaline myopathy but were absent in the muscles of seven patients with a benign course, in a study reported from the Departments of Neurology and Pathology, University of Rochester Medical Center, NY. (Rifai Z et al. Intranuclear rods in severe congenital nemaline myopathy. <u>Neurology</u> Nov 1993;<u>43</u>:2372-2377). The presence of intranuclear rods represents a marker for the severe form of congenital nemaline myopathy.

The clinical manifestations of three forms of nemaline myopathy are reported as follows: 1) *severe neonatal form,* with hypotonia, feeding and respiratory difficulties, and death in infancy; 2) *nonprogressive or slowly progressive form,* presenting in infancy or early childhood with delayed motor milestones and facioscapuloperoneal weakness; and 3) *adult-onset form,* with a progressive proximal weakness. The term "congenital nemaline myopathy" is applied to forms 1) and 2). The authors caution that the neonatal type is not invariably fatal, and improvement may occur, oralternatively, deterioration may follow an initial stable course. -Editor. *Ped Neur Briefs* Feb 1994.

DISTAL VACUOLAR MYOPATHY IN CYSTINOSIS

Distal vacuolar myopathy in 13 post-renal-transplant cystinosis patients, ages 17 to 27 years, and studied at multiple centers, is reported from the National Institute of Child Health and Human Development, Bethesda, MD. Among 54 untreated patients with cystinosis, 13 (24%) developed hand weakness and wasting, sometimes accompanied by facial weakness and dysphagia, and becoming progressively more generalized. Tendon reflexes were preserved, and sensory testing and nerve conduction velocities were normal. EMG of affected distal muscles showed reduced amplitude and brief duration voluntary motor unit potentials. Muscle biopsy revealed fiber size variability, acid phosphatase-positive vacuoles, and absent fiber grouping or inflammation. Muscle cystine content of clinically affected muscles was markedly elevated. The cause of the distal myopathy was unclear. Systemic complications of nephropathic cystinosis or its treatment were excluded. (Charnas LR et al. Distal vacuolar myopathy in nephropathic cystinosis. <u>Ann Neurol</u> Feb 1994;<u>35</u>:181-188). (Respond: Dr Charnas, NICII, NIH, Bethesda, MD 20892).

COMMENT. Distal myopathy is a relatively common late complication of nephropathic cystinosis. Cysteamine therapy may prove effective. -Editor. *Ped Neur Briefs* March 1994.

ACUTE RECTUS PALSY AND MYOSITIS

Orbital myositis as the cause of palsy of the extraocular rectus muscle is reported in 7 children presenting with acute ocular pain at the Scottish Rite Children's Hospital, Atlanta, GA. All had chemosis and erythema of the conjunctiva restricted to the quadrant overlying the involved muscle. All had ocular pain and some had redness and swelling of the lids with ptosis.

All were afebrile. The diagnosis was confirmed by CT demonstration of an enlarged lateral rectus muscle. All had a benign course and were immediately responsive to corticosteroids. A recurrence in 2 patients was attributed to abrupt withdrawal of steroids. (Pollard ZF. Acute rectus muscle palsy in children as a result of orbital myositis. <u>J Pediatr</u> February 1996;128:230-3). (Reprints: Zane F Pollard MD, 5455 Meridian Mark Road, Suite 220, Atlanta, GA 30342).

COMMENT. The differential diagnosis includes orbital cellulitis which is distinguished by fever and response to antibiotics. Reported isolated causes of orbital myositis include Lyme disease, cysticercosis, and a paraneoplastic syndrome. -Editor. *Ped Neur Briefs* March 1996.

IV IMMUNOGLOBIN THERAPY IN DERMATOMYOSITIS

Improved strength and functional abilities following IV immunoglobulin treatment for chronic dermatomyositis is reported in two children from the University of Mississippi Medical Center, Jackson, MS. Both patients had developed side effects during prior treatment with prednisone and immunosuppressive agents. The response to IVIG was slow and occurred in a stepwise fashion after repeated monthly courses (2 g/kg). The rash on the face and hands also resolved. (Vedanarayanan V et al. Treatment of childhood dermatomyositis with high dose intravenous immunoglobulin. <u>Pediatr Neurol</u> 1995;13:336-339). (Respond: Dr Vedanarayanan, Division of Pediatric Neurology, University of Mississippi Medical Center, Jackson, MS 39216).

COMMENT. The authors consider IVIG a useful adjuvant therapy for dermatomyositis, permitting reduction in steroid dosage and lessening of treatment morbidity. -Editor. *Ped Neur Briefs* March 1996.

NEUROPATHIES

GUILLAIN-BARRE SYNDROME AND *CAMPYLOBACTER JEJUNI* INFECTION

A case control study of patients with Guillain-Barre syndrome (GBS) in South East England, reported from Guy's Hospital, London, has uncovered a strong asociation between *C jejuni* infection and a pure motor GBS, characterized by axonal degeneration either alone or combined with demyelination. *C jejuni* were isolated from the stools of 4 of 36 (11%) patients compared to 1 of 49 (2%) controls. A strong serological evidence of recent infection was found in an additional 5 patients. Of the total of 9 (25%) infected patients, 8 had a recent history of diarrhea, and 7 (78%) had one or more antibodies to glycoconjugates. (Rees JH, Hughes RAC. *Campylobacter jejuni* and Guillain-Barre syndrome. <u>Ann Neurol</u> Feb 1994;<u>35</u>:248-249). (Respond: Dr JH Rees, Department of Neurology, UMDS, Guy's Hospital, London SE1 9RT, UK).

COMMENT. The combination of recent *C jejuni* infection and positive anti-ganglioside GM1 antibodies heralds a poor prognosis in patients with GBS. The association of antecendent infection with *C jejuni* and GBS is also reported from the University of Texas Health Science Center, Houston (Vriesendorp FJ et al) and Julius-Maximilians-Universitat, Wurzburg, Germany (Enders U et al) (<u>Ann Neurol</u> Feb 1994;<u>35</u>:249).

A role for *C jejuni* infection in the etiology of a Chinese paralytic syndrome (acute motor axonal neuropathy) which resembles GBS has been proposed. (Gordon N. <u>Arch Dis Childhood</u> 1994;<u>70</u>:64-65). This disease shares clinical and CSF findings with the demyelinating GBS, but electrophysiological tests indicate an axonal neuropathy. A febrile illness preceeded muscle weakness in 30% of patients, and some had diarrhea. Outbreaks of the Chinese paralytic syndrome associated with diarrhea and *C jejuni* infection have also occurred in Japan and Bangladesh.

Environmental waterborne infections may have serious neurological complications. (<u>Environmental Food Poisons</u>, PNB Publ).-Editor. *Ped Neur Briefs* March 1994.

MEDIAN MONONEUROPATHIES

The clinical and electromyographic characteristics of median mononeuropathy in 17 children, 6 girls and 11 boys, aged 5-17 years, are reported from the Departments of Neurology, Children's Hospital, Boston and the Lahey Clinic, Burlington, MA. EMG showed a lesion at the wrist in 7 children, including 3 with idiopathic carpal tunnel syndrome (CTS), 1 related to skiing. Proximal lesions were identified in 10 (59%), including 8 with trauma. Five had bilateral disease, 3 with CTS. Nontraumatic cases (7) presented with intermittent numbness characteristic of CTS, pain and weakness, and painless weakness and atrophy of the thenar eminence. Mucolipidosis III, scleroderma, cutaneous mucinosis, and osteoid osteoma at the elbow were etiological factors in 4. Symptoms improved in 4 patients. Traumatic cases (10) occurred mainly in boys (8). Five were secondary to an elbow injury and 2 to more distal fractures. A laceration was responsible in 2. Complete recovery occurred in 2 with nerve compression. The results of surgery were variable; of 5 who had surgical decompression for nerve entrapment 3 improved initially. (Deymeer F, Jones HR Jr. Pediatric median mononeuropathies: a clinical and electromyographic study. <u>Muscle & Nerve</u> July 1994;17:755-762). (Reprints: H. Royden Jones Jr, MD, Department of Neurology, Lahey CVlinic, 41 Mall Road, Burlington, MA 01805).

COMMENT. Carpal tunnel syndrome is more common in adults than children. A small thenar eminence in a child may be secondary to congenital thenar hypoplasia or congenital constriction bands.-Editor. *Ped Neur Briefs* July 1994.

PYRIDOXINE-INDUCED SENSORY NEUROPATHY

An 18-year-old man with seizures from birth was followed in the Department of Clinical Neurological Sciences, University of Western Ontario, London, and was found to have developed a sensory neuropathy by 2 years of age following treatment with pyridoxine in doses up to 2000 mg/day. The initial seizure at birth responded to pyridoxine 150 mg IV, after treatment with diazepam had failed. A sister had died in status epilepticus at age 9 days and had not received pyridoxine. Complex febrile seizures from 1 to 4 years, followed by recurrent afebrile convulsions, and at 13 years, complex partial seizures continued despite pyridoxine 2000 mg/day, phenytoin, and phenobarbital. At 18 years, following the addition of carbamazepine, seizures were controlled, and pyridoxine was decreased to 100 mg daily. MRI showed left mesial temporal sclerosis. Nerve conduction studies at 2 years revealed absent sensory action potentials and normal motor conduction. Sural nerve biopsy showed severe, axonal, sensory neuropathy. At 18 years, vibration sense in the feet was absent, position sense was decreased in the toes, pain sensation was impaired to the midcalf and in the fingers, tendon reflexes were absent, and plantar responses were flexor. His gait was ataxic. Sural, peroneal and median sensory nerve action potentials were absent. The sensory neuronopathy diagnosed at 2 years had not progressed or remitted at 18 years. (McLachlan RS, Brown WF. Pyridoxine dependent epilepsy with iatrogenic sensory neuronopathy. <u>Can J Neurol Sci</u> February 1995;22:50-51). (Reprints: Dr RS McLachlan, University Hospital, 339 Windermere Rd, London, Ontario N6A 5A5).

COMMENT. The authors explain the failure of pyridoxine to completely control the seizures in this patient by a combination of pyridoxine-dependent epilepsy with complex partial seizures due to mesial sclerosis. Unusually high doses of pyridoxine were prescribed in this patient. Doses as low as 50 mg/day have caused neuropathy when continued for months or years. Individual susceptibility is also a factor in the occurrence of this side effect. -Editor. *Ped Neur Briefs* Feb 1995.

CRITICAL ILLNESS NEUROMUSCULAR DISEASE

Four children with critical illness neuromuscular disease following prolonged dependency on a ventilator are reported from the Departments of Neurology and Pediatrics, West Virginia University Health Sciences Center, Morgantown, and the Department of Medicine (Neurology), Memorial University of Newfoundland, St John's, Canada. One patient, a 15-year-old boy with septic shock, required ventilatory support and intermittent vecuronium for neuromuscular blockade. Extubation on day 8 was unsuccessful because of quadriparesis, with diffuse muscle atrophy, and absent reflexes. Muscle strength gradually returned over 3 months, but hyporeflexia persisted for > 1 year. (Sheth RD, Bodensteiner JB et al. Critical illness neuromuscular disease in children manifested as ventilatory dependence. J Pediatr February 1995;126:259-61). (Reprints: Raj D Sheth MD, West Virginia University Health Science Center, Box 9180, Morgantown, WV 26506).

COMMENT. Critical-illness polyneuropathy, a complication of sepsis in adults, and a cause of difficulty in weaning from the ventilator, is covered in Progress in Pediatric Neurology II, 1994, pp275-276. The syndrome appears to be unusual in children. -Editor. *Ped Neur Briefs* Feb 1995.

ACQUIRED "PSEUDO" HYPERTROPHIC NEUROPATHY

A 9-year-old boy with chronic progressive motor-sensory neuropathy beginning in early infancy and reversed by corticosteroid therapy is reported from the Institute of Neurological Diseases, Hirosaki

University School of Medicine, Japan. The parents had noticed an awkward gait and frequent falling after learning to walk at 15 months of age. He was in a wheel chair at examination, and he complained of hand numbness. Limb muscles were severely weakened and atrophied, and intrinisic hand muscles totally paralysed. Pes cavus was bilateral. Tendon reflexes were absent. Nerves at elbows and knees and behind the ears were thickened and enlarged. CSF protein was 68 mg/dl. Biopsy of the sural nerve showed edematous swelling, and loss of myelinated fibers, but only occasional onion bulbs. One week after IV methylpredisolone (25 mg/kg/day) for 3 days, followed by oral prednisolone (2 mg/kg/day), numbness in the hands decreased, and sensation and muscle strength improved. Within four weeks, he was walking alone, and posterior auricular nerves were no longer visible. Comparison of EMG and NCS before and after steroids showed that the extremely slow conduction velocities of 2 m/s had increased to 7 to 16 m/s. (Baba M et al. "Pseudo" hypertrophic neuropathy of childhood. <u>J Neurol Neurosurg Psychiatry</u> Feb 1995;58:236-237). (Respond: Dr Masayuki Baba, Department of Neurology, Institute of Neurological Diseases, Hirosaki University School of Medicine, Zaifu-cho 5, Hirosaki 036, Japan).

COMMENT. Steroid responsive neuropathy in childhood (Byers and Taft. <u>Pediatrics</u> 1957;20:517) was cited as the first reference to this disorder.-Editor. *Ped Neur Briefs* March 1995.

OBSTETRIC BRACHIAL PLEXUS PALSY: OUTCOME

The functional outcome with conservative management of 186 patients with obstetrical brachial plexus palsy, evaluated between 1981 and 1993, is reviewed at the Children's National Medical Center, George Washington University, Washington, DC. The majority (88%) had impairment ratings of mild (63%) to moderate (25%); 12% had complete lesions involving C4-5 to T1 and were rated severe. The palsy was bilateral in 7 patients. Perinatal complications included fractures of the clavicle (8) and humerus (5), Horner's syndrome (8), respiratory distress (16), transient stridor with recurrent laryngeal nerve involvement (3), phrenic nerve palsy (3), and torticollis (11). Of 10 with complete lesions, 5 had MRIs of cervical spines, and all showed root avulsions. The initial (at <3 months) clinical impairment ratings correlated closely with those at the last follow-up exam and with the electrodiagnostic studies repeated at intervals. Only 6 (4%) of 149 patients showed complete recovery, and 92 (62%) had mild impairments, including winging of the scapula, restricted shoulder abduction and external rotation, forearm supination, but normal hand use and sensation. The original severity groups were unchanged at follow-up in 108 (72%) patients. In 41 (28%) patients with discrepant scores at follow-up, 31 had improved by one grade, 2 improved by 2 grades, and 8 deteriorated between the first and last exam. Of 46 patients with typical Erb's palsy, graded as moderate in severity at initial exam, 28 had persistent functional limitations at follow-up. Selection criteria for microsurgery in this population were not clearly defined. (Eng GD et al. Obstetrical brachial plexus palsy (OBPP) outcome with conservative management. <u>Muscle Nerve</u> July 1996;19:884-891). (Reprints: Gloria D Eng MD, Children's National Medical Center, 111 Michigan Avenue, NW, Washington, DC 20010).

COMMENT. The majority of patients with obstetrical brachial plexus palsies have mild to moderate upper plexus lesions. In this study, complete recovery was exceptional, and mild sequelae were the rule.

Alfonso I et al, Miami Children's Hospital, review the differential diagnosis and management of obstetric brachial plexus injury. (<u>Int Pediatr</u> 1995;10:208-213). Prenatal non-obstetric trauma produces a fixed anatomical deformity and EMG fibrillations present at or soon after birth. These authors recommend early EMG only in the exceptional cases without history of a difficult birth, those infants with a low birth weight, and with signs of congenital muscular atrophy or contractures indicative of prenatal pathology. Congenital chicken pox, amniotic bands, and pseudoparalysis due to fractures or osteomyelitis may mimic Erb's palsy. I have seen cases of congenital syphilitic osteochondritis that presented as pseudoparalysis and were treated initially as an obstetric Erb's palsy.

Caution is required in the interpretation of fibrillation potentials in the newborn infant. Transient spontaneous potentials, similar in amplitude, duration, and frequency to fibrillation potentials, have been reported in "essentially normal" premature and full-term infants. Jones HR, Bolton CF, Harper CM (Pediatric Clinical Electromyography, Philadelphia, Lippincott-Raven, 1996) have reviewed in detail the electromyography of newborns and reasons for inconclusive or erroneous EMG clinical correlations. Animal data suggest that fibrillation potentials may occur within 2 days after nerve section. EMG must be performed during the first 12 to 48 hours of life in order to attempt a distinction between prenatal and perinatal nerve injury. Further studies are needed to determine more accurately the temporal relationship of injury to onset of denervation potentials in the newborn. It might be imprudent to rely on EMG findings alone to assign cause of brachial plexus injury in obstetric litigation cases. -Editor. *Ped Neur Briefs* July 1996.

RADIAL MONONEUROPATHIES

Sixteen cases of radial mononeuropathy, presenting with wristdrop and seen in the EMG laboratory at Children's Hospital, Boston, during 16 years, 1979-95, were analysed. Eight were atraumatic, including 2 in newborns, related to compression in 6 and entrapment in 2. Eight were caused by fractures or lacerations. The lesions localized by EMG were in the distal main radial nerve trunk in 9 (56%), the posterior interosseous nerve in 5 (31%), and in the proximal main radial nerve trunk in 2 (13%). Demyelinating lesions in 4 cases improved within 6-12 weeks, and axonal injuries in 13 took between 6 weeks and 18 months to improve or recover. Two showed no improvement in 4 years, and 1 caused by sclerotherapy for a nevus was progressive. (Escolar DM, Jones HR Jr, Pediatric radial mononeuropathies: a clinical and electromyographic study of sixteen children with review of the literature. <u>Muscle Nerve</u> July 1996;19:876-883). (Reprints: H Royden Jones Jr MD, Department of Neurology, Lahey Hitchock Medical Center, 41 Mall Road, Burlington, MA 01805).

COMMENT. These authors have previously determined that an EMG taken within 1-2 days of birth and showing fibrillation potentials is required to support a diagnosis of intrauterine prenatal-onset neuropathy. (Jones HR et al. Intrauterine onset of a mononeuropathy: peroneal neuropathy in a newborn with EMG findings compatible with a prenatal onset. <u>Muscle Nerve</u> 1996;19:88-91). The precise temporal profile for signs of denervation in the neonate with birth injury has not been well defined, and an EMG performed later than 48 hours after birth may not distinguish prenatal from perinatal injuries. The *distribution* of the EMG abnormalities differentiates the radial neuropathies from the brachial plexus palsies. -Editor. *Ped Neur Briefs* July 1996.

CHRONIC INFLAMMATORY NEUROPATHIES

The clinical characteristics, response to therapy, and long-term prognosis in 13 children (1.5 to 16 years of age) with chronic inflammatory demyelinating polyneuropathy (CIDP) were reviewed from records of patients seen at Washington University Medical Center, St Louis, MO, and the Royal Children's Hospital, Melbourne, Australia, between 1979 and 1994. Boys were affected more often than girls in a ratio of 1.6:1. Antecedent events noted within one month of onset occurred in 7 children (54%), and included vaccinations (measles-mumps-rubella immunization in

2), intercurrent infections (URI or tonsillitis in 4), and chicken pox in 1. Lower extremity weakness, associated with difficulty in walking, was the most common presenting symptom, found in 85% of children. Motor symptoms predominated, but sensory symptoms were also noted by 85%. Deep tendon reflexes were diminished or absent in all patients. Facial weakness ocurred in 4. CSF protein was elevated (mean, 177mg/dL) in 92%, but cells were not increased. Electrodiagnostic studies showed F-wave abnormalities (92%) and slowing of nerve conduction velocities (77%). Nerve biopsies performed in 4 showed demyelination. Prednisone resulted in initial improvement in all 13 patients. Relapses required continued prednisone in 8, and other therapies, such as immunoglobulin, plasma exchange, or immuno-suppressive medications, were added. One group of patients (4) with weakness developing over a short period of 1 to 3 months showed a monophasic course with complete recovery in 3. A second group (9), with slower evolution of symptoms from 3 months to several years, had no complete recoveries and mild to severe residual weakness. (Nevo Y, Pestronk A et al. Childhood chronic inflammatory demyelinating neuropathies: clinical course and long-term follow-up. <u>Neurology</u> July 1996;47:98-102). (Respond: Dr Pestronk, Department of Neurology, Box 8111, 660 South Euclid Ave, St Louis, MO 63110).

COMMENT. Childhood onset chronic inflammatory demyelinating polyneuropathy (CIDP) has in general a poor long-term prognosis, the majority showing relapses and having residual weakness. After an initial improvement with prednisone therapy, attempts to withdraw steroids were often unsuccessful and the addition of immunosuppressive medications was rarely of benefit. The few children who recovered completely had an antecedent illness of URI or tonsillitis. Of two patients with CIDP associated with MMR immunization, none recovered and one had severe residual weakness. CIDP is a previously unreported side effect of MMR immunization. Transverse myelitis following MMR vaccine was reviewed in <u>Ped Neur Briefs</u> Sept 1995;9:65. -Editor. *Ped Neur Briefs* Aug 1996.

DYNAMICS OF MUSCLE MATURATION

A painless, non-invasive technique for measuring the effects of age on the relaxation of calf muscle in 22 healthy children is reported from the Departments of Paediatric Neurology and Physiology, Royal Hospital for Sick Children, Edinburgh. The study was undertaken as a prelude to investigations of contractile properties of muscles in children with cerebral palsy and other motor handicaps. Soleus muscle twitches were generated by a single Achilles tendon tap which caused a monosynaptic reflex muscle-twitch contraction, recorded by EMG. Half-relaxation times halved from about 90 ms at age 3 years to 40 ms at age 10. Compared to a 19-year-old healthy male, relaxation was prolonged in a 3-year-old boy. The younger the child, the slower the muscle-relaxation time. Muscle maturation rate-limits motor tasks, and modifies the effects of early brain or spinal cord damage. (Lin J-P, Brown JK, Walsh EG. Physiological maturation of muscles in childhood. <u>Lancet</u> June 4 1994;343:1386-89). (Respond: Dr J-P Lin, Paediatric Neurology, Great Ormond Street Hospital for Children, London, WC1N 3JH, UK).

COMMENT. Having attempted quantitative measurements of motor function and muscle tone and relaxation in children with cerebral palsy for the purpose of evaluation of muscle relaxant drugs, I am aware of the paucity of reliable measures of muscle function in children. (Millichap JG, Hadra R. Quantitative assessment of motor function in cerebral palsy, Evaluation of Zoxazolamine (Flexin), a new muscular relaxant drug. <u>Neurology</u> Dec 1956;6:843-852). Measurements of muscle tone by speed and height of hammer recoil were abandoned in favor of quantitative tests of muscle function involving range, rapidity, strength, and coordination of voluntary movements.

The Edinburgh method of measurement for muscle relaxation should be of value in assessment of various treatments of cerebral palsy. -Editor. *Ped Neur Briefs* June 1994.

CHAPTER 7

CONGENITAL MALFORMATIONS AND MENTAL RETARDATION SYNDROMES

OVERVIEW OF RECENT ADVANCES
Harvey B. Sarnat, M.D., F.R.C.P.C.
University of Washington School of Medicine, Seattle

Recent advances and data related to human cerebral dysgenesis include both new clinical and neuropathological observations and new molecular genetic information on normal and abnormal programming of embryonic neural development. The most exciting discovery relating molecular genetic programming of the embryonic neural tube to human cerebral malformations was the finding by Belloni et al and Roessler et al that mutations in the organizer gene

Sonic hedgehog (Shh) were involved in the pathogenesis of holoprosencephaly. The gene products of Shh are expressed early in embryogenesis by the notochord and by the floor plate, the ventral midline ependyma that are the first neural cells to differentiate from the neuroepithelial placode. Shh is a strong ventralizing gradient in the development of the neural tube and induces differentiation of motor neuroblasts in the neuroepithelium adjacent to the floor plate; it also induces the O2-A progenitor cells that will form oligodendrocytes, all of which develop in the ventral half of the neural tube. Though the notochord does not extend further rostrally than the midbrain, the prechordal mesenchyme assumes its function in the region of the forebrain and also secretes the Shh gene product.

Another major cerebral malformation linked to the abnormal genetic programming is X-linked dominant periventricular heterotopia, clinically expressed as refractory epilepsy and diagnosed by MRI. Markers in the distal Xq28 locus that are highly pH-sensitive were demonstrated by Eksioglu et al. Another X-linked malformation, mapped by linkage analysis to the Xq23 (DXS1059) locus by Illarioshkin et al, is a form of congenital cerebellar hypoplasia.

Morphological studies using immunohisto-chemistry and electron microscopy also provided new data on brain development and cerebral dysgenesis. Kendler and Golden demonstrated a population of progenitor cells outside the ventricular and subventricular zones during human brain development, using antibodies against a proliferating cell nuclear antigen. O'Kusky et al studied synaptogenesis in hemimegalencephalic brain tissue surgically resected for intractable epilepsy. Kato et al demonstrated localized epidermal growth factor in the affected hemisphere of these cases.

Clinical studies of malformations included unilateral cerebellar aplasia described by Boltshauser et al, who speculated that fetal infarction rather than primary genetically-determined dysgenesis was the cause. Williams et al also described cerebellar dysplasia in Marinesco-Sjogren syndrome, an autosomal recessive disease characterized by congenital cataracts, cerebellar ataxia, mental deficiency, and myopathy. Cases of cerebellar hypoplasia were reported by Shevell and Majnemer.

A true tethered hindbrain related to a Chiari III malformation was described in an 11-year old boy by Kernan et al. Deformities of the cervicomedullary junction and spinal cord in Chiari I malformation were described by Beuls et al. Evaluations of autonomic cardiovascular responses and cough syncope syndrome in patients with Chiari I and II malformations were presented by Ireland et al.

Cortez and Kinney provided further neuropathological documentation of tegmental infarcts of the brainstem in the perinatal period as a cause of congenital apnea and failure of central respiratory drive; the hypoplasia of the inferior olivary nuclei noted in this case could result from intrauterine ischemic atrophy rather than a primary developmental malformation.

A full-term neonate with Hirschsprung's disease, hypertrophic pyloric stenosis and agenesis of the corpus callosum was reported by Sayed and Al-Alaiyan. This case report suggests a possible programming factor and production of neural defects from neural crest tissue as well as callosal agenesis centrally. Hori published a provocative hypothesis, based upon neuropathological studies of four brains, that callosal agenesis is associated with precocious cerebral development in gyration, transiently in midfetal life; further development of the cerebral cortex compensates and obliterates the evidence by the end of gestation.

Finally, two major textbooks were published that should prove invaluable to the student of human neuroembryology and developmental malformations of the nervous system. O'Rahilly and Muller published an atlas of human neuroembryology in 1994, as a summary statement of their lifelong major contributions to this field. In late 1995, the thorough and extensive work by Margaret Norman and her colleagues on cerebral malformations was published, a laudable and mostly successful integration of neuropathological, clinical, genetic, and imaging data. *Harvey B. Sarnat, M.D.*

BIBLIOGRAPHY

Belloni E, Muenke M, Roessler E et al. Identification of *Sonic hedgehog* as a candidate gene responsible for holoprosencephaly. Nature Genet 1996;14:353-356.

Beuls EAM, Vandersteen M-AM, Vanormelingen LM et al. Deformation of the cervicomedullary junction and spinal cord in a surgically treated adult Chiari I hindbrain hernia associated with syringomyelia: a magnetic resonance microscopic and neuropathological study. J Neurosurg 1996;85:701-708.

Bertolino E, Wildt S, Richards G, Clerc RG. Expression of a novel murine homeobox gene in the developing cerebellar external granular layer during its proliferation. Dev Dynam 1996;205:410-420.

Boltshauser E, Steinlin M, Martin E, Deonna T. Unilateral cerebellar aplasia. Neuropediatrics 1996;27:50-53.

Cortez C, Kinney HC. Brainstem tegmental necrosis and olivary hypoplasia: a lethal entity associated with congenital apnea. J Neuropathol Exp Neurol 1996;55:841-849.

Eksioglu YZ, Scheffer IE, Cardenas P et al. Periventricular heterotopia: an X-linked dominant epilepsy locus causing aberrant cerebral cortical development. Neuron 1996;16:77-87.

Hori A. Precocious cerebral development associated with agenesis of the corpus callosum in mid-fetal life: a transient syndrome? Acta Neuropathol 1996;91:120-125.

Illarioshkin SN, Tanaka H, Markova ED et al. X-linked nonprogressive congenital cerebellar hypoplasia: clinical description and mapping to chromosome Xq. Ann Neurol 1996;40:75-83.

Ireland PD, Mickelsen D, Rodenhouse TG et al. Evaluation of the autonomic cardiovascular response in Arnold-Chiari deformities and cough syncope syndrome. Arch Neurol 1996;53:526-531.

Kato M, Mizuguchi M, Sakuta R, Takashima S. Hypertrophy of the cerebral white matter in hemimegalencephaly. Pediatr Neurol 1996;14:335-338.

Kendler A, Golden JA. Progenitor cell proliferation

outside the ventricular and subventricular zones during human brain development. J Neuropathol Exp Neurol 1996;55:1253-1258.

Kernan J, Horgan MA, Piatt JH. Tethered hindbrain. J Neurosurg 1996;85:713-715.

Norman MG, McGillivray BC, Kalousek DK, Hill A, Poskitt KJ. Congenital Malformation of the Brain. Pathological, Embryological, Clinical, Radiological and Genetic Aspects. New York: Oxford University Press. 1995. 452 pages.

O'Kusky JR, Akers M-A, Vinters HV. Synaptogenesis in hemimegalencephaly: the numerical density of asymmetric and symmetric synapses in the cerebral cortex. Acta Neuropathol 1996;92:156-163.

O'Rahilly R, Muller F. The Embryonic Human Brain. An Atlas of Developmental Stages. New York: Wiley-Liss. 1994. 342 pages.

Roessler E, Belloni E, Gaudenz K et al. Mutations in the human *Sonic hedgehog* gene cause holoprosencephaly. Nature Genet 1996;14:357-360.

Sayed M, Al-Alaiyan S. Agenesis of corpus callosum, hypertrophic pyloric stenosis and Hirschsprung disease: coincidence or common etiology? Neuropediatrics 1996;27:204-206.

Shevell MI, Majnemer A. Clinical features of developmental disability associated with cerebellar hypoplasia. Pediatr Neurol 1996;15:224-229.

Williams TE, Buchhalter JR, Sussman MD. Cerebellar dysplasia and unilateral cataract in Marinesco-Sjogren syndrome. Pediatr Neurol 1996;14:158-161.

CONGENITAL HYDROCEPHALUS

HYDROCEPHALUS IN OSTEOGENESIS IMPERFECTA

The neurological complications of osteogenesis imperfecta in 76 patients are reported from the Human Genetics Branch, National Institute of Child Health and Human Development, NIH, Bethesda, MD. The mean age was 8 years. Communicating hydrocephalus was diagnosed by MRI in 17 patients, macrocephaly in 11, and basilar invagination in 8, with brainstem compression in 3. Seizures occurred in 5 patients, and skull fracture in 10. The importance of detection and treatment of neurological features of osteogenesis imperfecta is noted. (Charnas LR, Marini JC. Communicating hydrocephalus, basilar invagination, and other neurologic features in osteogenesis imperfecta. Neurology Dec 1993;43:2603-2608). (Reprints: Dr Lawrence R Charnas, Building 10, Room 9S242, NIH, Bethesda, MD 20892).

COMMENT. The high frequency of basilar impression in severe cases of osteogenesis imperfecta (OI) was remarkable, in comparison with previous reports. Cervical syringohydromyelia is sometimes a concomitant abnormality with basilar impression.

Mosaic rarefaction of the parietal and occipital bones, a characteristic finding in OI in infancy, may persist throughout childhood, and these strips and linear streaks of diminished density of the calvarium must be distinguished from multiple skull fractures, a common complication of OI. (Caffey J. Pediatric X-Ray Diagnosis, Chicago, Year Book Publ, 1956). Editor. *Ped Neur Briefs* March 1994.

INTELLIGENCE OUTCOME IN SHUNTED HYDROCEPHALUS

The intelligence outcome of 44 children, tested between 2 and 17 years, and having a shunted hydrocephalus without tumor and with normal ventricular size, was evaluated at the Departments of Child Neurology and Neurosurgery, Instituto Nazionale Neurologico, Milan, Italy. IQ scores ranged from normal to highly defective. Verbal IQs were always higher than performance IQs. Variables without effect on IQ were: 1) site of obstruction; 2) number of shunt revisions; and 3) history of seizures. Verbal IQ was influenced negatively by antiepileptic therapy and motor deficits, and positively by an older age at time of shunting. Non-verbal, performance IQ was lower in patients with cerebral hemisphere malformations, those with more than one shunt, pre- and perinatal problems, and antiepileptic therapy. The side of shunt placement was significantly correlated with non-verbal IQ, insertion on the right ensuring a better outcome. Posterior fossa malformations were not correlated with IQ. (Riva D et al. Intelligence outcome in children with shunted hydrocephalus of different etiology. <u>Child's Nerv Syst</u> Jan 1994;<u>10</u>:70-73). (Respond: Dr Daria Riva, Dept of Child Neurology, Instituto Nazionale Neurologico "C Besta", Via Celoria, 11, I-20133 Milan, Italy).

COMMENT. Shunted hydrocephalic children have a preferential loss of non-verbal IQ. Verbal and Performance IQs are influenced by different factors. Verbal IQ is correlated mainly with antiepileptic therapy, while non-verbal IQ was dependent on several surgical and medical variables.

A study of long-term outcome of hydrocephalus at the Service de Neurochirurgie Pediatrique, Hopital Necker-Enfants Malades, Paris, France, showed that IQ was related more to etiology than to ventricular dilatation, and to time of treatment. IQs are higher in patients with meningomyeloceles than in those with brain parenchymal lesions, toxoplasmosis, hemorrhage, or meningitis. IQs were above 80 in 60% of those shunted before 2 months of age and in only 29% treated after 2 years. (Hirsch J-F. Consensus: long-term outcome in hydrocephalus. <u>Child's Nerv Syst</u> Jan 1994;<u>10</u>:64-69).

A unifying theory for the definition and classification of hydrocephalus is proposed by Raimondi AJ, University of Rome. (<u>Child's Nerv Syst</u> Jan 1994;<u>10</u>:2-12). Hydrocephalus is a pathological increase in intracranial CSF volume, either 1) intraparenchymal (cerebral edema), or 2) extraparenchymal (subarachnoid, cisternal, or intraventricular), and independent of hydrostatic or barometric pressure. Ventricular or subarachnoid dilatation occurs as a result of intermittent increases in extraparenchymal CSF volume. Hydrocephalus may be present in a child who does not yet have dilated ventricles but in whom both CSF volume and pressure are increased. Cerebral edema may cause the same volumetric changes as increases in intraventricular fluid volume, and the term internal hydrocephalus is of little significance. Editor. *Ped Neur Briefs* March 1994.

ACETAZOLAMIDE IN HYDROCEPHALUS MANAGEMENT

The efficacy of treatment with acetazolamide (100 mg/kg/day) without frusemide in arresting post-hemorrhagic ventricular dilatation was evaluated in 3 infants at the Hammersmith Hospital, London, UK. Treatment was begun at 21, 25, and 35 days of age. A decrease in ventricular size occurred after one week in all patients. Dilatation recurred when acetazolamide was withdrawn or reduced. Reintroduction of therapy was less effective and less well tolerated. Treatment was tailed off between 8 and 14 months of age. No patient has required shunting. In 2 additional infants, a severe and treatment-resistant acidosis required discontinuation of therapy after two days. Nephrocalcinosis was not a side-effect with monotherapy, whereas the combination of acetazolamide and frusemide is known to cause kidney damage. (Mercuri E, Dubowitz L et al. Acetazolamide without frusemide in the treatment of post-haemorrhagic hydrocephalus. <u>Acta Paediatr</u> Dec 1994;83:1319-21). (Respond: Dr L Dubowitz, Department of Paediatrics and Neonatal Medicine, Hammersmith Hospital, London W12 0NN, UK).

COMMENT. Huttenlocher first described the benefit of acetazolamide in 8 of 15 children with hydrocephalus due to various etiologies. Bergman, Shinnar, and colleagues recommended acetazolamide combined with frusemide. The report of nephrocalcinosis with the combined therapy in 1992 was cause for concern and a return to trials of monotherapy. Acetazolamide may reduce ventricular size and postpone or obviate the need for shunt insertion in neonates with hydrocephalus. The use of acetazolamide in hydrocephalus is discussed by Sarnat HB in <u>Progress in Pediatric Neurology II</u>, 1994, pp277-8.

The long-term prognosis for 42 children, born between 1963 and 1975, who underwent shunting for hydrocephalus, was reported from Oulu University Central Hospital, Finland. (Kokkonen J et al. <u>Child's Nerv Syst</u> 1994;10:384-387). Seven had died, 5 were in institutions for the mentally handicapped, one-half of the patients had neurological abnormalities or epilepsy, one-third were receiving vocational training, and one-quarter had no meaningful work. Shunts had been changed 103 times in 29 patients still alive. Encouragement and support for the families seemed essential in improving social development of patients in adolescence. Editor. *Ped Neur Briefs* Feb 1995.

MENINGOMYELOCELE AND EPILEPSY

The prevalence of seizures and epilepsy and the occurrence of other brain malformations or structural abnormalities were examined in 81 children with meningomyelocele followed at the multidisciplinary Children's Clinics for Rehabilitative Services, University of Arizona Health Sciences Center, Tucson, AZ. Seventeen (21%) had seizures during follow-up ranging from 1.3 to 16 years. Fourteen (17%) had epilepsy and 5 had seizures controlled by anticonvulsant drugs. CNS pathology in addition to the shunted hydrocephalus included encephalomalacia in 7, cerebral malformations in 2, and calcifications in 1. (Talwar D et al. Epilepsy in children with meningomyelocele. <u>Pediatr Neurol</u> July/August 1995;13:29-32). (Respond: Dr Talwar, Department of Pediatrics, University of Arizona Health Sciences Center, 1501 North Campbell Avenue, Tucson AZ 85724).

COMMENT. Although epilepsy in children with meningomyelocele occurs mainly in those with shunted hydrocephalus, structural cerebral abnormalities other than the shunt may be important causes. Editor. *Ped Neur Briefs* Aug 1995.

OTHER CNS MALFORMATIONS

SEPTO-OPTIC DYSPLASIA, CORPUS CALLOSUM AGENESIS, AND DIABETES INSIPIDUS

The clinical and endocrinological findings in 24 children with septo-optic dysplasia and/or agenesis of the corpus callosum are described with reference to posterior pituitary function in a report from the Institute of Child Health and The Hospital for Sick Children, London, UK. Congenital optic nerve hypoplasia, absent septum pellucidum, and pituitary deficiency, characteristic of the complete syndrome of septo-optic dysplasia, were present in 8 children, and 13 had incomplete forms. Five had agenesis of the corpus callosum. Growth hormone insufficiency was found in 20 (83%). Nine (38%) had diabetes insipidus, often complicated by hypernatremia. Management of fluid balance was difficult, even with vasopressin treatments, because of blindness, developmental delay, impairment of the sense of thirst, and dependence on the parents for food and water intake. (Masera N, Grant DB et al. Diabetes insipidus with impaired osmotic regulation in septo-optic dysplasia and agenesis of the corpus callosum. <u>Arch Dis Child</u> Jan 1994;<u>70</u>:51-53). (Respond: Dr DB Grant, The Hospital for Sick Children, Great Ormond Street, London WC1N 3JH, England).

COMMENT. The syndrome of septo-optic dysplasia appears to be a mild form of holoprosencephaly with single cerebral ventricle and agenesis of the corpus callosum, among other midline defects. Anterior pituitary deficiency is a frequent feature of the syndrome, whereas posterior pituitary disorders are less well documented. In the present study, diabetes insipidus is shown to be a relatively common complication. -Editor. *Ped Neur Briefs* March 1994.

CONGENITAL MIDLINE DEFECT IN PITUITARY DWARFS

MRI evaluations of pituitary volume, and clinical and endocrine findings in 101 pituitary dwarfs with congenital idiopathic growth hormone deficiency (CIGHD) are reported from the Departments of Neuroradiology and Pediatrics, Scientific Institute H San Raffaele, Milan, Italy. Ectopia of the posterior pituitary (PPE) was discovered in 59 patients and pituitary volume was reduced. Pituitary hormone deficiency, breech delivery, and other congenital brain anomalies occurred more frequently in PPE patients than in the 42 with normal posterior pituitary except for a narrowed stalk. Associated anomalies included septo-optic dysplasia, with septum pellucidum agenesis and/or hypoplastic optic chiasm, corpus callosum dysgenesis, and basilar impression. A congenital defect involving the pituitary and hypothalamus would account for the MRI abnormalities and the clinico-endocrinological features of CIGHD patients. Breech delivery is the result of the midline brain anomaly, rather than the cause. The hypothesis of a perinatal traumatic transection of the pituitary stalk is contradicted by the findings in this study. (Triulzi F et al. Evidence of a congenital midline brain anomaly in pituitary dwarfs: a magnetic resonance imaging study in 101 patients. <u>Pediatrics</u> March 1994;<u>93</u>:409-416). (Reprints: Dr Fabio Triulzi, Dept of Neuroradiology, Scientific Institute H S Raffaele, via Olgettina 60, 20132 Milano, Italy).

COMMENT. Major brain midline anomalies, including holoprosencephaly, corpus callosum dysgenesis, and septo-optic dysplasia may be associated with hypothalamo-hypophyseal deficiency. Pituitary gland hypoplasia and ectopia, demonstrated by MRI in this and other studies of CIGHD patients, is not correlated with breech delivery, but is related to an anatomical defect in hypothalamic-pituitary structures. -Editor. *Ped Neur Briefs* March 1994.

PRENATAL EVENTS AND CNS MIGRATION DISORDERS

The role of pre-, peri-, and postnatal environmental factors and genetic predisposition in the genesis of neuronal migration disorders (NMD) in 40 patients with epilepsy was determined by standardized questionnaires at the Montreal Neurological Institute and Hospital, Canada. Potentially harmful prenatal events (maternal trauma, medications, roentgenograms, infections) were reported in pregnancy histories of 58% of patients with NMD compared to 15% of 40 epileptic controls without NMD. In contrast, peri- and postnatal factors were present in only 22% of NMD patients compared to 50% of controls. Genetic factors (family history of epilepsy, mental retardation, or CNS malformation) occurred in 13 and 20% of families, respectively. Stillbirths occurred in 3% of NMD sibling pregnancies, but none in controls. Prenatal environmental factors are important in the cause of NMD. (Palmini A, Andermann E, Andermann F. Prenatal events and genetic factors in epileptic patients and neuronal migration disorders. <u>Epilepsia</u> Sept/Oct 1994;35:965-973). (Reprints: Dr E Andermann, Montreal Neurological Institute, 3801 University St, Montreal, Quebec H3A 2B4, Canada).

COMMENT. Maternal physical trauma in the first trimester was the most significant factor associated with neuronal migration disorders. Genetic factors are important in lissencephaly. Dr Harvey B Sarnat comments on advances in neuroblast migratory disorders in <u>Progress in Pediatric Neurology II</u>, PNB Publishers, 1994, pp279-280. Morphological and metabolic abnormalities of the ependyma, and congenital cytomegalovirus were documented as causes, as well as new experimental data on neuroblast migration mediated by radial glial cells. -Editor. *Ped Neur Briefs* Dec 1994.

PRENATAL CEREBRAL DYSGENESIS AND CEREBRAL PALSY

The MRIs of 70 cerebral palsy patients, aged 2 - 16 years, performed between 1989 and 1993 at Kansai Medical University Otokoyama Hospital, were analysed to evaluate the causative roles of pre-, peri-, and postnatal events. The CP was related to neuronal migration disorders in the embryonal stage in 26 patients. These included pachgyria and polygyria in 8, schizencephaly in 4, heterotopia in 4, agenesis of the corpus callosum in 4, cerebellar hypoplasia 3, and disorders of neuronal proliferation, differentiation and histiogenesis in 3. Vascular disorders were diagnosed in 30, intra-uterine infection in 5, and birth asphyxia in only 9. The authors conclude that CP of term infants is frequently the result of prenatal factors, either migration defects or cerebral infarction, and birth asphyxia is a relatively uncommon cause. (Sugimoto T et al. When do brain abnormalities in cerebral palsy occur? An MRI study. <u>Dev Med Child Neurol</u> April 1995;37:285-292). (Respond: Dr Tateo Sugimoto, Department of Paediatrics, Kansai Medical University Otokoyama Hospital, Izumi 19, Yawatashi, Kyoto 614, Japan).

COMMENT. The MRI may be used to identify causes of brain lesions underlying cerebral palsy, and birth asphyxia resulting from obstetrical factors is frequently excluded. In 31 of the 70 infants in this study the CP-related brain abnormalities were clearly developmental and prenatal in origin. In 10 of 30 with vascular lesions the damage had probably occurred in the prenatal period, and in 13 the time of damage was undetermined. The World Federation of Neurology cautions that the term birth asphyxia should be applied only to cases with definite evidence of an asphyxial origin for the neurological disability. Neonatal seizures are the most reliable evidence of intrapartum asphxia. The Apgar score is not the best indicator and most children with CP do not have low Apgar scores at birth. A possible causal relationship of perinatal asphyxia and CP should require the following: 1) severe newborn acidosis, 2) damage to other organs, and 3) severe neurologic abnormalities in the first 24-72 hours. (see Progress in Pediatric Neurology I, 1991, p333-6).-Editor. *Ped Neur Briefs* May 1995.

HIPPOCAMPAL CHANGES IN DOWN'S SYNDROME

Semiquantitative scales and quantitative computerized image analyses were used to determine the neurofibrillary tangle formation and AB amyloid deposition in the hippocampal formation and inferior temporal gyrus in 36 Down's syndrome cases, aged 4 to 73 years. Neuropathological material was collected from several sources in Great Britain and America, and results are reported from the Massachusetts General Hospital, Boston, and the University of Manchester, England. Neurofibrillary tangles (NFTs) accumulated in patients with Down's syndrome over the age range 35 to 75 years, in the same anatomic locale as individuals with sporadic Alzheimer's disease. The entorhinal cortex, area CA1/subiculum, and other hippocampal subfields were especially vulnerable. Amyloid deposition is more widespread, accumulating over the years 30 to 50, and then reaching a plateau. Inheritance of the apolipoprotein E (Apo E) e4 genotype predisposed to more than double the amount of amyloid burden and was associated with increased numbers of senile plaques in Down's syndrome individuals with Alzheimer's disease. (Hyman BT et al. Neuropathological changes in Down's syndrome hippocampal formation. Effect of age and apolipoprotein E genotype. Arch Neurol April 1995;52:373-378). (Reprints: Dr Bradley T Hyman, Neurology Service, Massachusetts General Hospital, Fruit Street, Boston, MA 02114).

COMMENT. In a study at Mount Sinai School of Medicine, NY, the University of Kentucky, and the University of Geneva, Switzerland, quantitative analyses of neuropathologic changes in cerebral cortex of 16 patients (aged 6 to 74 years) with Down's syndrome and in 10 elderly individuals with Alzheimer's disease showed a similar time course of neurofibrillary tangle formation. Older patients with Down's syndrome had more neurofibrillary tangles and senile plaques than patients with Alzheimer's disease. Amyloid deposition preceeded neurofibrillary tangle formation. (Hof PR et al. Age-related distribution of neuropathologic changes in the cerebral cortex of patients with Down's syndrome. Quantitative regional analysis and comparison with Alzheimer's disease. <u>Arch Neurol</u> April 1995;52:379-391). -Editor. *Ped Neur Briefs* May 1995.

LISSENCEPHALY TYPE III SYNDROME AND ARTHROGRYPOSIS MULTIPLEX CONGENITA

Arthrogryposis multiplex congenita (AMC), called fetal akinesia sequence (FAS) in this study of 5 lethal cases, was associated with a distinctive neuropathological pattern, named type III lissencephaly syndrome, as reported from the Hopital Henri Mondor, Creteil, and the Hopitals Port Royal and Saint Antoine, Paris, France. In this group of primary neurogenic FAS a diffuse neurodegenerative process affected the cerebrum and spinal cord, causing brain atrophy, hydrocephalus, microcephaly, and gyral reduction. Parental consanguinity was present in one case, and 2 cases occurred in sibs, suggesting a genetic, autosomal recessive, cause. Polyhydramnios, intrauterine growth retardation, severe arthrogryposis, and pulmonary hypoplasia was present in all 5 cases. The developmental abnormalities are thought to be secondary to fetal akinesia. (Razavi FE et al. Lethal familial fetal akinesia sequence (FAS) with distinct neuropathological pattern: Type III Lissencephaly syndrome. <u>Am J Med Genet</u> 1996;62:16-22). (Reprints: Ferechte Encha Razavi MD, Service Histo-Neuropathologie, Hopital Henri Mondor, 51 Bld de Ml de Lattre de Tassigny, Creteil, Cedex 94010, France).

COMMENT. In a prospective study of 89 infants with arthrogryposis multiplex congenita, Banker

(1986) found 84 neurogenic in type. The present authors emphasize the heterogeneous nature of the syndrome, with special attention to neurodegenerative familial cases. -Editor. *Ped Neur Briefs* May 1996.

BRAIN DEVELOPMENT MEASURED BY MRI

MRI data read as normal on 88 male and female patients aged 3 months to 30 years and on 73 healthy male volunteers aged 21 to 70 years were quantified and the volumes of cortical white matter, gray matter, and CSF were computed in a study at the Department of Veterans Affairs Medical Center, and the Department of Psychiatry and Behavioral Science, Stanford University School of Medicine, CA. *In the younger samples*, obtained from four California clinics, intracranial volume increased by about 300 ml from 3 months to 10 years. Head size of boys was larger than that of girls by about 70 mL, but both sexes followed the same growth trend. Cortical gray matter volume peaked at age 4 years and decreased thereafter; cortical white matter volume increased steadily until age 20 years: cortical and ventricular CSF volumes remained constant. *In the older sample*, cortical gray matter volume decreased curvilinearly by 0.7 mL/year, while white matter volume remained constant through 5 decades. Cortical CSF volume increased by 0.6 mL/y and ventricular volumes increased by 0.3 mL/y as cortical gray matter decreased. (Pfefferbaum A et al. A quantitative magnetic resonance imaging study of changes in brain morphology from infancy to late adulthood. <u>Arch Neurol</u> Sept 1994;51:874-887). (Reprints: Dr Pfefferbaum, Psychiatric Service (116A3), Palo Alto Department of Veterans Affairs Medical Center, 3801 Miranda Ave, Palo Alto, CA 94304).

COMMENT. Age-related changes in gray-white matter ratio suggest that growth in white matter exceeds that of gray during the first 5 years, continues to expand until age 20 years, whereas gray matter volume declines after age 5. Age 4 years marks the end of gray matter growth and the beginning of a consistent decline throughout the life span. A relation between head size and cortical gray matter is established early and persists into late adulthood. These quantitative studies of normal brain development, reflecting cell growth and death, myelination, and atrophy, provide important comparative data in the investigation of neurodegenerative processes. -Editor. *Ped Neur Briefs* Oct 1994.

NEURAL TUBE DEFECTS AND CHROMOSOME DELETIONS

Patients with neural tube defects (NTDs) complicated by congenital heart defects, facial anomalies, thymic hypoplasia, cleft lip or palate, or hypocalcemia and a family history of NTDs and other anomalies were tested for 22q11 deletions at the Departments of Pediatrics and Molecular Genetics, Oregon Health Sciences University, Eugene, Oregon. Of 295 patients identified with NTDs, 22 had at least one more clinical anomaly and/or a positive family history. Fetal alcohol and valproate syndromes were excluded. Cytogenetic analysis and molecular testing on 16 revealed 22q11 deletions in 3 and normal results in 13. Deletion of 22q11 was an infrequent cause of NTDs. (Nickel RE, Magenis RE. Neural tube defects and deletions of 22q11. <u>Am J Med Genet</u> Dec 1996;66:25-27). (Reprints: Dr Robert E Nickel, 901 East 18th Avenue, Eugene, OR 97403).

COMMENT. Cytogenetic testing for the 22q11 deletion is recommended in infants with neural tube defects complicated by congenital heart defects, particularly conotruncal defect, and in those with a family history of the heart defect, velo-cardio-facial syndrome, or DiGeorge sequence. -Editor. *Ped Neur Briefs* Dec 1996.

MENTAL RETARDATION SYNDROMES

SMITH-MAGENIS SYNDROME AND SELF-HUGGING BEHAVIOR

A self-hugging behavior is described in 11 patients with Smith-Magenis syndrome (SMS) examined at Elwyn, PA, and the Alfred I du Pont Institute, Wilmington, Delaware. Five were children ages 7 - 16, and 6 were adults of 19 - 51 years. All had chromosome deletion 17p11.2, characteristic of SMS, and were mentally retarded, with IQs of 40-50. The involuntary, tic-like movements consisted of crossing both arms across the chest and tensing the body or clasping the hands and squeezing the arms to the sides. The spasms lasted a few seconds and occurred in series or flurries, generally accompanied by facial grimacing and occasional grunting. They were expressions of happiness, affection or positive excitement and were most pronounced during transition periods, at the beginning or end of a class, in gym or during soccer. They were not observed in temper tantrums, at times of emotional upset, or during visits to the doctor's office. In contrast to the frequent negative, aggressive, and self-injurious behaviors characteristic of SMS, self-hugging was perceived as a favorable personality trait and a behavior of value as a diagnostic marker. (Finucane BM et al. The spasmodic upper-body squeeze: a characteristic behavior in Smith-Magenis syndrome. <u>Dev Med Child Neurol</u> Jan 1994;<u>36</u>:70-83). (Respond: BM Finucane, Elwyn Inc, Elwyn, PA 19063).

COMMENT. Smith-Magenis syndrome has specific physical as well as behavioral features. These include brachycephaly, midface hypoplasia, ear malformations, and brachydactyly. Mental retardation is usually moderate. Aggression and self-mutilation, head-banging and hand-biting, and sleep disorders are the most typical behaviors, causing management problems. Self-hugging is a more benign behavior and a welcome contrast to the self avulsion of fingernails, and insertion of foreign objects into bodily orifices (*polyembolokoilomania*), as sometimes described in patients with SMS and other mental retardation syndromes (<u>Ped Neur Briefs</u> Jan 1994;<u>8</u>:10). Self-hugging was considered distinct from the stereotypical hand movements of autism and Rett syndrome and a pathognomonic sign of Smith-Magenis syndrome. -Editor. *Ped Neur Briefs* Feb 1994.

RING 22 SYNDROME AND POLYEMBOLOKOILOMANIA

A 24 year-old severely retarded, hyperactive woman with a long history of foul smelling discharge from the nasal fossae, requiring removal under general anesthesia of foreign material (rocks, crayon, cotton, paper) on 9 separate occasions by an ENT surgeon, is reported from my own practice records in Chicago. The cumbersome term, *polyembolokoilomania,* has been applied to this behaviorism. The patient was referred from a residential home center where she was placed at 16 years because of violent and destructive behavior, eccentric habits, insomnia, refusal to eat, and self-injurious behavior, including body bruising and insertion of foreign bodies in her nose. She had occasional minor seizures. Her IQ was <20 on the Stanford-Binet. She did not speak but giggled frequently, often had a blank stare, and sometimes appeared catatonic. Her facial features were not dysmorphic. Attention to a visual object was poor. Hearing was intact. Her gait was uncoordinated, she was hypotonic and could not hop, but she had learned to swim. Deep tendon reflexes were hypoactive and plantar responses flexor. EEG showed a 8-9 Hz/sec basic rhythm, excess theta and low-voltage-fast activity, but no epileptiform discharges. CT scan was normal. Birth was normal, she walked late at 2 years, and never talked intelligibly. An older brother was normal; a paternal aunt was retarded. She had a febrile seizure at 2 years and minor partial seizures controlled with phenytoin up to 9 years. EEGs had shown bilateral independent spikes in temporoparietal areas. Chromosome examination revealed 46,XX, r(22), with ring 22 chromosome present in all cells. Fragile X was absent. Improvement followed behavioral modification and use of signs for communication. (Millichap JG. Ring 22 syndrome and self-injurious behavior. <u>Ped Neur Briefs</u> Feb 1994;<u>8</u>:10).

COMMENT. Syndrome-specific behavioral phenotypes receive increasing attention in the literature, and the proposal that certain stereotypic behaviors are pathognomonic of a distinct syndrome requires further examination. The above case report is presented to demonstrate that one form of self-injurious behavior, involving repeated insertion of foreign bodies in the nose or other bodily orifices, may be common to ring 22 syndrome and the 17p11.2 deletion syndrome of Smith-Magenis.

Ring 22 syndrome is characterized by severe mental retardation, often associated with muscular hypotonia, poor coordination, hyperactivity and aggressive behavior, and rarely seizures. Facial features are not consistently dysmorphic but may include epicanthal folds, bushy eye-brows and long lashes, broad nasal bridge, high-arched palate, clinodactyly and syndactyly, More than two thirds are female. The above case report emphasizes the indication for chromosomal analyses in girls with severe mental retardation and self- injurious behavior, despite the absence of facial dysmorphism.-Editor. *Ped Neur Briefs* Feb 1994.

RING CHROMOSOME 20 AND COMPLEX PARTIAL SEIZURES

A ring chromosome 20 mosaicism in an 11-year-old girl with complex partial seizures resistant to medication is reported from the Department of Paediatric Neurology, University Hospital of Turku, Finland. Early psychomotor development was normal, but speech was delayed. She attended special schools for dyslexia, writing difficulties, and a wide range of cognitive problems, which became progressively worse. She had no dysmorphic features. Her behavior was infantile and interrupted by uncontrolled bursts of laughter. Epilepsy began with absence attacks at 7 years of age. A prolonged partial status at 10 years was associated with fronto-temporal focal seizure activity and bilateral spikes on the EEG, compatible with partial, secondarily generalized epilepsy. MRI was normal. Control of absence attacks with valproate was incomplete, and trials of oxcarbazepine and clobazam for complex partial seizures were only partially effective. The karyotype was mosaic 46,XX/46,XX,r(20)(p13q13). (Holopainen I et al. Ring chromosome 20 mosaicism in a girl with complex partial seizures. <u>Dev Med Child Neurol</u> Jan 1994;<u>36</u>:70-83). (Respond: Irma Holopainen MD, PhD, Department of Paediatric Neurology, University Hospital of Turku, Kiinamyllynk, 1-3, SF-20500 Turku, Finland).

COMMENT. Chromosome analysis may be indicated in a child with drug refractory idiopathic epilepsy and learning disabilities, despite the absence of dysmorphic features or other congenital anomalies.

Ring chromosome 20 syndrome is characterized by progressive cognitive impairments, behavior disorders and epilepsy resistant to conventional medications.

Trials of newer antiepileptic medications with specificity against partial seizures (eg gabapentin) should provide more complete seizure control. (US Gabapentin Study Group No 5. Gabapentin as add-on therapy in refractory partial epilepsy: A double-blind, placebo-controlled, parallel-group study. <u>Neurology</u> Nov 1993; <u>43</u>:2292-2298). Unlike many antiepileptic agents, gabapentin does not affect serum concentrations of AEDs and may be used as concurrent therapy. It had no hematologic, hepatic, pancreatic, or hypersensitivity adverse effects in this 12-week study of 306 patients. -Editor. *Ped Neur Briefs* Feb 1994.

GOLDBERG-SHPRINTZEN SYNDROME AND CEREBRAL DYSGENESIS

A 5-year-old girl with Goldberg-Shprintzen syndrome and an abnormal CT scan suggesting neuronal migration defect or brain dysgenesis is reported from the Departments of Pediatrics, Asahikawa Habilitation Center, and Kitami Red Cross Hospital, Japan. Hirschsprung disease was diagnosed at age 4 days, and congenital heart disease with heart failure at 3 months. Clonic convulsions developed at 5 years. Motor development was severely delayed; she sat at 15 months and was unable to stand at 5 years. She had microcephaly, hypertelorism, broad nasal bridge, high-arched palate, thick eyebrows, and an IQ of 25. CT showed frontal and temporal lobe atrophy. The clinical findings in 8 additional patients are summarized from published reports. No chromosomal abnormalities were detected. (Tanaka H et al. Hirschprung disease, unusual face, mental retardation, epilepsy, and congenital heart disease: Goldberg-Shprintzen syndrome. <u>Pediatr Neurol</u> Nov/Dec 1993;<u>9</u>:479-81). (Respond: Dr Tanaka, Department of Pediatrics, Asahikawa Habilitation Center for Disabled Children, Shunkodai 2-1, Asahikawa 078, Japan).

COMMENT. *Waardenburg* (congenital deafness, white forelock and depigmented, joined eyebrows, heterochromia iridum, broad nasal bridge) and *Smith-Lemli-Opitz* (micrognathia, microcephaly, retardation, broad nose and anteverted nostrils, skeletal and urogenital abnormalities) *syndromes* have similar facial features to those of G-P syndrome and are sometimes complicated by Hirschprung disease. -Editor. *Ped Neur Briefs* Feb 1994.

WIEDEMANN SYNDROME

A boy, aged 2 years 5 months, with microcephaly, large anterior fontanelle, delayed psychomotor development, micropenis, and anomalies of thumbs and halluces is reported from the Department of Medical Genetics, Belfast City Hospital, Northern Ireland. From 9 months of age, he had generalized clonic convulsions, and at 18 months he developed minor seizures. An EEG at 13 months showed prominent delta activity and runs of low voltage fast, but no hypsarryhthmia or other seizure patterns. He was never able to sit and he had no speech. Muscle tone was increased, reflexes were hyperactive, and plantar responses extensor. Eye movements were roving. Fundi were normal. Head circumference was normal (50th centile) at birth and fell to below the 2nd centile within a year. Chromosome analysis showed a 46, XY karyotype. Renal ultrasound revealed an absent left kidney. CT of head at 22 months showed enlargement of all ventricles and cisterns and hypoplasia of the vermis. At 2 years 9 months he became comatose and he died at 3 years. Autopsy was refused. A maternal aunt had short broad thumbs, but no other congenital or genetic disorders were found in the family. Using the criteria microcephaly, short thumbs, micropenis, and mental retardation, the London Dysmorphology Database selected only Wiedemann's syndrome in diagnosis. Smith-Lemli-Opitz syndrome was also considered. (Nevin NC et al. Microcephaly with large anterior fontanelle, generalized convulsions, micropenis, and distinct anomalies of the hands and feet. Another example of Wiedemann syndrome? <u>Clin Genet</u> Aug 1994;46:205-208). (Respond: Professor NC Nevin, Department of Medical Genetics, Floor A, Lisburn Road, Belfast BT9 7AB, UK).

COMMENT. Wiedemann and associates (1985) described 2 males, first cousins, with similar characteristics, whose mothers and maternal grandfather had short broad thumbs and halluces. The present case, the second report of this syndrome, had normal parents. Autosomal or X-linked dominant inheritance was thought to be most consistent with the findings. -Editor. *Ped Neur Briefs* Oct 1994.

SILVER-RUSSELL SYNDROME AND COGNITIVE DISORDERS

Cognitive abilities of 20 boys and 5 girls, aged 6 to 11 years, with Silver-Russell syndrome were investigated at the Prince of Wales Hospital, Shatin, Hong Kong, the Institute of Child Health, and Middlesex Hospital, London, UK. The mean full scale IQ was 86, and 32% scored <70. Reading comprehension was 24 months below chronological age in 40%. Speech therapy was required in 48%. IQ scores were positively correlated with growth in head circumference. (Lai KYC et al. Cognitive abilities associated with the Silver-Russell syndrome. <u>Arch Dis Child</u> Dec 1994;71:490-496). (Respond: Professor D Skuse, Institute of Child Health, London, UK).

COMMENT. Features of Silver-Russell syndrome include low birth weight, short stature, body asymmetry, clinodactyly, and craniofacial dysmorphism - small triangular face, large forehead, small chin, shark's mouth, and low set ears. The present study adds cognitive disorders to the list of features. Intrauterine growth retardation of Silver-Russell syndrome beginning early in pregnancy results in reduction in both birth weight and length. In this "symmetrical" type of growth retardation, in utero brain development is more likely to be affected than when growth retardation begins late in pregnancy. -Editor. *Ped Neur Briefs* Jan 1995.

MICHELIN TIRE BABY SYNDROME VARIANT

A syndrome of multiple congenital anomalies, mental retardation, and symmetrical circumferential skin creases of arms and legs in a 4.5-year-old male is reported from the Montreal Children's Hospital, Quebec, Canada. Craniofacial anomalies included a high forehead, microphthalmia, optic nerve hypoplasia, telecanthus, and micrognathia. CT showed dilated lateral ventricles. Chromosomes were normal. (Elliott AM, Ludman M, Teebi AS. New syndrome?: MCA/MR syndrome with multiple circumferential skin creases. <u>Am J Med Genet</u> 1996;62:23-25). (Reprints: Dr AS Teebi, Division of Medical Genetics, Montreal Children's Hospital, 2300 Tupper Street, Montreal, Quebec, Canada H3H 1P3).

COMMENT. This mental retardation syndrome

resembles the "Michelin tire baby syndrome" but has some additional unique anomalies. -Editor. *Ped Neur Briefs* May 1996.

SMITH-LEMLI-OPITZ SYNDROME

Clinical features as specific indicators in the diagnosis of Smith-Lemli-Opitz syndrome (SLOS) and the reliability of ultraviolet spectrophotometry (UVS) as a biochemical screening test were examined by an Italian SLOS Collaborative Group of investigators. Of 20 patients with clinical suspicion of SLOS, referred to 11 Italian pediatric and clinical genetic centers in 1994, the diagnosis was confirmed biochemically by gas chromotography/mass spectrometry analysis (GC/MS) of serum sterols in 10, and serum sterols were normal in 10. Comparison of clinical signs in confirmed cases and biochemically negative patients did not reveal a specific group of manifestations of SLOS. UVS measurement of 7-dehydrocholesterol, which accumulates in the plasma in SLOS, correlated with GC/MS profiles. Serum bile acid concentrations were lower than normal in 4 of 5 patients with the syndrome. (Guzzetta V, Andria G et al. Clinical and biochemical screening for Smith-Lemli-Opitz syndrome. <u>Acta Paediatr</u> Aug 1996;85:937-942). (Respond: Dr G Andria, Department of Pediatrics, Federico II University, Via Pansini 5, 80131 Naples, Italy).

COMMENT. The "gestalt" impression formed by an experienced clinician examining the facial appearance of a child is perhaps the most practical and reliable method of diagnosis of Smith-Lemli-Opitz syndrome. Signs and symptoms of the syndrome are variable and non-specific and include mental retardation, failure to thrive, feeding difficulties, hypotonia, microcephaly, ptosis and epicanthal folds, anteverted nostrils, micrognathia, low set ears, syndactyly, simian creases, and hypospadias. Ultraviolet spectrophotometry determination of serum 7-DHC levels is 100% sensitive, relatively inexpensive, and specific for the biochemical diagnosis of SLOS. -Editor. *Ped Neur Briefs*

Sept 1996.

MYOCLONUS IN ANGELMAN SYNDROME

A clinical and electroencephalographic study of 11 unrelated patients with Angelman syndrome (AS), confirmed by genetic analysis, is reported from the University of Pisa, Italy. All patients showed the jerky, tremulous, or dystonic motor pattern typical of AS. Using long-term video-EEG and polygraphic monitoring, these abnormal movements were shown to be a form of fast-bursting cortical myoclonus. Antimyoclonic treatment with piracetam in 5 patients produced a marked functional improvement. (Guerrini R, De Lorey TM, Bonanni P, et al. Cortical myoclonus in Angelman syndrome. <u>Ann Neurol</u> July 1996;40:39-48). (Respond: Dr Guerrini, Institute of Child Neurology and Psychiatry, University of Pisa, Via dei Giacinti 2, 56018 Calambrone, Pisa, Italy).

COMMENT. The diagnostic features of Angelman syndrome include ataxia, developmental delay, paroxysmal laughter, microcephaly, and seizures. The "puppetlike" movement disorder is related to a cortical myoclonus. -Editor. *Ped Neur Briefs* Oct 1996.

PSYCHIATRIC DISORDERS IN MENTALLY RETARDED, EPILEPTIC CHILDREN

The prevalence and types of psychiatric disorders in 98 school-age children with mental retardation (MR) and active epilepsy were investigated in the Departments of Child and Adolescent Psychiatry and Pediatrics, University of Goteborg, Sweden. At least 1 psychiatric diagnosis was uncovered in 53 (59%) patients, and symptoms could not be classified because of profound MR in 30 (33%). Autistic disorder was diagnosed in 24 (27%), and autistic-like disorder in 10 (11%). ADHD was present in 11, and Angelman syndrome in 4. In those with autism the most common seizures were complex partial, absence, myoclonic, and tonic-clonic. A history of infantile spasms occurred in 12 (13%). Many of the psychiatric disorders had not previously been diagnosed despite parental concern. (Steffenburg S et al. Psychiatric disorders in children and adolescents with mental retardation and active epilepsy. <u>Arch Neurol</u> Sept 1996;53:904-912). (Respond: Dr Suzanne Steffenburg, Department of Child and Adolescent Psychiatry, University of Goteborg, Annedals Clinic, S-413 45 Goteborg, Sweden).

COMMENT. Autism or autistic-like disorder are common in children with mental retardation and epilepsy and are frequently undiagnosed. Neurologists and psychiatrists might work in closer collaboration for optimal management of these patients. -Editor. *Ped Neur Briefs* Sept 1996.

NEUROLOGICAL ASSESSMENT OF DEVELOPMENTAL DELAY

The etiologic or diagnostic yield of the neurologic examination in 60 children referred to a pediatric neurologist for evaluation of global developmental delay was determined at the Montreal Children's Hospital-McGill University, Quebec, Canada. Examination at a mean age of 3.58 years revealed mild delay in development in 25, moderate delay in in 23, and severe delay in 12. EEG, MRI, metabolic screens, fragile X test and karyotype established an etiologic diagnosis in 38 (63%), including cerebral dysgenesis (17%), HIE (10%), chromosomal anomalies (10%), toxins (8%), and metabolic disorders (5%). (Majnemer A, Shevell MI. Diagnostic yield of the neurologic assessment of the developmentally delayed child. <u>J Pediatr</u> August 1995;127:193-199). (Reprints: Annette Majnemer PhD, Montreal Children's Hospital, 2300 Tupper St, Room A-509, Montreal, Quebec H3H 1P3, Canada).

COMMENT. Optimal management of children with developmental delay should include a neurologic examination and selected laboratory tests. An etiologic diagnosis provides physician and family with important information regarding risks of recurrence and choice of therapeutic intervention. -Editor. *Ped*

Neur Briefs Sept 1995.

CHAPTER **8**

PRENATAL AND PERINATAL DISORDERS

INTRODUCTION
Israel Alfonso, M.D.
Miami Children's Hospital, Miami, FL.

The role of pediatric neurologists in the neonatal intensive care units has changed from one of a passive observer, ill equipped to predict the outcome in most neurologically affected neonates, to one of an active participant, able to contribute to the diagnosis and treatment of many disorders that affect the neonatal nervous system. This change in roles is due, in large part, to the dedication of pediatric neurologists who submit their experiences for publication, and the willingness of neuroscience editors to disseminate current research in the neurological literature.

Progress in Pediatric Neurology III presents abstracts of articles gathered from the world literature and provides editorial comments. The abstracts were published in the monthly journal review, **Pediatric Neurology Briefs**© (PNB), during the last three years. This series of well-selected and abstracted articles and commentaries summarizes the most significant advances in neonatal neurology during this period. The topics of the articles include neonatal seizures, hypoxic-ischemic encephalopathy, CNS infection, teratogenicity, and peripheral nerve lesions. The commentary after each article adds practical application with an emphasis on the three most common reasons a pediatric neurologist is consulted: 1) to help manage a specific problem, 2) to solve a mystery, and 3) to predict the future outcome.

Pediatric neurologists are often consulted to help manage neonatal seizures. Although the appropriate management of neonatal seizures continues to be an area of debate, several tentative conclusions have become apparent in the last three years: 1) most seizures, especially in neonates receiving antiepileptic drugs, are subclinical (PNB Oct 1995), making continuous EEG recording (PNB Oct 1995) or, at least, 60 min recording after the clinical seizure ends (PNB Jan 1996) a necessity in guaging success of AEDs; 2) neonatal seizures have a restricted electrical field that requires a full-neonatal montage for their detection (PNB Oct 1995); 3) a loading dose of phenobarbital 20 mg/kg does not cause significant cardiovascular changes (PNB Sept 1994); 4) focal pathology, with its potential for surgical intervention may be detected by SPECT in young patients with non-focal ictal EEG recording (PNB Dec 1994); 5) the presence of structural brain anomalies (enlarged ventricles etc) does not exclude the possibility of pyridoxine-responsive seizures (PNB June 1994; Dec 1996); 6) neonatal seizures do not raise the baseline prolactin level (PNB July 1995); 7) early AED withdrawal is recommended in most cases of neonatal seizures (PNB April 1995); and 8) neonates with hypomagnesemia and seizures should have a cardiac evaluation (PNB Sept 1994).

Besides neonatal seizures, other management

problems discussed in this chapter include a new type of congenital myasthenia successfully treated with pyridostigmine and predisone (PNB Jan 1994), the need to search for antepartum factors in neonates with encephalopathy (PNB Oct 1995), and the possible use of indomethacin to prevent grade IV hemorrhage in neonates (PNB April 1994).

Several abstracts address the issue of an unexplained clinical or radiological finding that can be solved by a pediatric neurology consultation. Increased motor activity and decreased visual and auditory attention occur in neonates exposed to cocaine during pregnancy (PNB July 1996). Microcephaly and dysmorphic features may be explained by fetal exposure to valproic acid (PNB May 1994) or toluene (PNB Feb 1994). Intracranial bleeding in neonates may be caused by maternal aspirin (PNB Jan 1994) or alcohol ingestion (PNB Jan 1995). Hyperexcitability may occur in neonates exposed to valproic acid during pregnancy, especially at high doses (PNB July 1996).

Pediatric neurologists are often consulted on clinical outcome of a disease process. This subject is also well represented in this Volume III of **Progress in Pediatric Neurology.** Neonates with enteroviral meningitis may later develop language problems (PNB July 1996). A progressive encephalopathy is likely to occur in HIV neonates affected with AIDS but not in those without AIDS (PNB Dec 1994, June 1995). Decreased head growth during the first four months of life following HIE carries a poor neurodevelopmental prognosis (PNB May 1994). Symmetrical parieto-occipital cysts on ultrasound are predictors of cerebral palsy in low birth weight infants (PNB June 1994). Infants born with middle cerebral artery stroke may be asymptomatic at birth and later develop hemiparesis (PNB April 1995). Moderate Erb's palsy is followed by significant functional incapacity in 28% of cases (PNB July 1996). Intranuclear rods in nemaline myopathy predict a poor prognosis (PNB Feb 1994). It is hoped that my brief synopsis of neonatal neurology topics will encourage readers to study the abstracts and commentaries in more detail.   *Israel Alfonso, M.D.*

MICROCEPHALY AFTER HYPOXIC-ISCHEMIC ENCEPHALOPATHY

The development of microcephaly after hypoxic-ischemic cerebral injury in the full-term newborn was studied at the University of British Columbia, Vancouver, Canada. Serial head circumference measurements obtained at 4, 8, and 18 months of age in 54 newborns suffering from acute, hypoxic-ischemic encephalopathy showed that a decrease in head circumference ratios of >3.1% between birth and 4 months of age was highly predictive of the development of microcephaly before 18 months. Head circumference ratios were actual head circumference/mean head circumference x 100%. They were correlated with severity of neonatal HIE and outcome at 18 months. (Cordes I et al. Early prediction of the development of microcephaly after hypoxic-ischemic encephalopathy in the full-term newborn. Pediatrics May 1994;93:703-707). (Reprints: Dr Alan Hill, Division of Neurology, British Columbia's Children's Hospital, 4480 Oak St, Vancouver, BC, Canada V6H 3V4).

COMMENT. A decreased rate of head growth in the first 4 months after acute, intrapartum HIE correlates with the later development of microcephaly and neurological sequelae in the full-term neonate as well as very low birth weight infants. -Editor. *Ped Neur Briefs* May 1994.

LIFE EXPECTANCY WITH CEREBRAL PALSY

The life expectancy of children with idiopathic cerebral palsy born during 1966-84 to mothers resident in Mersey region has been analysed at the Department of Public Health, University of Liverpool, UK. Among 1251 subjects traced, one third had quadriplegia, one third hemiplegia, a quarter had diplegia, and the remainder dyskinesia and ataxia. A quarter had severe ambulatory disability, a fifth severe manual disability, and a third an IQ of 50 or less; 11% had died. One third had a birth weight of 2500 g or less, and one third a gestational age of 37 weeks or less. Those with normal birth weight had the highest proportion of severe disabilities. About 85-90% of subjects with CP survived to 20 years compared to 97% 20 year survival in the general population in 1970-2. Subjects with mild functional disabilities (ambulation, manual dexterity, and IQ deficits) had 20 year survival of 99%, while those severely disabled had a 50% 20 year survival. Birth weight and gestational age were less predictive of survival than functional disability. (Hutton JL et al. Life expectancy in children with cerebral palsy. BMJ 13 August 1994;309:431-435). (Respond: Professor Peter OD Pharoah, Department of Public Health, University of Liverpool, Liverpool L69 3BX, UK).

COMMENT. One-half of severely disabled cerebral palsied children survived to age 20, and the life expectancy to 20 years of mild to moderately disabled children was not much lower than that of unaffected children. As more severely affected low birth weight infants survive with advances in neonatal care, future cohorts may show a higher proportion of severely disabled with CP and a life expectancy approaching that of the normal birth weight CP children. The social, educational, health service, and medico-legal aspects of these findings are noted. A much shorter life expectancy is reported in US studies. -Editor. *Ped Neur Briefs* Oct 1994.

PRENATAL CEREBRAL DYSGENESIS AND CEREBRAL PALSY

The MRIs of 70 cerebral palsy patients, aged 2 - 16 years, performed between 1989 and 1993 at Kansai Medical University Otokoyama Hospital, were analysed to evaluate the causative roles of pre-, peri-, and postnatal events. The CP was related to neuronal migration disorders in the embryonal stage in 26 patients. These included pachgyria and polygyria in 8, schizencephaly in 4, heterotopia in 4, agenesis of the corpus callosum in 4, cerebellar hypoplasia 3, and disorders of neuronal proliferation, differentiation and histiogenesis in 3. Vascular disorders were diagnosed in 30, intra-uterine infection in 5, and birth asphyxia in only 9. The authors conclude that CP of term infants is frequently the result of prenatal factors, either migration defects or cerebral infarction, and birth asphyxia is a relatively uncommon cause. (Sugimoto T et al. When do brain abnormalities in cerebral palsy occur? An MRI study. <u>Dev Med Child Neurol</u> April 1995;37:285-292). (Respond: Dr Tateo Sugimoto, Department of Paediatrics, Kansai Medical University Otokoyama Hospital, Izumi 19, Yawatashi, Kyoto 614, Japan).

COMMENT. The MRI may be used to identify causes of brain lesions underlying cerebral palsy, and birth asphyxia resulting from obstetrical factors is frequently excluded. In 31 of the 70 infants in this study the CP-related brain abnormalities were clearly developmental and prenatal in origin. In 10 of 30 with vascular lesions the damage had probably occurred in the prenatal period, and in 13 the time of damage was undetermined.

The World Federation of Neurology cautions that the term birth asphyxia should be applied only to cases with definite evidence of an asphyxial origin for the neurological disability. Neonatal seizures are the most reliable evidence of intrapartum asphxia. The Apgar score is not the best indicator and most children with CP do not have low Apgar scores at birth. A possible causal relationship of perinatal asphyxia and CP should require the following: 1) severe newborn acidosis, 2) damage to other organs, and 3) severe neurologic abnormalities in the first 24-72 hours. (see <u>Progress in Pediatric Neurology I</u>, 1991, p333-6). -Editor. *Ped Neur Briefs* May 1995.

ENCEPHALOPATHY: ANTEPARTUM CAUSES

Adverse factors in the family and maternal history, pregnancy, and birth related to the occurrence of neonatal encephalopathy (NE) in full term newborn infants were evaluated in a matched case-control study at the Institute for Child Health Research, West Perth, and the Department of Neonatology, Princess Margaret Hospital for Children, Subiacco, Western Australia. Of 89 cases studied, 42 met criteria for moderate or severe neonatal encephalopathy: *severe* NE -mechanical ventilation required for >24 hours, multiple anticonvulsants, coma, or death; *moderate* NE: -neurologic abnormalities or seizures requiring anticonvulsants, but resolving before discharge. The estimated incidence of NE in the first week of life was 3.75 per 1000 full term live births, and a case fatality of 8%. Intrapartum hypoxia was the cause of NE in only 5 cases, and antepartum factors were more significant and frequent. Maternal vaginal bleeding in pregnancy, physical trauma during pregnancy, maternal thyroxine treatment, and congenital abnormalities were significantly more frequent in NE patients than in controls. Maternal alcohol consumption, smoking during pregnancy, and gestational diabetes were not related to NE. (Adamson SJ et al. Predictors of neonatal encephalopathy in full term infants. BMJ 2 September 1995;311:598-602). (Respond: Professor Fiona Stanley, Institute for Child Health Research, PO Box 855, West Perth 6872, Western Australia, Australia).

COMMENT. Antepartum factors and preexisting neurologic abnormalities are important in the cause of neonatal encephalopathy occurring in full term infants. Intrapartum hypoxia is significant in only 6% of cases.

Problems with definitions and classifications of newborn encephalopathy are reviewed in Progress in Pediatric Neurology II, 1994, pp321-2. The clinical features of hypoxic-ischemic encephalopathy are not specific, and similar symptoms may be caused by metabolic disorders, infection or cerebral malformations. -Editor. *Ped Neur Briefs* Oct 1995.

INFANTILE MACROCRANIA AND SUBARACHNOID FLUID COLLECTIONS

Macrocrania caused by subarachnoid fluid

collections (SFC) in 12 very low birth weight (VLBW) infants is reported from the Department of Pediatrics, University of Manitoba, and the Newborn Follow-up Program, Health Sciences Centre, Winnipeg, Manitoba, Canada. Ultrasound had shown grade II and III intraventricular hemorrhages in 7 infants in the neonatal period. The prevalence of SFC in VLBW infant survivors attending this clinic was 2.6%. SFC accounted for 30% of cases of macrocrania in VLBW infants. The incidence of SFC was 3.3 per 1000 VLBW survivors annually. The occipitofrontal circumference was at 5 to 50th percentile at birth and >95th percentile at age of diagnosis (mean, 7.7 months). A frontal subarachnoid space 6 mm or more, an interhemisperic fissure 8mm or more, and normal ventricles on ultrasound were required for diagnosis of SFC. Head growth stabilized along a curve above and parallel to the 95th percentile by age 15 to 18 months. Transient neurodevelopmental abnormalities (hypertonia and hyperreflexia) found in 5 infants at 6 to 8 months had disappeared by 18 months, and all had normal findings at 25 month follow-up. No infant had cerebral palsy or retardation <70, and none required neurosurgery. (Al-Saedi SA et al. Subarachnoid fluid collections: a cause of macrocrania in preterm infants. <u>J Pediatr</u> February 1996;128:234-6). (Reprints: Oscar G Casiro MD, FRCPC, Director, Newborn Follow-up Program, Children's Hospital, 840 Sherbrook Street, Winnipeg, Manitoba R3A 1S1, Canada).

COMMENT. Various names used to describe benign SFC include "external hydrocephalus," and "benign subdural collection of infancy." If sonograms are normal except for SFC the infant may be followed with periodic head circumference measurements and clinical evaluation. An abnormal ultrasound may require follow-up with CT. The prognosis is usually favorable without intervention. Fukuyama Y et al have provided norms for age-specific CT measurements of subarachnoid spaces up to 1 year. (<u>Dev Med Neurol</u> 1979;21:425). The abnormal measurements by ultrasound used for diagnosis of SFC in the above study exceeded the Fukuyama upper limits of CT norms: >5.7mm sa spaces and >7.6 mm ih fissures.

Cerebral ventricular enlargement in female adolescents with anorexia nervosa corelated with the degree of malnutrition and returned to normal after refeeding and weight gain in an MRI quantitative study at the Schneider Children's Hospital, Albert Einstein College of Medicine, New Hyde Park, NY. (Golden NH et al. <u>J Pediatr</u> February 1996;128:296-301). Body mass and ventricular volume were inversely correlated. -Editor. *Ped Neur Briefs* March 1996.

INTRAVENTRICULAR HEMORRHAGE AND COGNITION

The effects of premature birth-related subependymal and mild intraventricular hemorrhage (S/IVH) on specific cognitive abilities in 2-year-old children were investigated at the Perinatology Center, New York Hospital, and Cornell and New York University Medical Colleges. Of 82 children included in the study, 27 had premature births complicated by Grade I or II hemorrhages, 28 prematurely born children had normal neonatal ultrasound, and 27 were born at term without complications. The premature group with S/IVH at birth performed significantly less well than children without hemorrhage on a measure of memory for location and on ability to change response set. Both groups of prematurely born children performed less well than full term children on systematic search for an object when the order of hiding was reversed. All groups performed equally on a visual attention task and on the global Bayley mental ability scores. (Ross G, Boatright S, Auld PAM, Nass R. Specific cognitive abilities in 2-year-old children with subependymal and mild intraventricular hemorrhage. <u>Brain Cogn</u> Oct 1996;32:1-13). (Reprints: Dr Gail Ross, Perinatology Center, New York Hospital, 525 East 68th Street, New York, NY 10021).

COMMENT. Prior testing of these prematures at age 10 months had shown that S/IVH affected global mental ability and habituation to visual patterns, and prematurity was associated with poorer memory for location. When reevaluated at 2 years, the premature groups with or without hemorrhage did not differ on the visual attention task, but prematures with S/IVH did poorly on the memory for location task and ability to change response set. Memory for location is a function of the caudate nucleus and thalamus and frontal cortex, areas affected by subependymal and intraventricular hemorrhage of prematurity. Fronto-striatal structural changes in the MRI have been demonstrated in patients with ADHD. (Denckla MB. In: Progress in Pediatric Neurology II, Chicago, PNB Publ, 1994:173-176). At a later age, the incidence of ADHD in the S/IVH affected children will be of interest.

Indomethacin prophylaxis against IVH in very low birth weight infants did not result in adverse cognitive or motor outcomes at 36 months, in a study at Yale University School of Medicine. (Ment LR et al. <u>Pediatrics</u> Oct 1996;98:714-718). The authors suggest that the early administration of intravenous low-dose indomethacin to neonates weighing 1250 g or less is beneficial and does not cause neurodevelopmental delay. However, Dr Henrietta Bada, University of Tennessee, Memphis, advises caution, and slow infusion, because of reported acute cerebral effects. (Commentary. Routine indomethacin prophylaxis: has the time come? <u>Pediatrics</u> Oct 1996;98:784-785). -Editor. *Ped Neur Briefs* Nov 1996.

EARLY DETECTION OF CEREBRAL PALSY

An Early Motor Pattern Profile (EMPP), consisting of 15 tests of muscle tone, reflexes; and movement, organized in a standardized format, was used to identify children with cerebral palsy (CP) in the first year of life at the University of Illinois at Chicago, College of Medicine at Peoria. The items evaluated included head lag, hip abduction, tonic neck reflex, fisting, scissoring, and toe-walking, and a three-point scoring system was applied to each item. In 1247 high-risk infants from a neonatal intensive care unit followed for 36 months, the EMPP identified children at risk for CP by 6 to 12 months of age. The optimal cutoff score of points at 6 months was 10, and at 12 months it was 4. The predictive value was approximately 90%. (Morgan AM, Aldag JC. Early identification of cerebral palsy using a profile of abnormal motor patterns. <u>Pediatrics</u> Oct 1996;98:692-697). (Reprints: Dr Andrew M Morgan, Department of Pediatrics, St Francis Medical Center, 530 NE Glen Oah Ave, Peoria, IL 61637).

COMMENT. The authors emphasize that the EMPP is not a method of diagnosis, but only a step toward more formal evaluation by a pediatric neurologist. False positive and negative results are always a problem with screening procedures of this type, and their sensitivity is dependent on the skill and expertise of the examiner.

Progressive deterioration of dyskinetic cerebral palsy in adult life is reported in the majority of 20 patients examined between 20 and 40 years of age at the Institute of Neurology, London. (Fletcher NA, Marsden CD. Dyskinetic cerebral palsy: a clinical and genetic study. <u>Dev Med Child Neurol</u> Oct 1996;38:873-880). Genetic heterogeneity with autosomal recessive and dominant variants was suggested by familial cases, casting doubt on the perinatal hypoxic-ischemic etiology of this form of CP. -Editor. *Ped Neur Briefs* Nov 1996.

NON-PROGRESSIVE ATAXIAS

A population-based study of 78 Swedish children with non-progressive ataxia is reported from the Department of Paediatrics, Malarsjukhuset, Eskilstuna; Department of Neuroradiology, Karolinska Institute, Stockholm; and Department of Paediatrics, University of Goteborg, Sweden. Criteria for inclusion were an ataxic gait, dyssynergia, dysmetria and intention tremor, resulting from prenatal (45%) or perinatal events (4%), and excluding patients with spasticity (51% were unclassifiable). The prevalence was 0.13 per thousand of 6- to 22-year-old children and adolescents. CT or MRI, available in 70 patients (90%), showed infratentorial pathology in 27%, including focal maldevelopments of the cerebellum: Dandy-Walker (2), Joubert syndrome (1), encephalocele (1), and hypoplasia (1). A genetic anomaly was found in 18 patients, including Angelman syndrome in 3. Forty-seven patients (60%) had mental retardation, severe in 25 and mild in 22; sixty nine (88%) had delayed speech development; 58% had visual dysfunction; and only 17 (22%) had normal cognitive function. (Esscher E et al. Non-progressive ataxia: origins, brain pathology and impairments in 78 Swedish children. <u>Dev Med Child Neurol</u> April 1996;38:285-296). (Respond: Dr Eva Esscher, Department of Paediatrics, Malarsjukhuset, Eskilstuna, S-633 88, Sweden).

COMMENT. Simple non-progressive ataxias comprise less than 10% of cases of cerebral palsy. Of 50% with known pathologies, the majority were prenatal in origin, many with a genetic background. No abnormality was revealed by imaging studies in 61%. -Editor. *Ped Neur Briefs* June 1996.

●●●●●●●●●●●●●

Additional articles pertaining to Prenatal and Perinatal Disorders are included in other chapters: neonatal seizures in Chap. 1, congenital neuromuscular disorders (*see* Chap. 6), congenital malformations (Chap. 7), and neonatal metabolic disorders (*see* Chap. 15). *Editor.*

CHAPTER 9

CNS NEOPLASMS

OVERVIEW OF RECENT ADVANCES

Cerebral tumors associated with neurofibromatosis-1 (NF-1) have been the subject of intensive study in the past three years, and neurologists at one center found that 4 per cent of their NF-1 clinic population had tumors located in the brainstem.

The single most important factor predictive of recurrence of craniopharyngioma is the extent of surgical resection, according to a retrospective analysis of patients. Surveillance MRI scanning in children with medulloblastoma has limited clinical value and carries risk of complications from sedation or anesthesia. Children with neuroblastoma and opsoclonus-myoclonus have an excellent surgical outcome.

Infantile spasms complicate brain tumors in two

studies, and signs of brain tumors in infants are analysed in one report. The diagnosis of intracranial tumor presenting in infancy may be difficult, and a high index of suspicion is advisable in patients with vomiting, unsteadiness, and enlarged head. A follow-up study of intracranial ependymomas reveals a poor prognosis; long-term survival is achieved only after complete resection followed by radiotherapy.

Complications of tumor therapy, especially cranial irradiation, include cognitive deficits, cerebellar atrophy, migraine episodes, meningioma, stroke, somnolence syndrome, seizures, and effects on puberty and growth. Language dominance does not usually transfer to the contralateral hemisphere in young children with low grade left hemisphere tumors.

Symptoms and signs of pseudotumor in children are described, and results of therapy with acetazolamide and furosemide are satisfactory, even when monitored clinically and without repeated spinal tap.

J. Gordon Millichap, M.D., Editor.

OPTIC PATHWAY TUMORS AND NF-1

The natural history of 33 optic pathway tumors (OPT) diagnosed in 227 children with neurofibromatosis type 1 (NF-1) seen in a specialty clinic was evaluated in a prospective, longitudinal study at Children's Memorial Hospital and Northwestern University Medical School, Chicago. OPTs were found in 19% of 176 who had CT or MRI at a median age of 4.2 years. No OPT developed on later follow-up in children who had not received an MRI. In those without ophthalmological complaints at diagnosis, the incidence of OPT was 15%. The median age of children with ophthalmologic complaints such as proptosis or glaucoma (1.9 years) was significantly lower than that of children without such complaints (5.3 years). Only 8 tumors were discovered because of visual complaints or precocious puberty; 25 (76%) children were asymptomatic at time of diagnosis, and 21 (64%) had normal eye findings. Six with chiasmal tumors had decreased visual acuity without proptosis. At follow-up of 0.2 - 8 years, only 3 (9%) showed progressive tumor growth on MRI or deteriorating vision after diagnosis. Symptomatic OPT were diagnosed before the age of 6 years. (Listernick R, Charrow J, Greenwald M, Mets M. Natural history of optic pathway tumors in children with neurofibromatosis type 1: A longitudinal study. <u>J Pediatr</u> July 1994;125:63-66). (Reprints: Robert Listernick MD, Div Gen Acad & Emergency Peds, Children's Memorial Hospital, 2300 Children's Plaza, Chicago, IL 60614).

COMMENT. The child with NF-1 is at greatest risk for symptomatic optic pathway tumor during the first 6 years of life. Tumor growth after 6 years is unusual. Progressive abnormalities and precocious puberty occurred only with chiasmatic tumors. Tumors confined to the optic nerve discovered by screening with MRI were not accompanied by decreased visual acuity or evidence of progression. The authors advocate serial ophthalmologic examinations in young children with neurofibromatosis type 1, but find that serial MRI is of limited value in asymptomatic patients. The frequency and indications for neurological and neurosurgical consultations in these patients would be of interest. -Editor. *Ped Neur Briefs* Aug 1994.

OPTIC PATHWAY TUMORS, PRECOCIOUS PUBERTY, AND NEUROFIBROMATOSIS 1

The prevalence of precocious puberty and its relationship to optic pathway tumors (OPTs) have been examined in 219 children with neurofibromatosis 1 (NF-1) seen between Jan 1985 and April 1993 at Children's Memorial Hospital, Chicago. Of seven (3%) with precocious puberty, all had OPTs which involved the optic chiasm and all had abnormal luteinizing hormone-releasing hormone (LH-RH) stimulation tests. They represented 39% of children with NF-1 and chiasmal tumors. Seventy-six percent of OPTs were detected by screening with neuroimaging rather than by clinical symptoms. Biochemical evidence of premature hypothalamic-pituitary-gonadal axis activation may be demonstrated by LH assay, without provocative testing, before overt signs of puberty appear. (Habiby R, Silverman B, Listernick R, Charrow J. Precocious puberty in children with neurofibromatosis 1. <u>J Pediatr</u> March 1995;126:364-7). (Reprints: Joel Charrow MD, Division of Genetics, Children's Memorial Hospital, 2300 Children's Plaza, Chicago, IL 60614).

COMMENT. Precocious puberty associated with neoplastic invasion of the hypothalamus has been reported with gliomas, hamartomas, infundibulomas, and supracellar cysts. Ford FR, in his classic textbook, Diseases of the Nervous System in Infancy, Childhood and Adolescence, 4th ed (Springfield Illinois, CC Thomas, 1960), refers to precocious puberty seen occasionally in cases of tuberous sclerosis and von Recklinghausen's disease. The association with optic pathway tumors and NF-1, emphasized in the present Chicago study, was noted in a 1979 article cited by the authors (Tertsch D et al. Pubertas praecox in neurofibromatosis of the optic chiasm. <u>Acta Neurochir (Wien)</u>;28(suppl):413). -Editor. *Ped Neur Briefs* April 1995.

BRAINSTEM TUMORS AND NEUROFIBROMATOSIS I

Seventeen children with neurofibromatosis type 1 (NF1) and MRI evidence of brainstem tumor are reported from the Children's Hospital of Philadelphia, PA. The mean age of diagnosis of NF1 was 55 months, and of brainstem tumor, 101 months. Headache was the most frequent complaint affecting 53%, motor incoordination (41%), cranial neuropathies (35%), dysarthria (29%), hemiparesis (12%), papilledema (12%), ataxia (12%), head tilt (12%), and seizures occurred in 6%. The primary tumor site was in the medulla in 82%, in contrast to the pontine location in non-NF1 patients with brainstem tumor. Shunt placement for hydrocephalus was required in 41%, more frequent than in non-NF1 patients. Only 18% had clinical signs of progression. At a median follow-up of 52 months, 15 of 17 were alive. (Molloy PT et al.

Brainstem tumors in patients with neurofibromatosis type 1: a distinct clinical entity. <u>Neurology</u> October 1995;45:1897-1902). (Reprints: Dr Patricia T Molloy, Division of Neurology, Children's Hospital of Philadelphia, 324 South 34th Street, Philadelphia, PA 19104).

COMMENT. Brainstem tumors in children with NF1 present with headache and cranial nerve palsies, they are often complicated by symptomatic hydrocephalus, are usually located in the medulla, and pathologically are benign or malignant astrocytomas, with variable outcome but usually prolonged survival. They can be distinguished from the typical NF-1 high-intensity foci on T2-weighted MRI (UBOs) by their mass effect and enhancement with gadolinium. Therapeutic intervention should be withheld pending evidence of progression, as determined by periodic neurologic examination and MRI. The authors estimated that 4% of their NF1 clinic population had a brainstem tumor. -Editor. *Ped Neur Briefs* Nov 1995.

CERVICOMEDULLARY TUMORS

The perioperative course and outcome of 17 children who underwent surgical resection of an intra-axial cervicomedullary tumor between 1980-1992 are reported from the Departments of Pediatrics and Neurology, University of Michigan Medical Center, Ann Arbor, MI, and New York University Medical Center, New York, NY. One group of 11 with no treatment before surgery was compared to 6 who had signs of progression following previous radiotherapy. Surgical resection was total in 2 and partial in 15. Low-grade glial tumors were found in 15 and anaplastic gangliogliomas in 2. Symptoms were present for a mean of 2.1 years before diagnosis. They were medullary in 11, including nausea, vomiting, head tilt, dysarthria, and dysphagia; and consistent with cervical cord involvement in 8. Four-year progression-free rates for newly diagnosed and radiation-relapsed patients were 70% and 41%, respectively. The prognosis was superior to that of typical pontine brainstem tumors not amenable to surgery. (Robertson PL, Allen JC et al. Cervicomedullary tumors in children: A distinct subset of brainstem gliomas. Neurology Oct 1994;44:1798-1803). (Reprints: Dr Patricia L Robertson, R 6060 Kresge II, Box 0570, University of Michigan Medical Center, Ann Arbor, MI 48109).

COMMENT. Cervicomedullary tumors are a distinct sub-group of brainstem tumors with a slowly progressive course and low-grade malignancy. They appear to be amenable to surgery, and a favorable prognosis is expected in two thirds. Patients who have relapsed following prior radiotherapy have a higher morbidity. Preliminary results of chemotherapy in recurrent intrinsic brainstem gliomas of childhood are encouraging.

Five children with brainstem gliomas (1 cervicomedullary type) were treated with tamoxifen (80 mg/m^2), a nonsteroidal, antiestrogen chemotherapy, at Children's Mercy Hospital, Kansas City, MO. Four have shown objective shrinkage as measured by MRI during treatment from 6 to 30 months. Side-effects were described as minimal. (Pons M et al. Ann Neurol Sept 1994;36:514 [abstr]). -Editor. *Ped Neur Briefs* Nov 1994.

CRANIOPHARYNGIOMA: RECURRENCE FACTORS

Factors predictive of recurrence and functional outcome were determined in a retrospective clinicopathological analysis of 56 patients (26 children and 30 adults) operated on for craniopharyngioma since 1981 at New York University Medical Center. Children underwent gross total resection (GTR) of tumor more frequently than adults (77% cf 27%). Tumors were almost all adamantinomatous in children, whereas in adults, two thirds were adamantinomatous and one third were squamous papillary. Brain invasion was most frequent with the adamantinomatous craniopharyngiomas; invasion had occurred in 46% of the children compared with 17% of adults. Subtotal resection was associated with a higher rate of recurrence compared with total resection. Brain invasion had no effect on recurrence rate in totally resected cases. Functional, visual, and endocrine outcomes were not sacrificed by total resection of tumor. (Weiner HL et al. Craniopharyngiomas: a clinicopathological analysis of factors predictive of recurrence and functional outcome. <u>Neurosurgery</u> December 1994;35:1001-1011). (Reprints: Howard L Weiner MD, Dept of Neurosurgery, New York University Medical Center, 550 First Ave, New York, NY 10016).

COMMENT. The single most important factor predictive of craniopharyngioma recurrence is the extent of surgical resection. Total compared to subtotal resection has a significantly lower recurrence rate without affecting functional outcome. Brain invasion does not predict higher recurrence provided the tumor is totally resected.

Estogen Receptor Gene Expression. Craniopharyngiomas are histologically benign neoplasms of the sellar region that frequently show local invasion of brain tissue. In a collaborative study at the University of Toronto, Canada, the Mayo Clinic, and the University of Virginia, Charlottesville, 23 surgically removed craniopharyngiomas uniformally expressed the estrogen receptor gene. A possible hormonal component to the genesis and progression of craniopharyngiomas and investigation of hormonal therapy are suggested. -Editor. *Ped Neur Briefs* Dec 1994.

MEDULLOBLASTOMA SURVEILLANCE SCAN

The value of surveillance scanning, compared to periodic history taking and physical examination, in detection of asymptomatic recurrent tumors was examined in 86 children with posterior fossa medulloblastoma followed regularly between 1980 and 1991 at the Children's Hospital of Philadelphia. Recurrences were diagnosed in 23 (27%); 4 were detected by scanning only and 19 were associated with symptoms that developed at a median of 4 months after the last scan. No patient survived after a recurrence. (Torres CF et al. Surveillance scanning of children with medulloblastoma. <u>N Engl J Med</u> March 31, 1994;<u>330</u>:892-5). (Reprints: Dr Beverly J Lange, Division of Oncology, Dept of Pediatrics, Children's Hospital of Philadelphia, University of Pennsylvania School of Medicine, Philadelphia, PA 19104).

COMMENT. The authors conclude that surveillance scanning in children with medulloblastoma has limited clinical value. General anesthesia was required for MRI in 10% of children under 4 years of age, and sedation was requested or required by most children under the age of 7 years. More frequent scanning has the disadvantages of morbidity from sedation or anesthesia and increased cost, and earlier detection of recurrence is unlikely to change the outcome. Regular clinical evaluation and scanning are recommended to determine response and change in status after therapy. After a maximal response is achieved, scanning should be based on clinical symptoms and signs. These investigators had reached these conclusions more than 18 months ago and had presented their findings in Oct 1992: Torres C et al. <u>Ann Neurol</u> Sept 1992;<u>32</u>:458(abstract). (see <u>Ped Neur Briefs</u> Dec 1992;<u>6</u>:94). -Editor. *Ped Neur Briefs* April 1994.

MOLECULAR GENETICS OF TURCOT'S SYNDROME WITH MEDULLOBLASTOMA

Genetic abnormalities in 13 of 14 families with concurrent primary brain tumors and multiple colorectal adenomas (Turcot's syndrome) are reported from the Johns Hopkins University School of Medicine and other centers. Germ-line adenomatous polyposis coli (APC) mutations were present in 10 families. The predominant brain tumor in the families with APC was medulloblastoma, present in 11 of 14 patients (79%). The relative risk of cerebellar medulloblastoma in patients with familial APC was 92 times that in the general population. In the group from birth to 29 years, the risk of brain tumor was increased by a factor of 23. The brain tumor presented after the diagnosis of polyposis in 4 patients and before polyposis was detected in 6. The brain tumor was the cause of death in 7 of the 8 patients who died. Patients with glioblastoma multiforme and colorectal tumors, identified in 4 families, including the original family studied by Turcot, had DNA replication errors characteristic of hereditary nonpolyposis colorectal cancer (HNPCC), or Lynch syndrome. Two families with HNPCC had germline mutations in nucleotide mismatch-repair genes. Patients with Turcot's syndrome can be classified by genetic tests for APC gene mutations and for mutant DNA mismatch-repair genes in peripheral blood lymphocytes, and by evaluating tumor DNA for errors of replication. (Hamilton SR et al. The molecular basis of Turcot's syndrome. <u>N Engl J Med</u> March 30, 1995;332:839-47). (Reprints: Dr Hamilton, Department of Pathology, Ross Bldg, Rm 632, Johns Hopkins University School of Medicine, 720 Rutland Ave, Baltimore, MD 21205).

COMMENT. These molecular genetic studies can distinguish the phenotypic characteristics of two types of Turcot's syndrome, those in whom brain tumor is associated with familial APC and those with HNPCC.

Medulloblastoma represents a pleiotropic manifestation of the germ-line APC mutation. Glioblastoma mutiforme, cafe-au-lait spots and colorectal carcinoma in childhood may be associated with HNPCC.

Glioblastoma in patients with colorectal cancer has a more favorable prognosis and longer survival than usual. Familial clustering occurs in families with APC, 40% of families having two members with brain tumors. Tumor DNA testing for the incidence of mutations in APC genes in sporadic cases of medulloblastoma would be of interest (Groden J. Colon-cancer genes and brain tumors. <u>N Engl J Med</u> March 30;332:884-5). -Editor. *Ped Neur Briefs* April 1995.

OPSOCLONUS WITH NEUROBLASTOMA
The neurologic and developmental outcomes in

10 children with opsoclonus-myoclonus ("dancing eyes syndrome") and neuroblastoma were reviewed by examination of records at Northwestern University Medical School and Children's Memorial Hospital, and the University of Illinois Hospital, Chicago. Ages ranged from 8 months to 30 months. Opsoclonus and ataxia had been present from 6 days to 1 year before diagnosis of neuroblastoma. All had localized disease and 50% had extraabdominal tumors. All are alive and without recurrence of tumor 8 months to 111 months after resection. All had opsoclonus-myoclonus or ataxia for at least 5 months after surgery, but eventually responded to ACTH therapy. Two were symptom-free 12 months after surgery, and 3 remitted after 36 months. Nine relapsed and had chronic deficits, including cognitive and motor delays, reading and language deficits, and behavioral abnormalities. Factors precipitating recurrences of opsoclonus-myoclonus or ataxia included discontinuance or reduction of ACTH, febrile illness, and immunizations. (Koh PS, Raffensperger JG et al. Long-term outcome in children with opsoclonus-myoclonus and ataxia and coincident neuroblastoma. <u>J Pediatr</u> Nov 1994;125:712-716). (Reprints: John G Raffensperger MD, Pediatric Surgery, Children's Memorial Hospital, 2300 Children's Plaza, Chicago, IL 60614).

COMMENT. All children with neuroblastoma and opsoclonus-myoclonus and ataxia had an excellent surgical outcome and their eye movement disorder eventually responded to ACTH. The majority have long-term learning and behavioral problems, requiring special remedial education and behavioral intervention. Immunizations should be delayed or withheld when possible to avoid relapse of opsoclonus and ataxia. -Editor. *Ped Neur Briefs* Dec 1994.

BRAIN TUMORS AND INFANTILE SPASMS

Two patients, aged 6 and 7 months, with brain tumors who presented with infantile spasms and hypsarrhythmia are reported from Sapporo and

Asahikawa Medical Universities, Japan. One had a hypothalamic hamartoma and the other a oligoastrocytoma with calcification in the right temporal lobe. ACTH controlled spasms and EEG seizure discharges. (Asanuma H et al. Brain tumors associated with infantile spasms. <u>Pediatr Neurol</u> May 1995;12:361-364). (Respond: Dr Asanuma, Department of Pediatrics, Sapporo Medical University, School of Medicine, S1 W16, Cho-ku, Sapporo, 060, Japan).

COMMENT. The authors cite 9 additional reports in the literature of brain tumors associated with infantile spasms. Focal brain lesions may underly the origin of infantile spasms.

Brain tumor was not listed as a cause of infantile spasms in an epidemiological study involving 57 patients treated in Sweden for the period 1987-1991. (Sidenvall R, Eeg-Olofsson O. <u>Epilepsia</u> July 1995;36:572-574). -Editor. *Ped Neur Briefs* July 1995.

PINEAL AND EPENDYMAL CYSTS AND INFANTILE SPASMS

A 3-month-old infant with infantile spasms and hypsarrhythmia associated with multiple pineal cysts and an ependymal cyst is reported from Marmara University Medical Center, Istanbul, Turkey. Despite total surgical resection of the cysts, spasms persisted. (Ozek E et al. Multiple pineal cysts associated with an ependymal cyst presenting with infantile spasms. <u>Child's Nerv Syst</u> April 1995;11:246-249). (Dr E Ozek, Department of Pediatrics, Marmara University Medical Center, Tophanelioglu cad No 13-15, TR-81190 Altunizade-Istanbul, Turkey).

COMMENT. The authors considered the cysts to be coincidental and not the cause of the infantile spasms. ACTH was administered post-operatively but the response was not noted. -Editor. *Ped Neur Briefs* July 1995.

SIGNS OF BRAIN TUMORS IN INFANTS

The presenting symptoms and signs of intracranial tumors diagnosed before the age of 2 years in 21 children treated at the University Hospital of Wales are reported from the Department of Child Health, Cardiff, UK. Nine of the tumors were supratentorial and 12 were infratentorial. The commonest tumor types were astrocytoma in 5, ependymoma 4, and medulloblastoma in 4. The interval between onset of symptoms and diagnosis ranged from less than 1 day to 7 months. Nine had symptoms for at least 3 months before diagnosis. CT or MRI and biopsies were performed in all cases. The commonest presenting symptoms were vomiting in 9, and unsteadiness in 8. The commonest presenting sign was enlarged head circumference in 16. Meningitis was suspected initially and a spinal tap was performed before neuroimaging in 5 of the cases with raised intracranial pressure. Only one had neck stiffness. One received antituberculous treatment before a diagnostic CT was prompted by a rapidly deteriorating state. Multiple diagnoses were considered other than tumor and the significance of the head enlargement was not recognized in cases diagnosed late. (Gordon GS, Wallace SJ, Neal JW. Intracranial tumours during the first two years of life: presenting features. <u>Arch Dis Child</u> 1995;73:345-347). (Respond: Dr Wallace, University Hospital of Wales, Heath Park, Cardiff CF4 4XW, Wales, UK).

COMMENT. The diagnosis of intracranial tumor presenting in infancy may be difficult. A high index of suspicion is advisable in infants presenting with vomiting, unsteadiness, and enlarged head circumference. CT or MRI should precede consideration of spinal tap in infants with the above presenting features, especially if the diagnosis of meningitis is clinically indefinite. Not only is a spinal tap hazardous in the presence of raised intracranial pressure but a CSF pleocytosis and elevated protein, frequently found with tumors, may be misleading and lead to incorrect treatment and delay. Seizures are an uncommon presenting symptom in this age group of brain tumor patients whereas in children of all ages, seizures occur in 17% of cases, especially with supratentorial tumors. (Backus RE, Millichap JG. <u>Pediatrics</u> June 1962;29:978-984). See <u>Progress in Pediatric Neurology II</u>, 1994, pp344-5. -Editor. *Ped Neur Briefs.* Dec 1995.

INTRACRANIAL EPENDYMOMA FOLLOW-UP STUDY

The management and outcome of 24 children with intracranial ependymomas (22 benign and well differentiated) treated over a 10-year period, 1979-1988, and with a minimum 5-year follow-up were analysed at Great Ormond Street Hospital, London, UK. Of 16 with infratentorial ependymomas, 4 were alive, all 4 having total resection and 3 having craniospinal radiotherapy in addition. Of 12 who died, 5 had total resections and 4 had radiotherapy. All 7 with incomplete resections had died within 5 years despite radiotherapy and chemotherapy as well in some. Ventriculo-peritoneal shunting for hydrocephalus was required in 8 of 17 patients with posterior fossa ependymomas. In the supratentorial group of 7 patients, only one was alive and tumor-free at 5 years. No metastases were detected by myelography in 9 patients examined. (Jayawickreme DP, Hayward RD, Harkness WFJ. Intracranial ependymomas in childhood: a report of 24 cases followed for 5 years. <u>Child's Nerv Syst</u> July 1995;11:409-413). (Respond: Mr RD Hayward, Department of Neurosurgery, Great Ormond Street Hospital, Great Ormond Street, London WC1 3JH, UK).

COMMENT. In posterior fossa ependymomas an apparent total resection is associated with a better outcome but may be followed by local recurrence. Partial resection carries a very poor outcome, even with radiotherapy. Supratentorial ependymomas have a worse prognosis than the infratentorial group. In general, intracranial ependymomas in childhood have a very poor prognosis. Long-term survival may be achieved only after complete resection followed by radiotherapy, with its known effects on intellectual function and school achievement. Spinal metastases are unusual and prophylactic spinal irradiation in benign ependymoma is not recommended. Multicenter studies including chemotherapy are indicated. -Editor. *Ped Neur Briefs* Sept 1995.

INTRACRANIAL EPENDYMOMAS: GRADING, LOCALIZATION, AND PROGNOSIS

Grading and localization of 67 intracranial ependymomas operated on in children less than 15 years of age from 1951 to 1990 were correlated with prognosis in a retrospective study at the University of Koln, Germany. Grade II ependymomas (38) were located in the IV ventricle and supratentorial midline, making complete removal impossible. The majority of grade III anaplastic, malignant tumors (28) were in the cerebral hemispheres and were totally removed. Operative mortality was higher in grade II than grade III. Median progression-free survival time was 120 months for grade II and 18 months for grade III ependymomas. (Ernestus R-I, Schroder R, Stutzer H, Klug N. Prognostic relevance of localization and grading in intracranial ependymomas of childhood. Child's Nerv Syst Sept 1996;12:522-526). (Respond: Dr Ralf-Ingo Ernestus, N Klug Klinik fur Neurochirurgie der Universitat zu Koln, Joseph-Stelzmann-Strasse 9, D-50924 Koln, Germany).

COMMENT. As might be expected, the progression-free survival time is longer for the grade II ependymomas than the anaplastic grade III tumors, despite incomplete operative removal of the less malignant type.

Prognosis of cerebral oligodendrogliomas is studied in 15 children operated on at the Hopital Pierre Wertheimer, Lyon, France. Two groups were recognized: 1). Seven presenting with epilepsy had benign tumors and all survived at 72-month follow-up; 2). Eight presenting with intracranial hypertension had malignant anaplastic tumors, and 6 died within 17 months despite postoperative radiotherapy and chemotherapy. Clinical presentation and histology were correlated with survival time. (Rizk T, Mottolese C, Bouffet E et al. Cerebral oligodendrogliomas in children: an analysis of 15 cases. Child's Nerv Syst Sept 1996;12:527-529). -Editor. *Ped Neur Briefs* Nov 1996.

PRIMITIVE NEUROECTODERMAL TUMOR PROGNOSIS

Biological factors of prognostic significance in primitive neuroectodermal tumors (PNETs) were evaluated in tumor specimens of 86 children examined at the Children's Hospital of Philadelphia and University of Pennsylvania. Immunochemical evidence of glial differentiation (glial fibrillary acidic protein, GFAP) or neuronal differentiation (neurofilament proteins, NFPs) was associated with a 6.7-fold greater risk of relapse than tumors that did not express GFAP or NFPs. These biological characteristics of PNETs were as significant as tumor location and metastatic stage in predicting rate of relapse. (Janss AJ et al. Glial differentiation predicts poor clinical outcome in primitive neuroectodermal brain tumors. Ann Neurol April 1996;39:481-489). (Respond: Dr Janss, Division of Neurology, Children's Hospital of Philadelphia, 3400 Civic Center Blvd, Philadelphia, PA 19104).

COMMENT. The authors suggest that children with PNETs, especially cerebellar medulloblastoma, that express large amounts of glial fibrillary acidic protein (GFAP) are at increased risk for relapse and should be treated aggressively. Tumors should be classified as low or high risk based on both clinical factors, tumor location and metastatic stage, and biological factors, including GFAP expression.

The Mayo Clinical Update (12;1:1996) notes that malignant brain tumors in children are increasing in incidence at a rate of 1.4% per year. For medulloblastoma, after radical resection followed by cisplatin and craniospinal irradiation, 5-year survival rate is 75%. A protocol involving gene therapy is about to be opened for the treatment of recurrences of some malignant tumors. The tumor is injected with cells that secrete a retroviral vector containing thymidine kinase gene isolated from herpes simplex virus. This therapy should result in killing of tumor cells with sparing of normal brain. New therapies are needed for PNETs since no effective treatment for children with recurrent medulloblastoma has been identified. Intensive therapies presently employed result in complications, including second malignancies, endocrine and growth dysfunction, and cognitive impairments. Basal-cell carcinoma, discussed below, is an example of a secondary malignancy induced by spinal irradiation for medulloblastoma. Low risk tumors, identified by the biological method, may be spared unnecessary aggressive and disabling therapy. -Editor. *Ped Neur Briefs* May 1996.

NEVOID BASAL-CELL CARCINOMA (GORLIN) SYNDROME

A unique case of a 15-year-old girl with nevoid basal-cell carcinoma (NBCCS), who presented with uncontrolled temporal lobe epilepsy due to neuronal heterotopia, is reported from the Royal Melbourne Hospital, Australia. Seizures began at age 13 months, often precipitated by fever. She had a dermoid cyst removed from her nose, multiple dental cysts, and seborrheic keratosis of the scalp. Growth increased dramatically at age 9 years, and seizures became refractory to treatment. Chest X-ray showed cervical spina bifida occulta and fused ribs. Head CT showed calcification of falx cerebri and tentorium. MRI showed a lesion in the left anterior temporal lobe. EEG recorded seizure activity in the left frontotemporal areas. Temporal lobectomy specimen showed neuronal heterotopias and cortical dysplasia. After surgery, she was seizure free at 6 months follow-up. (Hogan RE et al. Epilepsy in the nevoid basal-cell carcinoma syndrome (Gorlin syndrome): Report of a case due to a focal neuronal heterotopia. <u>Neurology</u> Feb 1996;46:574-576).

(Reprints: Dr R Edward Hogan, Department of Neurology, St Louis University, 3635 Vista Ave at Grand Blvd, PO Box 15250, St Louis, MO 63110).

COMMENT. Nevoid basal-cell carcinoma syndrome presents at puberty with multiple basal-cell carcinomata, palmar and plantar pits, odontogenic painful cysts of the mandible, facial paresthesia, macrocephaly, large stature, frontal bossing, broad nasal bridge, narrow shoulders, fused ribs, polydactyly, bone cysts, calcified falx, cervical spina bifida occulta, odontoid agenesis, corpus callosum agenesis, meningioma, and medulloblastoma. Medulloblastoma, occurring in 3-5% of cases, may precede the development of other manifestations of the syndrome, and may have a better prognosis than general. Patients with seizures should be investigated for neuronal heterotopias, which may be treated surgically. The syndrome is autosomal dominant and the gene is localized to chromosome 9q22. -Editor. *Ped Neur Briefs* May 1996.

INTRACRANIAL GERM-CELL TUMORS

Prognosis of 26 children with intracranial germ-cell tumors (17 germinomas and 9 teratomas) treated in a 10 year period is reported from the University Hospital Hamburg-Eppendorf, Germany. Median age at diagnosis was 11.5 years (range 1.5-16.8 years). Tumor location was in the pineal region in 69% and suprasellar/hypothalamic in 31%. Symptoms were increased intracranial pressure, Parinaud's syndrome, and endocrine deficits. Surgical resection was attempted in 22 patients, 25 were irradiated, and 8 received additional chemotherapy. Long-term survival rate was 88% for germinomas and 43% for malignant teratomas; 57% had no and 37% had mild neurologic deficits, and 24% had neuro-endocrine dysfunction. Neuropsychological function was normal or only mildly impaired in 53%, and 69% had no change in their level of education. (Haupt C et al. Intracranial germ-cell tumours - treatment results and residuals.

<u>Eur J Pediatr</u> March 1996;155:230-236). (Respond: Dr C Haupt, Departments of Paediatrics and Neurosurgery, University Hospital Hamburg-Eppendorf, D-20251 Hamburg, Germany).

COMMENT. In this center, primary intracranial germ-cell tumors (PGCT) accounted for 8.5% of childhood brain tumors, while other series report a frequency of less than 5%. Germinomas arising in the pineal or suprasellar region are the most common form (65%) of PGCT and have a good prognosis, with 88% long-term survival after surgical removal and radiation. Severe residual complications, including cognitive deficits, are uncommon, despite post-operative craniospinal axis irradiation. Malignant teratomas have a less favorable prognosis. The younger age at which medulloblastomas are treated with irradiation accounts for the higher incidence of cognitive deficits in these tumor patients. -Editor. *Ped Neur Briefs* May 1996.

CEREBELLAR GANGLIOGLIOMA AND INFANTILE HEMIFACIAL SEIZURES

A female infant with cerebellar ganglioglioma who developed hemifacial seizures from the first day of life is reported from the Miami Children's Hospital, FL. When investigated at 6 months of age there were daily episodes of left hemifacial contraction, resistant to medication, head and eye deviation to the right, nystagmoid jerks to the right, autonomic dysfunction, while consciousness was retained. MRI at 2 months showed a mass in the left cerebellar hemisphere. The scalp EEG recordings were normal, while interictal and ictal intracranial EEGs revealed focal spikes, confirming seizures arising in the region of the left cerebellar mass. Partial resection of a ganglioglioma at 3 months was accompanied by remission of seizures. Six previous reports of infants with hemifacial spasms and cerebellar mass lesions are cited in the literature and reviewed, 3 having gangliogliomas. (Harvey AS, Jayakar P, Duchowny M, Resnick T, Renfroe JB et al.

Hemifacial seizures and cerebellar ganglioglioma: an epilepsy syndrome of infancy with seizures of cerebellar origin. <u>Ann Neurol</u> July 1996;40:91-98). (Respond: Dr Jayakar, Neuroscience Center, Miami Children's Hospital, 3100 SW 62nd Ave, Miami, FL 33155).

COMMENT. The authors describe a syndrome of infantile focal facial seizures associated with cerebellar ganglioglioma. Seizures associated with cerebellar tumors in infants and children have been described previously. The term "ictus infratentorialis" was coined by Penfield and Jasper for attacks of opisthotonus, syncope, vertigo, and focal clonic movements occurring in patients with infratentorial tumors. In a study at the Mayo Clinic of 291 children with intracranial tumors, seizures occurred in 17% of the total group, in 25% of those with supratentorial and in 12% of infratentorial tumors. None had gangliogliomas. (Backus RE, Millichap JG. The seizure as a manifestation of intracranial tumor in childhood. <u>Pediatrics</u> June 1962;29:978-984). -Editor. *Ped Neur Briefs* Aug 1996.

COMPLICATIONS OF TUMOR THERAPY

CEREBELLAR ATROPHY AND COGNITIVE DEFICITS IN LEUKEMIA SURVIVORS

MRI changes in the cerebellum and cognitive function of 13 survivors of childhood acute lymphoblastic leukemia (ALL) treated with cranial radiation of 24 Gy and intrathecal methotrexate were studied at the University of New Mexico, Albuquerque, Manitoba Cancer Foundation, Winnipeg, and University of Alberta, Edmonton. Age at diagnosis was a mean of 3 yrs 3 mos (range, 2 yrs - 4 yrs 10 mos), and age at testing was 11 yrs 8 mos (9 - 14 yrs). Hypoplasia of the cerebellar vermis and cognitive deficits involving visual-spatial-motor coordination and memory were observed in patients compared to controls. (Ciesielski KT et al. Hypoplasia of the cerebellar vermis and cognitive deficits in survivors of childhood leukemia.

<u>Arch Neurol</u> Oct 1994;51:985-993). (Reprints: Dr Ciesielski, Department of Psychology, University of New Mexico, Logan Hall, Albuquerque, NM 87131).

COMMENT. The neurotoxic effects of prophylactic cranial irradiation in children with acute lymphoblastic leukemia are well documented. As in this study, deficits in visual-motor skills and right brain involvement have been more pronounced than language and verbal deficits - evidence of left brain sparing. A causal relationship between the structural cerebellar abnormalities and the neuropsychological dysfunction is unproven. Children treated before 5 years of age are more susceptible to post-irradiation cognitive deficits than those diagnosed at or later than 5 years. Children in families of higher educational status who receive more attention and academic stimulation have a lower incidence of cognitive deficit than those with sensory-motor learning deprivation.

The dose of cranial irradiation, 2400 rads, used in this study is highly toxic in young patients. In the 1980s, most leukemia protocols limited the prophylactic dose to 1800 rads for use only in high risk patients. Reliance on intrathecal methotrexate chemotherapy for the majority of ALL patients is not known to result in significant intellectual or coordination deficits. (Personal communication: Dr David O. Walterhouse, Oncology Service, Children's Memorial Hospital, Chicago). -Editor. *Ped Neur Briefs* Nov 1994.

COGNITIVE EFFECTS OF CRANIAL IRRADIATION

The effects of cranial irradiation on neuropsychological test performance, 9 months after diagnosis of acute lymphoblastic leukemia (ALL), were evaluated in 74 children aged 3 to 6 years included in the Children's Cancer Group cooperative treatment trials. Children who received cranial irradiation (18 Gy divided in 10 fractions) plus intrathecal methotrexate had significantly lower scores on the McCarthy Motor Scale and the Token Test of receptive language and auditory comprehension, when compared to children receiving intrathecal methotrexate alone. Performance of tests of general cognition, visual motor integration, and receptive language requiring verbal recognition and visual recognition (Peabody Picture Vocabulary Test-R) showed no differences among the treatment groups. (MacLean WE Jr et al, for the Children's Cancer Group. Neuropsychological effects of cranial irradiation in young children with acute lymphoblastic leukemia 9 months after diagnosis. <u>Arch Neurol</u> February 1995;52:156-160). (Reprints: Dr D Hammond, Children's Cancer Group, PO Box 60012, Arcadia, CA 91066).

COMMENT. In the past nine months, issues of *Ped Neur Briefs* have included two previous reports of the adverse effects of cranial irradiation in children treated for acute lymphoblastic leukemia. In a study from the Institute of Child Health, University of London, children who received a second course of cranial radiotherapy for relapsing lymphoblastic leukemia suffered from neurologic deficits, growth impairment, ventricular enlargement on MRI, and impairments of tests of verbal comprehension, attention, and memory. Girls were affected more than boys. (<u>Ped Neur Briefs</u> June 1994;8:47).

Hypoplasia of the cerebellar vermis and cognitive deficits involving visual-spatial-motor coordination and memory were reported at 9 year follow-up in 13 children who received 24 Gy cranial radiation and intrathecal methotrexate at the University of New Mexico and centers in Canada. (<u>Ped Neur Briefs</u> Nov 1994;8:82).

The late morbidity associated with cranial radiotherapy has been recognized for some time. The Children's Cancer Group study demonstrates that cognitive deficits may become evident as early as 9 months after treatment, even with more moderate levels of irradiation. Whole-brain radiotherapy for brain tumors may also result in significant IQ deficits in children treated before age 7. (<u>Progress in Pediatric Neurology II</u>, 1994, p199). -Editor. *Ped Neur Briefs* Feb

1995.

RADIOTHERAPY FOR LOW-GRADE ASTROCYTOMAS

The effect of radiotherapy on the survival of 143 children with low-grade (grade 1 or 2) astrocytomas was evaluated at the Royal Manchester Children's Hospital, and Christie Hospital and Holt Radium Institute, Manchester, UK. The 5-year survival was 85%, 10-year 79%. and 15-year 72%. Children over 3 years of age had a better prognosis than younger children. Peripherally located tumors, with their easier access and more complete resection, have a significantly better survival outcome than deep-seated tumors. In 68 children whose tumors were completely resected and who required no radiation, the 15-year survival rate was 90%; if radiotherapy was given for some reason the 15-year survival fell to 75% for this peripheral tumor group. All 9 children with deep-seated tumors died when treated with surgery alone; a 15-year survival rate of 64% was obtained in patients who received radiation after surgery for deep tumors. (West CGH et al. Radiotherapy in the treatment of low-grade astrocytomas. I. A survival analysis. <u>Child's Nerv Syst</u> August 1995;11:438-442). (Respond: Mr Charles GH West, Department of Neurological Surgery, Royal Manchester Children's Hospital, Manchester M27 1HA, UK).

COMMENT. Radiation therapy had no benefit and in some cases, an adverse effect in children with superficial tumors that were amenable to complete or near complete resection. In deep seated tumors incompletely resected, radiation after surgery resulted in a significant improvement in survival rates. While radiotherapy may improve the survival rate in children with deep tumors, it can adversely affect the quality of life by causing long-term cognitive dysfunction. -Editor. *Ped Neur Briefs* Sept 1995.

COGNITIVE SEQUELAE OF RADIOTHERAPY

Long-term neurological and neuropsychological outcome in 25 irradiated children <15-years of age and 25 treated with surgery alone for low-grade astrocytoma was evaluated by two neurosurgeons and two psychologists independently at the Royal Manchester Children's Hospital, UK. Neurological function was not different in the irradiated group compared to the non-irradiated patients. In all neuropsychological tests used to assess intelligence, word reading, memory, learning and information processing, the performance of children with cranial radiation therapy was worse than those treated by surgery alone, and significant changes occurred in tests of IQ and information processing. Special education was required more frequently in the irradiated group. Both supratentorial tumor radiotherapy and local field irradiation to the posterior fossa for cerebellar tumors produced significant cognitive impairments. (Chadderton RD et al. Radiotherapy in the treatment of low-grade astrocytomas. II. The physical and cognitive sequelae. Child's Nerv Syst August 1995;11:443-448). (Respond: Mr CGH West, Department of Neurological Surgery, Royal Manchester Children's Hospital, Manchester M27 1HA, UK).

COMMENT. This study confirms previous reports of cognitive impairments following irradiation for supratentorial tumors in children. Additionally, even local field irradiation to the posterior fossa can result in learning and academic problems. Children receiving cranial radiation therapy, locally or to the whole brain, should be followed with neuropsychological testing for longer than 3 years to determine effects on IQ and the need for special education. -Editor. *Ped Neur Briefs* Sept 1995.

MIGRAINE EPISODES FOLLOWING CRANIAL IRRADIATION

Complicated migraine-like episodes occurring 1.2 to 2.8 years after cranial irradiation and chemotherapy for brain tumor are reported in four children treated at the Children's National Medical Center, Washington, DC. Three had neuroectodermal tumors and one an ependymoma in the posterior fossa. Headaches lasted 2 to 24 hours and were intermittent, unilateral, and associated with nausea, visual loss, hemiparesis, aphasia, or hemisensory loss. MRIs were unchanged, and CSF, EEGs, EKGs, and MR angiograms were normal. Cerebral angiograms in 3 children were normal but caused recurrence of temporary migraine-like episodes complicated by delirium. Response to propranolol and aspirin was good in 1 and partial in 3. (Shuper A, Packer RJ et al. 'Complicated migraine-like episodes' in children following cranial irradiation and chemotherapy. <u>Neurology</u> Oct 1995;45:1837-1840). (Reprints: Dr Roger J Packer, Department of Neurology, Children's National Medical Center, 111 Michigan Ave, NW, Washington, DC 20010).

COMMENT. Clinical manifestations of cranial irradiation toxicity can occur in three stages: 1) acute increase in intracranial pressure related to brain edema; 2) subacute 'somnolence syndrome' developing after a 1 to 3 month interval and related to demyelination; and 3) chronic focal neurologic deficits, seizures, and cognitive, developmental, and endocrine deficiencies, caused by vascular damage and tissue necrosis and appearing months to years after radiation therapy. The delayed-onset headaches reported in the above patients were vascular in type but were unassociated with demonstable vascular damage. The authors caution that cerebral angiography may exacerbate the migraine-like episodes.

Stroke as a late sequela of cranial irradiation for childhood brain tumors was reported in 11 children treated at the Southern California School of Medicine, Los Angeles (Mitchell WG et al. 1991). The addition of chemotherapy may potentiate damage to endothelial cells produced by irradiation causing a mineralizing microangiopathy. For a review of adverse effects of cranial irradiation and chemotherapy in the treatment of brain neoplasms, see <u>Progress in Pediatric Neurology II</u>, PNB Publishers, 1994, pp339-344). -Editor. *Ped Neur Briefs* Nov 1995.

RADIATION-INDUCED MENINGIOMA

A case of radiation-induced meningioma that appeared in a 27-year-old woman, 12 years after treatment of a childhood-onset posterior fossa medulloblastoma, is reported from the Department of Neurosurgery, Bretonneau Hospital, Tours, France. She was admitted with a left facial neuralgia and transitory aphasia. MRI showed a large left temporal mass which was removed surgically. Histopathological examination was consistent with a meningotheliomatous meningioma. Eight months later the patient was readmitted with ataxia, memory disturbances, and left lower limb paresis. CT showed multiple intracerebral tumors in the left temporal area, posterior fossa, and interhemisperic area. Removal of the largest tumor showed a medulloblastoma recurrence. Despite chemotherapy, the patient deteriorated and died. (Dweik A et al. Radiation-induced meningioma. <u>Child's Nerv Syst</u> 1995;11:661-663).

COMMENT. Glial and meningeal cells are most commonly involved in radiation-induced neoplasms. Meningiomas may occur after low-dose, intermediate, or high-dose irradiation of the head. The meninges of children are particularly susceptible. The majority of radiation-induced meningiomas are situated in the falx and parasagittal area or over the convexity of the skull. The temporal and sphenoidal location of the above reported meningioma folowing irradiation is unusual. -Editor. *Ped Neur Briefs* Jan 1996.

CNS IRRADIATION EFFECTS ON PUBERTY AND GROWTH

The relation between age at irradiation, sex, and age at puberty onset was determined in 36 children treated with high-dose irradiation for tumors anatomically distant from the hypothalamic-pituitary region at the New York University Medical Center, St Luke's/Roosevelt Hospital, and Memorial Sloan Kettering Cancer Center, New York. Twenty six also received chemotherapy. Age at onset of puberty and pubarche was significantly earlier in girls but not in boys. The mean age at onset of puberty in both boys and girls was linearly correlated with age at diagnosis and irradiation, and was inversely related to body weight. (Oberfield SE et al. Age at onset of puberty following high-dose central nervous system radiation therapy. <u>Arch Pediatr Adolesc Med</u> June 1996;150:589-592). (Reprints: Sharon E Oberfield MD, New York University Medical Center, 550 First Ave, New York, NY 10016).

COMMENT. High dose cranial irradiation may cause precocious puberty in girls, particularly in those who are overweight.

High-dose methotrexate for acute lymphocytic leukemia in young children did not cause neurological abnormalities or MRI changes in a study of 12 children treated at the University Hospital of Tronheim, Norway. (Seidel H et al. <u>Acta Paediatr</u> April 1996;85:450-3). Some previous studies have demonstrated reversible acute and subacute neurotoxicity following methotrexate (MTX) therapy for ALL. The possible role of folinic acid rescue in avoiding MTX toxicity needs further study. -Editor. *Ped Neur Briefs* June 1996.

LANGUAGE DOMINANCE WITH LEFT HEMISPHERE TUMORS

Hemispheric language dominance in 12 children with slow growing tumors near left hemisphere language areas was studied at the Cleveland Clinic, OH. Complex partial seizures began at or under 6 years of age. Tumor resection was performed at ages 5 to 20 years, an average of 8 years after seizure onset. Neurologic exam was normal in 11 patients. Ten (83%) had amobarbital tests indicating left hemisphere language dominance, confirmed by cortical stimulation in 6. Eleven with complete tumor resection were seizure-free at follow-up. Most had developmental neoplasms, often congenital. Paired *t* tests found no differences between pre- and postoperative performance of language tests, and a tendency for improved language function after operation. (DeVos KJ et al. Language dominance in patients with early childhood tumors near left hemisphere language areas. Neurology February 1995;45:349-356). (Reprints: Dr Elaine Wyllie, Pediatric Epilepsy Program, The Cleveland Clinic Foundation, 9500 Euclid Ave, Cleveland, OH 44195).

COMMENT. Language dominance does not usually transfer to the contralateral hemisphere in young children with low-grade left frontal and temporal tumors. Successful tumor resection is accomplished by using cortical stimulation studies and sparing of the language areas in close proximity to the tumor. -Editor. *Ped Neur Briefs* Feb 1995.

SYMPTOMS AND SIGNS OF PSEUDOTUMOR

A review of charts of 30 children with idiopathic intracranial hypertension, seen in a 30 year period between 1960 and 1990, is reported from the University of Iowa Hospital and Clinics. Common presenting symptoms included headache (63%), vomiting (43%), diplopia (36%), blurred vision (26%), and nausea (23%). The majority were heavier than the 50th percentile. All had bilateral papilledema, 30% had retinal hemorrhage, and 53% enlarged blind spots. CTs and MRIs were normal. Associated illnesses were URIs in 16%, otitis in 16%, head trauma in 6%; 46% were otherwise healthy. Six had taken antibiotics, and 4 were on vitamins, including vitamin A. Neurologic signs included VIth nerve palsy in 14, and ataxia in 4. Steroids were used in 9 and acetazolamide in 8. (Babikian P et al. Idiopathic intracranial hypertension in children: The Iowa experience. J Child Neurol April 1994;9:144-149). (Respond: Dr James J Corbett, Dept Neurology, UMC, 2500 North State Street, Jackson, MS 39216).

COMMENT. Abnormalities on neurologic examination are more common in children than in adults. The infrequent occurrence or recognition of the syndrome in infants and young children is noteworthy. A review of the literature before 1960 and prior to the period examined in the Iowa study showed that 84 (37%) of 224 patients were children and of these 75 (90%) were between 5 and 15 years of age. (Millichap JG. Benign intra-cranial hypertension and otitic hydrocephalus. <u>Pediatrics</u> Feb 1959;<u>23</u>:257). Antecedent otitis media was reported in 65 (29%), and mild head injury or infection other than otitis in 66 (29%). The 93 (41%) cases classified as idiopathic occurred principally in adults in this earlier series whereas approximately one half the pediatric cases in the later Iowa report were unassociated with otitis or other infection, trauma, or predisposing illness. The advent of antibiotics and virtual abolition of mastoiditis and "otitic hydrocephalus" accounts for the change in frequency of predisposing causes and the increase in "idiopathic" cases. For a recent major review of pediatric pseudotumor cerebri, see Lessell S. <u>Survey of Ophthalmology</u> 1992;<u>37</u>:155-166).

Combined therapy with acetazolamide (37 - 100 mg/kg/daily) and furosemide (1 mg/kg/daily) was effective in treating raised intracranial pressure in 8 children with pseudotumor cerebri at the Department of Pediatrics, University of Stellenbosch and Tygerberg Hospital, Republic of South Africa (Schoeman JF. <u>J Child Neurol</u> April 1994;<u>9</u>:130-134). Repeated lumbar cerebrospinal fluid pressure monitoring was used to evaluate response to therapy, but clinical monitoring correlated well and would be adequate in most children. -Editor. *Ped Neur Briefs* May 1994.

PSEUDOTUMOR CEREBRI WITHOUT EDEMA

The pathologic findings in two adult patients with idiopathic intracranial hypertension (IIH) who died unexpectedly are reported from the University of Iowa College of Medicine, Iowa City. Patient 1 died of cardiac arrest during operation for duodenal ulcer, and patient 2 died in her sleep of unknown cause. No histologic evidence of either intracellular or interstitial brain edema was found at autopsy. Arachnoid granulations were not available for study. (Wall M et al. Idiopathic intracranial hypertension. Lack of histologic evidence for cerebral edema. <u>Arch Neurol</u> Feb 1995;52:141-145). (Reprints: Dr Wall, Department of Neurology, University of Iowa, College of Medicine, 200 Hawkins Dr, Iowa City, IA 52242).

COMMENT. The absence of cerebral edema was in agreement with the report of 3 patients studied by Greer and in contrast to a finding of interstitial and intracellular edema in cortical biopsies of 10 patients reported by Sahs and Joynt. A review of tissue from 3 of the Sahs and Joynt cases, one a girl aged 17 years, showed artifactual changes and no convincing evidence of edema on re-examination of slides. The authors recommend measures of brain water content of frozen tissue and examination of arachnoid granulations when available, in future investigations of pathogenesis of pseudotumor cerebri.

The MRI has been used to clarify the pathophysiology of pseudotumor in 7 children, aged 6 months to 13 years. Normal signal intensity in the white matter was in keeping with absence of brain edema, as reported in the Iowa autopsy specimens. (Connolly MB et al. 1992; see <u>Progress in Pediatric Neurology II</u>, 1994, pp 336-7). -Editor. *Ped Neur Briefs* Feb 1995.

CHAPTER 10

NEUROCUTANEOUS SYNDROMES

INTRODUCTION

Joel Charrow, M.D.
Section of Clinical Genetics,
Children's Memorial Hospital,
Northwestern University Medical School, Chicago, IL.

Our understanding of the neurocutaneous syndromes (ataxia telangiectasia, tuberous sclerosis, neurofibromatosis, von Hippel-Lindau syndrome, and Sturge-Weber syndrome) continues to benefit from the explosive advances in molecular genetics. Most of what we know about the basic genetic and biochemical processes underlying these disorders has been learned in the last five years. Ataxia-telangiectasia (AT) apparently results from a disturbance in the cell cycle, which results in failure of DNA repair. Tuberous sclerosis, neurofibromatosis type 1 (NF1), and von

Hippel-Lindau (VHL) syndrome all appear to be caused by dominant mutations in tumor suppressor genes. Sturge Weber syndrome is usually not inherited, and its etiology remains obscure.

The discovery of tumor suppressor genes has provided insight into the genetic alterations which contribute to the development of neoplasia. These recessive genes appear to play a role in cell growth and differentiation. They contribute to tumorigenesis only when *both* alleles have been inactivated. Many of the inherited disorders in which there is a predisposition to neoplasia result from dominantly inherited mutations in a tumor suppressor gene, in which only one of the alleles is inactivated. This by itself is insufficient to cause tumor development; a "second hit" (somatic mutation), inactivating the *other* allele, is required. In non-inherited tumors, both "hits" are somatic mutations.

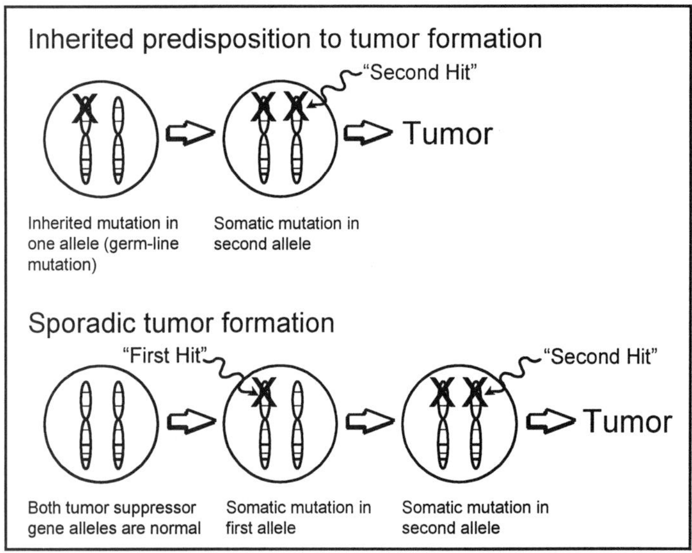

It is now clear that tuberous sclerosis is a genetically heterogeneous disorder, with approximately 40% of cases related to mutations in the TSC1 gene on chromosome 9 (9q34), and most of the remaining cases associated with alteration of the TSC2 gene on chromosome 16 (16p13.3). Little is known about the function of the gene products encoded by these genes, although substantial evidence has been presented that they are both tumor suppressor genes, with evidence of a second hit (by demonstration of loss of heterozygosity) at these loci in angiomyolipomas, rhabdomyomas, giant cell astrocytomas, and cortical tubers.

Although the gene responsible for neurofibromatosis type 1 was identified in 1990, progress toward understanding the function of the gene product, neurofibromin, has been slow. Nonetheless, it appears to be a tumor suppressor gene, and a role for neurofibromin in down-regulating cell growth has been postulated. While the mapping of the gene opened the door to presymptomatic and prenatal diagnosis in families with at least one affected individual, laboratory diagnosis of sporadic cases continues to be elusive. More than 90 mutations in the NF1 gene have been identified, and no mutation has been found to be common among affected individuals. Mutation detection by "standard" methods has been fruitful in only a minority of patients. However, the recently developed protein truncation assay is very promising. This test uses the patient's gene sequence to direct synthesis of neurofibromin fragments *in vitro*. Absence of an expected fragment or alteration of the size of any of the fragments is indicative of a mutation in the corresponding region of the gene. Using this method it is expected that 70-80% of NF1 mutations will be detectable (because this is the frequency of known premature termination mutations), and early experience with the test has been consistent with this expectation.

Von Hippel-Lindau syndrome research has advanced at both the clinical and basic levels. Although perceived by many as a rare disorder, the incidence (at least in the northwest of England) has been estimated at 1 in 40-50,000 live births. The most common presenting manifestation is cerebellar hemangioblastoma (present in 35%), with a mean age of onset of symptoms of approximately 25 years. Sixty percent of patients develop cerebellar hemangioblastomas, 40% retinal angiomas, 25% renal cell carcinomas, and 15% each spinal hemangioblastomas and pheochromocytomas. Mean age at death is 40 years, with the majority related to cerebellar hemangioblastomas.

The VHL gene has been mapped to the short arm of chromosome 3 (3p26-p25), and the complete sequence has been reported. It does not demonstrate sequence homology to any other known gene, although several lines of evidence indicate that it, too, is a tumor suppressor gene. The gene product is probably a nuclear protein which is a component of multiprotein compexes, perhaps functioning as an inhibitor of transcription elongation. A variety of types of mutations have been demonstrated in patients with VHL, and the type of mutation appears to correlate somewhat with the clinical manifestations of the disorder. Deletions, insertions, and nonsense mutations (which are generally expected to result in an absent or truncated protein) were found in more than half of patients with VHL type 1 (renal cell carcinoma *without* pheochromocytoma), while missense mutations (which may result in an abnormal gene product) were found in almost all patients with VHL type 2 (renal cell carcinoma *with* pheochromocytoma). In more than 40% of VHL type 2 patients, the mutations occurred in a single codon, at position 238. These observations may greatly aid presymptomatic diagnosis, prognosis, and prenatal diagnosis of pregnancies when one of the parents has VHL.

Recent progress in ataxia-telangiectasia research has been especially exciting, because the disorder appears to be related to altered regulation of the cell cycle. The AT gene (known as ATM, for AT 'mutated') has been mapped to chromosome 11 (11q22.3), and the full sequence determined. Although evidence for a second AT locus, also on chromosome 11, has been presented, all of the classical complementation groups are thought to represent allelic variants, i.e. different mutations at the same locus. ATM has significant homology with genes in *Drosophila,* yeast, the mouse and a variety of other mammals, suggesting that the gene product has a critically important function which has been conserved phylogenetically.

AT cells are abnormally sensitive to killing by ionizing radiation, and unlike normal cells, continue to synthesize DNA following irradiation. Associated with these phenomena are unusual numbers of chromosome breaks and gaps. These observations have long suggested that AT results from a defect in DNA repair. It is now apparent that the ATM gene product is an important regulator of the cell cycle, contributing to the control of the transition from G1-phase to S-phase. The "checkpoint" is necessary to allow repair of DNA before the cell enters S-phase, when DNA is replicated prior to cell division. If DNA repair does not occur, the alteration in DNA would be perpetuated. It is believed that this checkpoint permits "surveillance" of DNA to detect damage, and initiates other pathways that alter cell division or even repair the DNA damage. The mutation in ATM appears to abolish this G1-S checkpoint.

Although these exciting breakthroughs have begun to elucidate the molecular pathology of the neurocutaneous disorders, therapeutic strategies are still very limited. The development of novel therapies, therapies which alter the basic defects, and gene therapies are still in the future, but may come to light through further research on the natural history and molecular biology of these conditions.

Joel Charrow, M.D.

NEUROFIBROMATOSIS

OPTIC PATHWAY TUMORS AND NF-1

The natural history of 33 optic pathway tumors (OPT) diagnosed in 227 children with neurofibromatosis type 1 (NF-1) seen in a specialty clinic was evaluated in a prospective, longitudinal study at Children's Memorial Hospital and Northwestern University Medical School, Chicago. OPTs were found in 19% of 176 who had CT or MRI at a median age of 4.2 years. No OPT developed on later follow-up in children who had not received an MRI. In those without ophthalmological complaints at diagnosis, the incidence of OPT was 15%. The median age of children with ophthalmologic complaints such as proptosis or glaucoma (1.9 years) was significantly lower than that of children without such complaints (5.3 years). Only 8 tumors were discovered because of visual complaints or precocious puberty; 25 (76%) children were asymptomatic at time of diagnosis, and 21 (64%) had normal eye findings. Six with chiasmal tumors had decreased visual acuity without proptosis. At follow-up of 0.2 - 8 years, only 3 (9%) showed progressive tumor growth on MRI or deteriorating vision after diagnosis. Symptomatic OPT were diagnosed before the age of 6 years. (Listernick R, Charrow J, Greenwald M, Mets M. Natural history of optic pathway tumors in children with neurofibromatosis type 1: A longitudinal study. J Pediatr July 1994;125:63-66). (Reprints: Robert Listernick MD, Div Gen Acad & Emergency Peds, Children's Memorial Hospital, 2300 Children's Plaza, Chicago, IL 60614).

COMMENT. The child with NF-1 is at greatest risk for symptomatic optic pathway tumor during the first 6 years of life. Tumor growth after 6 years is unusual. Progressive abnormalities and precocious puberty occurred only with chiasmatic tumors. Tumors confined to the optic nerve discovered by screening with MRI were not accompanied by decreased visual acuity or evidence of progression. The authors advocate serial ophthalmologic examinations in young children with neurofibromatosis type 1, but find that serial MRI is of limited value in asymptomatic patients. The frequency and indications for neurological and neurosurgical consultations in these patients would be of interest. -Editor. *Ped Neur Briefs* Aug 1994. (*see also* Chap 9)

INFANTILE SPASMS AND NF-1

Two patients, ages 7 and 2 years, with neurofibromatosis type 1 complicated by infantile spasms are reported from the Pediatric Institutes, Siena and Catania, Italy. ACTH and anticonvulsants were ineffective. Both children were mentally retarded and one had UBOs on MRI. The authors believe that the association of NF-1 and infantile spasms is not a coincidence and infantile spasms should be included among the clinical manifestations of NF-1. (Fois A, Tine A, Pavone L. Infantile spasms in patients with neurofibromatosis type 1. <u>Child's Nerv Syst</u> 1994;10:176-179). (Respond: Dr A Fois, Pediatric Institute, University of Siena, I-53100 Siena, Italy).

COMMENT. The authors cite 7 additional cases of infantile spasms with NF-1 in the literature, the first reference to this association originating from Japan (Kurokawa T et al. <u>Pediatrics</u> 1980;65:81). They include a report by Motte et al of 15 cases, all responsive to steroids and having a good mental outcome (1992, unpublished data). A reference to 2 cases reported in a population study of 135 patients with NF-1 in Wales was omitted (Huson SM et al. In: <u>Progress in Pediatric Neurology I</u>, 1991, Chicago, PNB Publ, p 372). Infantile spasms and hypsarrhythmia occur much less frequently with NF-1 than in tuberous sclerosis, but the association is more prevalent than expected. -Editor. *Ped Neur Briefs* Aug 1994. (see Chap 1)

LEARNING DISABILITIES AND NF-1: MRI ABNORMALITIES

The significance of abnormalities on MRI was evaluated in 40 children with NF-1, aged 8 to 16 years, at the Children's Hospital, Sydney, Australia. The distribution of Full Scale IQ scores was bimodal, one group *with* and a second group *without* cognitive impairment. Children with areas of increased signal intensity on MRI (unidentified bright objects, UBO+), accounting for 62.5% of the study population, had lower IQs than those without these lesions. Language function, visuomotor integration, academic achievement, and coordination were also impaired in the UBO+ group. IQ and achievement in the UBO- group were similar to the general population. (North K et al.

Specific learning disability in children with neurofibromatosis type 1: Significance of MRI abnormalities. <u>Neurology</u> May 1994;44:878-883). (Reprints: Dr Kathryn North, Genetics Division, Fegan 10, Children's Hospital, 300 Longwood Ave, Boston, MA 02115).

COMMENT. UBOs in children with neurofibromatosis-1, representing areas of developmental dysplasia and aberrant myelination, are associated with cognitive deficits. Patients identified with UBOs should be managed separately from the UBO-negative group in determining the need for special education services.

Similar findings have been reported from the Johns Hopkins Hospital, Baltimore, MA (Hofman KJ, Denckla MB et al. Neurofibromatosis type 1: The cognitive phenotype. <u>J Pediatr</u> April 1994;124:S1-8). In a study of 12 families, children with NF-1 compared to unaffected siblings had a lower Full Scale IQ, multifocal cognitive deficits, reading disability, and neuromotor deficit. Paired cognitive differences correlated with the number of brain lesions on MRI. -Editor. *Ped Neur Briefs* Aug 1994. (*see also* Chap 4)

For additional articles on intelligence and MRI findings, including UBOs, in neurofibromatosis 1, see Chapter 4, pp 291-294.

PRESYMPTOMATIC DIAGNOSIS OF NEUROFIBROMATOSIS 2

The clinical spectrum of neurofibromatosis 2 (NF2) at the time of presymptomatic DNA diagnosis in at-risk first-degree relatives in five families were studied at the Cedars-Sinai Medical Center, UCLA School of Medicine, Los Angeles, and the Neurofibromatosis Institute, La Crescenta, CA. With molecular genetic analysis, 11 first-degree relatives were predicted to be at high risk, and 20 at low risk of carrying an NF2 mutation. Five mutation carriers, including a 31-year-old, had no clinical manifestations, while 4, including a 7-year-old, had vestibular schwannomas (VS), early-onset cataracts, or both. The identification of presymptomatic NF2 mutation carriers by DNA diagnosis permits improved genetic counselling and clinical management in at-risk subjects. The early detection of VS by gadolinium-enhanced MRI can improve surgical outcome. (Blaser ME, Mautner VF, Ragge NK et al. Presymptomatic diagnosis of neurofibromatosis 2 using linked genetic markers, neuroimaging, and ocular examinations. <u>Neurology</u> Nov 1996;47:1269-1277). (Reprints: Dr Michael E Blaser, 11746 Bellagio Rd, #308, Los Angeles, CA 90049 or Dr Stefan-M Pulst, Division of Neurology, Rm 8920 South Tower, Cedars-Sinai Medical Center, 8700 Beverly Blvd, Los Angeles, CA 90048).

COMMENT. In NF2 mutation carriers, DNA testing may lead to early diagnosis, and optimal treatment and counselling. However, ethical factors must be considered in testing children because of health insurance and other discriminating issues. -Editor. *Ped Neur Briefs* Dec 1996.

TUBEROUS SCLEROSIS, AUTISM AND ADHD

In a population-based psychiatric study of 28 patients with tuberous sclerosis (TS) at the University of Goteborg, Sweden, 24 had autistic symptoms and 17 met all DSM-III-R criteria for autistic disorder (AD). Of the 17 with AD, 7 were severely mentally retarded, 7 had mild retardation, 3 were near average IQ, and 11 had ADHD. One girl of average IQ had Asperger syndrome. Only 3 were free of psychiatric/behavioral problems, all having average IQs. Of the 24 with autistic behavior, 14 had a history of infantile spasms. Infantile spasms were not specifically associated with later development of autistic behavior. TS predisposes to both autism and infantile spasms. Nine per cent of all children and 20% of females with autism may have TS. Autistic behavior in children < 5 years of age has a stronger correlation with TS than facial angiofibromas, a sign often not clearly defined until later childhood. (Gillberg IC et al. Autistic behavior and attention deficits in tuberous sclerosis: a population-based study.

<u>Dev Med Child Neurol</u> Jan 1994;<u>36</u>:50-56). (Respond: Christopher Gillberg MD, Annedal Clinics, Child Neuropychiatry Clinic, University of Goteborg, S-413 45 Goteborg, Sweden).

COMMENT. An epidemiological study of TS in Western Sweden by the same authors showed a peak prevalence of 1 in 6800 in the 11 to 15 year-old age group, almost double that reported in earlier studies. In the whole cohort, ages 0-20 years, the prevalence was 1 in 12900. (Ahlsen G,Gillberg IC et al. Tuberous sclerosis in Western Sweden. <u>Arch Neurol</u> Jan 1994;<u>51</u>:76-81). -Editor. *Ped Neur Briefs* Feb 1994.

DECIDUOUS TEETH IN TUBEROUS SCLEROSIS

The diagnostic significance of enamel pits in shed deciduous teeth from 20 patients with tuberous sclerosis was investigated at the University of Copenhagen, Denmark. Examination with a surface microscope found enamel pits in all 87 teeth obtained from 20 tuberous sclerosis patients, but none in 253 deciduous teeth from 142 patients with cerebral palsy, phenylketonuria and Down syndrome, as well as healthy controls. The facial surfaces of the central incisor, lateral incisor and canine teeth were most frequently affected. (Russell BG, Russell MB, Praetorius F, Russell CA. Deciduous teeth in tuberous sclerosis. <u>Clin Genet</u> July 1996;50:36-40). (Respond: Dr Bjorn G Russell, Copenhagen County Dental Clinic for Handicapped, Bank Mikkelsens Vej 1, 2820 Gentofte, Denmark).

COMMENT. The occurrence of enamel pits in deciduous and permanent teeth may be a useful diagnostic criterion for tuberous sclerosis. Examination of the labial surfaces of the cleaned central and lateral incisors and canine teeth, using a magnifying glass, may be as important as the search for hypopigmented macules on the skin. -Editor. *Ped Neur Briefs* Oct 1996.

HYPOPIGMENTED MACULES: PREVALENCE

The prevalence of hypopigmented macules

among 423 white individuals and their significance in the diagnosis of tuberous sclerosis (TS) were evaluated at the University of Washington School of Medicine and Children's Hospital, Seattle, WA. Twenty (4.7%) had at least one macule, 4 of these had more than one macule, and none had more than three. Two (8%) of 25 hypopigmented macules were identified only with a Wood lamp. Of the 20 individuals with macules, 13 had ophthalmoscopic exams and none showed retinal changes of tuberous sclerosis. A few hypopigmented macules on the skin of otherwise healthy individuals without a family history of TS do not warrant a search for other signs of the disorder. (Vanderhooft SL, Francis JS, Pagon RA, Smith LT, Sybert VP. Prevalence of hypopigmented macules in a healthy population. J Pediatr Sept 1996;129:355-61). (Reprints: Sheryll L Vanderhooft MD, University of Utah Health Sciences Center, Department of Dermatology, 50 North Medical Dr, Salt Lake City, UT 84132).

COMMENT. Hypopigmented macules are apparently more common than previously determined, occurring in close to 5% of the general population under 45 years of age. The presence of one to three macules is not by itself a significant risk factor for tuberous sclerosis. As a secondary feature of TS, at least one other manifestation must be present to establish a diagnosis. -Editor. *Ped Neur Briefs* Oct 1996.

FAMILIAL KERATODERMA AND LEUKOENCEPHALOPATHY

A new familial neurocutaneous syndrome consisting of palmoplantar keratoderma (PPK) and adult-onset leukoencephalopathy is reported in four siblings from Hadassah University Hospital, Jerusalem, Israel. The proband, a 41-year-old woman, had a progressive gait disorder and cognitive impairment of 3 years' duration. Skin abnormalities had been present from early childhood: thick hyperkeratotic skin with numerous papules, most prominent over the palmar and plantar areas. Neurologic exam revealed cognitive impairments, generalized weakness with symmetric hyperreflexia, hypertonia, and Babinski signs. CSF protein was 1.18 g/L. MRI showed periventricular hyperintensity of white matter, brain atrophy, and thinning of the corpus callosum. Arylsulfatase A pseudodeficiency carrier state was identified by molecular analysis. Sural nerve biopsy showed loss of myelinated fibers. Bone X-rays showed osteochondritis dissecans of the talus. (Lossos A et al. Hereditary leukoencephalopathy and palmoplantar keratoderma: A new disorder with increased skin collagen content. <u>Neurology</u> Feb 1995;45:331-337). (Reprints: Dr A Lossos, Dept Neurol, Hadassah Univ Hosp, Jerusalem 91120, Israel.

COMMENT. Neurologic complications of familial palmoplantar keratoderma are rare and late in onset. -Editor. *Ped Neur Briefs* Feb 1995.

CHAPTER 11

VASCULAR DISORDERS AND MALFORMATIONS

OVERVIEW OF RECENT ADVANCES

Neck trauma as a cause of vertebral artery dissection and stroke in both boys and girls is reported from three different centers. Although the prognosis for survival is excellent, some may have residual paralysis.

Neonatal intracranial hemorrhage is frequently followed by cognitive and motor delay. Late onset of epilepsy, spastic hemiparesis, and thalamic atrophy may follow an apparent early favorable outcome in term neonates with middle cerebral artery infarcts. Developmental delay is also reported after surgery for hypoplastic left heart syndrome in infants. Indomethacin prophylaxis against intraventricular hemorrhage in very low birth weight infants does not result in adverse cognitive and motor outcome, according to some authorities, whereas others caution against its routine use. An increased frequency of stroke in HIV infected infants is anticipated because of longer survival.

Rapid clinical deterioration due to cardiac failure is the common presenting feature of cerebral arteriovenous malformation associated with ectasia of the vein of Galen in the newborn. Transarterial endovascular occlusion is the treatment of choice, with limitations. In moyamoya disease, surgery to revascularize ischemic brain tissue by collateral pathways is favored. The postoperative mortality of cerebral arteriovenous malformation in children is about 10%, versus 20-50% using conservative management.

Headache is the chief presenting symptom of cerebral venous thrombosis complicating systemic lupus erythematosus. A severe, persistent, throbbing headache, unresponsive to analgesics, points to a possible cerebral venous thrombosis, and is an indication for CT or MRI. In young women with migraine, especially those who smoke or use oral contraception, the risk of ischemic stroke is increased threefold, compared to nonmigraineurs. The ingestion of ginseng may be associated with headache and cerebral arteritis.   *J. Gordon Millichap, M.D.,* Editor.

STROKES AND VERTEBRAL ARTERY TRAUMA

Three boys, ages 11, 8, and 7 years, with strokes from vertebral artery lesions resulting from neck trauma are reported from Indiana University School of Medicine, Indianapolis, and Baylor College of Medicine, Houston, TX. The 11 year-old woke with left-leg ataxia and sore neck, the morning after being tackled at a football game. He had continued playing to finish the game. Brain stem and cerebellar signs, including left exotropia with nystagmus, impaired adduction of the left eye in convergence, and deviation to the left in compass gait test, were explained by a linear filling defect of the left vertebral artery at C1-2 level consistent with intimal dissection, documented by a 4-vessel cerebral arteriogram. CT and brain and cervical spine MRIs were normal. He recovered rapidly and was discharged to take one aspirin daily and avoid contact sports. The 8-year-old also recovered after minor neck trauma followed by recurrent episodes of ataxia, hemiparesis, and visual field defect with left VA thrombus at C-2 and multiple emboli in posterior cerebral arteries. The 7-year-old sustained a traumatic pseudoaneurysm with persistent hemiparesis and ataxia. Clinical data are summarized of 16 cases culled from the literature. (Garg BP, Fishman MA et al. Strokes in children due to vertebral artery trauma. <u>Neurology</u> Dec 1993;<u>43</u>:2555-2558). (Reprints: Dr Bhuwan P Garg, Section of Child Neurology, Department of Neurology, Riley Children's Hospital, Rm 1757, 702 Barnhill Drive, Indianapolis, IN 46202).

COMMENT. Fortunately, the prognosis for survival in vertebral artery stroke in children is generally excellent. Only one of 19 patients died. Two had residual quadriplegia, 9 had mild to moderate residual hemiparesis, ataxia, and/or dysarthria, and 7 (37%) recovered. -Editor. *Ped Neur Briefs* Jan 1994.

TRAUMATIC VERTEBRAL ARTERY DISSECTION

A girl, aged 9 years, with cerebellar infarction following minor neck injury sustained while ice-skating is reported from West Virginia University, Morgantown, WV. Symptoms began 12 hours after the fall, with vomiting that awakened her from sleep and recurred hourly. She complained of a throbbing occipital headache, stiff neck, photophobia, dizziness on standing, and ataxia. She had horizontal nystagmus, dysmetria bilaterally, and she stood and walked only with support. CT and MRI revealed a cerebellar vermian lesion extending into both hemispheres. Posterior fossa decompression and biopsy showed coagulative necrosis and no neoplasm. Vertebral angiography revealed a traumatic aneurysm within the distal right cervical vertebral artery and recanalization of an embolus in the right posterior inferior cerebellar artery with a narrowed lumen. She was treated with aspirin and recovery was complete after 3 months, with no recurrence at 1 year follow-up. (Sheth RJ, Bodensteiner JB et al. Stroke due to a traumatic vertebral artery dissection in a girl. <u>Clin Pediatr</u> Aug 1994;33:503-505). (respond: Raj D Sheth MD, Dept Neurology, Box 9180, West Virginia University, Health Science Center, Morgantown, WV 26506).

COMMENT. Childhood traumatic vertebral artery stroke was previously thought to affect boys only.(Garg BP et al. <u>Neurology</u> 1993;43:2555). With the increased participation of girls in contact sports, more female cases may be expected.

A further case of vertebral-artery dissection occurring in an 11-year-old boy following a judo session is reported from Besancon, France. (Lannuzel A, Rumbach L et al. <u>Neuropediatrics</u> 1994;25:106-108). CT showed a left thalamic infarct, and angiography revealed fibromuscular dysplasia ("string of beads" lesion) of the left vertebral artery with probable dissection. With anticoagulation, bed rest, and a cervical soft collar, symptoms of headaches, vomiting, left ptosis and diplopia, dysphasia, and ataxia resolved, and the boy was discharged taking aspirin after 2 weeks. -Editor. *Ped Neur Briefs* Sept 1994.

OUTCOME OF NEONATAL STROKE

Evaluations, including MRI, MR angiography, and neuropsychological tests, at 1.5-8.4 years, of 8 infants after neonatal stroke involving the middle cerebral artery are reported from the University of Heidelberg, Mannheim, Germany. Seven had mental and motor retardation and hemiparesis and 4 had epilepsy. Major deficits in cognitive function were found in 4 older children. One patient with normal development showed only a localized temporal lobe lesion on MRI and unremarkable MRA. Children with marked disorders of motor and cognitive development had defects of temporo-parietal lobes, basal ganglia, thalamus and internal capsule on MRI and recanalization of the middle cerebral artery shown on MRA. Those without recanalization had a poorer prognosis. (Koelfen W et al. Results of parenchymal and angiographic magnetic resonance imaging and neuropsychological testing of children after stroke as neonates. <u>Eur J Pediatr</u> Dec 1993;<u>152</u>:1030-1035). (Respond: Dr W Koelfen, Department of Pediatrics, Faculty of Clinical Medicine Mannheim, University of Heidelberg,Theodor Kutzer Ufer, D-68167 Mannheim, Germany).

COMMENT. Magnetic resonance angiography (MRA) images intracranial blood vessels without necessity for invasive contrast media. Children with neonatal stroke, seizures, and abnormalities shown on MRA have severe cognitive delays and the least favorable prognosis on long-term follow up. -Editor. *Ped Neur Briefs* Jan 1994.

ASPIRIN-INDUCED NEONATAL INTRACRANIAL HEMORRHAGE

A term newborn infant with intracranial hemorrhage associated with maternal acetylsalicylic acid ingestion before delivery is reported from the Departments of Pediatrics and Neurology, Eastern Virginia Medical School, Norfolk, VA. Pregnancy was complicated by alcohol abuse. Alka-Seltzer, 6 tablets daily, had been taken for 2 weeks for relief of hangover. The infant's serum salicylate level at 8 hours was 5.4 mg/dL. Hematocrit decreased from 29% at birth to 15% at 6 hours of age. Prothrombin time was >100 sec. Cranial ultrasound showed hemorrhage in the tentorium and hydrocephalus. CT also revealed a large cerebellar hemorrhage. Clinical findings included multiple ecchymoses, gastric hemorrhage, hematuria, a tense fontanelle, head circumference at the 95th percentile, hypotonia, and ocular bobbing and nystagmus. Transfusion, a second injection of vitamin K, and ventriculoperitoneal shunt were followed by recovery and discharge in care of grandmother on day

23. (Karlowicz MG, White LE. Severe intracranial hemorrhage in a term neonate associated with maternal acetylsalicylic acid ingestion. <u>Clin Pediatr</u> Dec 1993;<u>32</u>:740-743). (Respond: M Gary Karlowicz MD, Department of Pediatrics, Eastern Virginia Medical School, Children's Hospital of The King's Daughters, 601 Children's Lane, Norfolk, VA 23507).

COMMENT. Maternal salicylate ingestion should be considered in the etiology of neonatal intracranial hemorrhage without birth trauma. The infant's relatively low salicylate level is not inconsistent with chronic toxicity.

Surfactant therapy for respiratory distress syndrome in newborns of 600-750 g birth weight caused an increased risk of grades I and II intracranial hemorrhage compared to controls, in analyses of the literature by researchers at Ross Laboratories, Columbus, OH (Gunkel JH, Banks PLC. <u>Pediatrics</u> Dec 1993;<u>92</u>:775-786). -Editor. *Ped Neur Briefs* Jan 1994.

INDOMETHACIN FOR PREVENTION OF INTRAVENTRICULAR HEMORRHAGE

Results of a multicenter randomized trial of low-dose indomethacin (0.1 mg/kg IV) in prevention of intraventricular hemorrhage (IVH) in very low birth weight infants are reported from Yale New Haven Hospital, CT; Brown University, Providence, RI; and Maine Medical Center, Portland, ME. The incidence and severity of IVH were significantly lowered. Of 431 neonates enrolled, 25 (12%) treated and 40 (18%) controls developed IVH. Grade 4 IVH occurred in only 1 indomethacin-treated neonate and in 10 placebo-treated controls. (Ment LR et al. Low-dose indomethacin and prevention of intraventricular hemorrhage: a multicenter randomized trial. <u>Pediatrics</u> April 1994;<u>93</u>:543-550). (Reprints: Dr Laura R Ment, Dept of Pediatrics, Yale University School of Medicine, 333 Cedar St, New Haven, CT 06510).

COMMENT. Volpe JJ, Harvard Medical School, and

Reynolds EOR and Meek J, University College, London, are concerned about the cerebral vasoconstrictor effects of indomethacin and the dangers of periventricular ischemic injury. (Commentaries. <u>Pediatrics</u> April 1994;<u>93</u>:673-677, 677-678). These authorities are reluctant to endorse wholesale treatment of low birth weight newborns with indomethacin. -Editor. *Ped Neur Briefs* April 1994.

INTRAVENTRICULAR HEMORRHAGE AND COGNITION

The effects of premature birth-related subependymal and mild intraventricular hemorrhage (S/IVH) on specific cognitive abilities in 2-year-old children were investigated at the Perinatology Center, New York Hospital, and Cornell and New York University Medical Colleges. Of 82 children included in the study, 27 had premature births complicated by Grade I or II hemorrhages, 28 prematurely born children had normal neonatal ultrasound, and 27 were born at term without complications. The premature group with S/IVH at birth performed significantly less well than children without hemorrhage on a measure of memory for location and on ability to change response set. Both groups of prematurely born children performed less well than full term children on systematic search for an object when the order of hiding was reversed. All groups performed equally on a visual attention task and on the global Bayley mental ability scores. (Ross G, Boatright S, Auld PAM, Nass R. Specific cognitive abilities in 2-year-old children with subependymal and mild intraventricular hemorrhage. <u>Brain Cogn</u> Oct 1996;32:1-13). (Reprints: Dr Gail Ross, Perinatology Center, New York Hospital, 525 East 68th Street, New York, NY 10021).

COMMENT. Prior testing of these prematures at age 10 months had shown that S/IVH affected global mental ability and habituation to visual patterns, and prematurity was associated with poorer memory for location. When reevaluated at 2 years, the premature groups with or without hemorrhage did not differ on the visual attention task, but prematures with S/IVH did poorly on the memory for location task and ability to change response set. Memory for location is a function of the caudate nucleus and thalamus and frontal cortex, areas affected by subependymal and intraventricular hemorrhage of prematurity. Fronto-striatal structural changes in the MRI have been demonstrated in patients with ADHD. (Denckla MB. In: Progress in Pediatric Neurology II, Chicago, PNB Publ, 1994:173-176). At a later age, the incidence of ADHD in the S/IVH affected children will be of interest.

Indomethacin prophylaxis against IVH in very low birth weight infants did not result in adverse cognitive or motor outcomes at 36 months, in a study at Yale University School of Medicine. (Ment LR et al. <u>Pediatrics</u> Oct 1996;98:714-718). The authors suggest that the early administration of intravenous low-dose indomethacin to neonates weighing 1250 g or less is beneficial and does not cause neurodevelopmental delay. However, Dr Henrietta Bada, University of Tennessee, Memphis, advises caution, and slow infusion, because of reported acute cerebral effects. (Commentary. Routine indomethacin prophylaxis: has the time come? <u>Pediatrics</u> Oct 1996;98:784-785). -Editor. *Ped Neur Briefs* Nov 1996.

TREATMENT OF AVM AND VEIN OF GALEN ECTASIA

Optimal methods of evaluation and treatment of newborns with cerebral arteriovenous malformation associated with ectasia of the vein of Galen are outlined along with a case report of an inoperable malformation from the Dept of Pediatrics, Malarsjukhuset, Eskilstuna, and Dept of Neuroradiology, Karolinska sjukhuset, Stockholm, Sweden, and Centre Hospitalier Universitaire de Bicetre, France. The infant developed a general seizure at 10 min of age. She had a loud bruit over the skull and neck and congestive heart failure. Neurosonography showed a mass in the midline of the brain. CT confirmed a A-V malformation and ectasia of the vein of Galen, complicated by in utero encephalomalacia and more recent ischemic injury. Endovascular occlusive treatment was not appropriate and the child died at 15 days of age. Transarterial embolization of feeding arteries using bucrylate (isobutyl cyanoacrylate) is now considered the treatment of choice, in the absence of contraindications such as brain damage, prenatal cardiomegaly, or evidence of multi-organ failure. A free interval between birth and development of cardiac failure are factors of favorable prognostic value. (Swanstrom S et al. Conditions for treatment of cerebral arteriovenous malformation associated with ectasia of the vein of Galen in the newborn. Acta Pediatr March 1994;83:255-7). (Respond: Dr S Swanstrom, Dept of Pediatrics, Malarsjukhuset, S-631 88 Eskilstuna, Sweden).

COMMENT. Rapid clinical deterioration due to cardiac failure is the common presenting feature of this syndrome. Transarterial endovascular occlusive treatment is available only in specialized centers. The rapid evaluation of patients suited for intervention is essential for successful outcome. The authors caution against the use of contrast material for CT and advise against any form of angiography unless therapy is contemplated at the same time. -Editor. *Ped Neur Briefs* May 1994.

VASCULAR MALFORMATIONS AND INTRACTABLE EPILEPSY

A retrospective study of 20 consecutive patients with cerebral vascular malformations who were treated surgically for medically refractory partial epilepsy is reported from the Departments of Neurology and Neurologic Surgery, Mayo Clinic, Rochester, MN. MRI was more sensitive than CT and showed 36 vascular malformations (32 cavernous and 4 A-V malformations). Previous hemorrhage was verified in 18 patients. After complete resection of the lesion, 15 patients were free of seizures and 3 had a 90% control. Age of onset and duration of seizures did not affect outcome. A focal corticectomy in addition to lesionectomy was necessary in 11 patients with MRI-disclosed ipsilateral medial temporal lobe atrophy. (Dodick DW, Cascino GD, Meyer FB. Vascular malformations and intractable epilepsy: Outcome after surgical treatment. <u>Mayo Clin Proc</u> Aug 1994;69:741-745). (Reprints: Dr GD Cascino, Department of Neurology, Mayo Clinic, 200 First Street SW, Rochester, MN 55905).

COMMENT. The authors advocate early surgical intervention and excision of the lesion in patients with refractory partial seizures associated with vascular malformations. Corticectomy may be necessary in patients with dual temporal lobe pathologies. -Editor. *Ped Neur Briefs* Aug 1994.

SURGERY OF MOYAMOYA DISEASE

The manifestations of moyamoya disease in children and adults and the results of various surgical procedures are reviewed from the Department of Neurological Surgery and Section of Child and Adolescent Neurology, Mayo Clinic, Rochester, MN. Onset is in the first or the fourth decades of life. Of 518 patients registered in Japan, 155 were children <15 years, and 234 were adolescents or adults. In children, recurrent ischemic attacks (in 39%), strokes (in 39%), and seizures (14%) were the most common features, whereas in adults, hemorrhage (65%), and strokes (18%) were most frequent. Mortality was 7.5% for the total series; 10% for adults and 4.3% for children. Intracranial bleeding was the cause of death in 5 of 9 children (55%) and in 19 of 30 adults (63%). Of 27 children with only TIAs who were untreated, the TIAs gradually resolved but more than one-half showed cognitive impairment at 5 to 10 year follow-up. Ischemic symptoms diminished in 10 Mayo patients treated surgically at 13.5 years (mean age), using STA-MCA anastomosis (5), EDAS (2), and EDAS/EMS (3). Most published reports find surgical intervention of benefit in children but not in adults. (Ueki K, Meyer FB, Mellinger JF. Moyamoya disease: The disorder and surgical treatment. <u>Mayo Clin Proc</u> Aug 1994;69:749-757). (Reprints: Dr FB Meyer, Department of Neurologic Surgery, Mayo Clinic, 200 First Street SW, Rochester, MN 55905).

COMMENT. The natural history of moyamoya disease is characterized by neurologic deterioration, strokes and hemorrhage, seizures, and mental deterioration. Current evidence favors surgery to revascularize ischemic brain tissue by collateral pathways, especially in children with ischemic symptoms.

An 11 year-old girl with acute unilateral chorea as the presenting manifestation of moyamoya disease is reported from Hospital Plaza de Cruces, Vizcaya, Bilbao, Spain (Garaizar C, Prats JM et al. <u>Acta Neuropediatr</u> June 1994;1:59-64). Chorea resolved after 15 days haloperidol therapy, and no further ischemic episodes had occurred in 16 months during treatment with nicardipine. The authors cite two previous reports of moyamoya and chorea. -Editor. *Ped Neur Briefs* Aug 1994.

STROKE, CEREBRAL INFARCTS, AND GIANT ANEURYSM IN HIV INFECTION

Four out of 380 HIV-infected children followed in a 10 year period at the Hopital Bicetre, France, had acute hemiparesis and stroke with MRI and CT evidence of cerebral infarcts. Two patients had giant aneurysms and multiple thromboses, a history of frequent infections, a severe clinical course, and poor or fatal outcome. Two had an isolated thrombosis or necrotic area, a less progressive disease, and a more favorable outcome. In two additional patients, stroke was secondary to a massive cerebral hemorrhage and thrombocytopenia, and to sickle cell disease. (Philippet P, Tardieu M et al. Stroke and cerebral infarcts in children infected with human immunodeficiency virus. <u>Arch Pediatr Adolesc Med</u> Sept 1994;148:965-970).

(Reprints: Dr Tardieu, Neurologie Pediatrique, Hopital Bicetre, 94275 Le Kremlin, Bicetre Cedex, France).

COMMENT. Stroke in HIV infected children is rare but variable in underlying pathology and prognosis. The authors anticipate a more frequent incidence of this complication because of improved management and longer survival of patients with HIV. -Editor. *Ped Neur Briefs* Sept 1994.

CEREBRAL ARTERIOVENOUS MALFORMATIONS

A retrospective analysis of 62 children with cerebral arteriovenous malformations (AVM) seen over 17 years is reported from Hospital B, Lille, France. Ages ranged from 3 months to 14 years. Seven had a previous history of headache, and 5 (8%) had been treated for epilepsy. Intracranial hemorrhage and stroke was the presenting manifestation in 54 (87%). AVMs were supratentorial in 41 and infratentorial in 11. Total excision of the AVM was achieved in 47 of 52 operated. At follow-up, 50 had a good clinical outcome based on the Glasgow scale, 6 mild, 2 poor, and 4 died. Recurrent hemorrhage occurred in 3, fatal in 1. AVM recurrences in 2 were treated successfully by radiosurgery. Of ten with aphasia before surgery; 5 had improved. Of 25 with hemiparesis on admission, 12 recovered function and 7 have severe deficits. Two developed deficits after surgery. Of 7 with residual epilepsy after surgery, 6 are controlled with AEDs. (Hladky JP et al. Cerebral arteriovenous malformations in children: report on 62 cases. <u>Child's Nerv Syst</u> July 1994;10:328-333).

COMMENT. In reviewing the literature the authors report a postoperative mortality in children ranging from 8.5% to 11%, versus 23% to 57% following conservative management. Surgery is considered the most reliable treatment, combining teams experienced in neurosurgery, embolization, and radiosurgery. The smaller the AVM, the higher the risk of hemorrhage, and the greater the indication for surgery after diagnosis is established. The authors view angiography as superior to CT and MRI in diagnosis and management of AVM. Postoperative angiography after 2 years is advised to exclude enlarging residual microshunts or recurrence of AVM. -Editor. *Ped Neur Briefs* Sept 1994.

CEREBRAL BLOOD FLOW IN NEONATES WITH HIE: SAFETY OF PHENOBARBITAL

Phenobarbital treatment (20 mg/kg iv) had no significant effect on cerebral blood flow or blood pressure and heart rate, measured 60 min after a loading dose, in 7 term newborn infants with mild to moderate hypoxic ischemic encephalopathy examined in the Dept of Paediatrics, Alborg Hospital, Denmark. Phenobarbital imposed no risk of cerebrovascular damage in newborns with fetal distress. (Andersen K et al. The effect of phenobarbital on cerebral blood flow in newborn infants with foetal distress. Eur J Pediatr Aug 1994:153:584-587).

COMMENT. Phenobarbital is the most commonly used anticonvulsant in neonates and has been advocated in the prevention of periventricular hemorrhage in preterm infants. This demonstration of the safety of phenobarbital in neonates with HIE is encouraging and should offset in part the poor rating the drug has received in some febrile seizure studies. -Editor. *Ped Neur Briefs* Sept 1994.

NEONATAL MIDDLE CEREBRAL ARTERY STROKE

The presentation, EEG, imaging studies, and outcome of six term neonates with middle cerebral artery infarcts are reported from Mannheim Hospital, University of Heidelberg, Germany. Birth was by cesarean section in 5 cases. Apgars were normal in 4. Seizures occurred in 4 within 1 to 3 days and in 2 at the 5th and 9th days. EEGs showed focal slowing followed by focal spike-wave activity, correlating with the structural lesion defined by neuroimaging. EEG abnormalities sometimes antedated a positive ultrasound. A late intra-uterine event was suggested.

Only 2 had obvious hemiparesis at discharge, but all children showed developmental delay and spastic hemiparesis at 3 to 10 year follow up. One had infantile spasms and hemihypsarrhythmia, relieved only after drainage of a cyst and shunt procedure. Four developed epilepsy late. (Koelfen W, Freund M, Varnholt V. Neonatal stroke involving the middle cerebral artery in term infants: Clinical presentation, EEG and imaging studies, and outcome. <u>Dev Med Child Neur</u> March 1995;37:204-212). (Respond: Dr Wolfgang Koelfen, Kinderklinik Mannheim, Theodor Kutzer Ufer, 68127 Mannheim, Germany).

COMMENT. This study confirms previous reports of late onset of epilepsy and development of spastic hemiparesis and cognitive deficits following an apparent early favorable outcome in term neonates suffering middle cerebral artery infarcts.

Late Progressive Thalamic Atrophy in four children with neonatal middle cerebral artery infarction is reported from the Centre Hospitalo-Universitaire, Dijon, France. (Giroud M, Dumas R et al. <u>Child's Nerv Syst</u> March 1995;11:133-136). -Editor. *Ped Neur Briefs* April 1995.

DEVELOPMENTAL DELAY AFTER HEART SURGERY AND CIRCULATORY ARREST

The developmental and neurologic status of 155 children were evaluated one year after heart surgery for D-transposition of the great arteries, comparing those randomly assigned to circulatory arrest or low-flow cardiopulmonary bypass, at Children's Hospital, Boston, MA. Circulatory arrest was associated with lower scores on the Bayley Scales of Infant Development, and the Psychomotor Development Index was inversely related to the duration of circulatory arrest. Risk of neurologic abnormalities also increased with the duration of circulatory arrest. A ventricular septal defect, present in 35 (23%), and seizure activity detected by continuous EEG monitoring in the early postoperative period were independent risk factors for a poor outcome. MRI abnormalities, and mental development and visual memory test scores were not correlated with the method of circulatory support. (Bellinger DC, Newburger JW et al. Developmental and neurologic status of children after heart surgery with hypothermic circulatory arrest or low-flow cardiopulmonary bypass. <u>N Engl J Med</u> March 2, 1995;332:549-55). (Reprints: Dr Newburger, Department of Cardiology, Children's Hospital, 300 Longwood Ave, Boston, MA 02115).

COMMENT. This report is a follow up of the perioperative neurologic effects of hypothermic circulatory arrest compared to low-flow cardiopulmonary bypass in 171 patients operated within the first three months of age at the Children's Hospital, Boston. (Newburger JW et al. <u>N Engl J Med</u> 1993;329:1057-64). Circulatory arrest was associated with a higher incidence of clinical and EEG seizures in the first 6 hours after surgery, but the incidence of neurologic abnormalities was similar in the two groups at time of discharge. (See <u>Progress in Pediatric Neurology II</u>, 1994, p386). It now appears that the technical advantages of total circulatory arrest may be outweighed by delayed motor development and neurologic abnormalities at one year and potential cognitive deficits at school age.

Neurodevelopmental Outcome of 11 Infants with Surgery for Hypoplastic Left Heart Syndrome is reported from the State University of New York and Children's Hospital of Buffalo. (Rogers BT et al. <u>J Pediatr</u> March 1995;126:496-8). Testing at a mean age of 38 months showed microcephaly in 8 (73%), mental retardation in 7 (64%), gross motor delays in 5 (45%), and severe cerebral palsy in 2 (18%). The quality of life is obviously seriously impaired in these patients, a factor to be considered in treatment options. -Editor. *Ped Neur Briefs* April 1995.

CEREBRAL VEIN THROMBOSIS, SYSTEMIC LUPUS, AND HEADACHE

Three girls, ages 11, 14, and 17, with systemic lupus erythematosus, who had headache and were diagosed with cerebral vein thrombosis are reported from the Hospital for Sick Children, University of Toronto, and the Children's Hospital, McMaster University, Hamilton, Canada. Diagnosis was established by CT and MRI without need of angiography. Cerebral infarct occurred in one patient when diagnosis was delayed. All patients received low-dose oral anticoagulation and treatment for lupus and none had further thrombotic events during 10-18 month follow-up. (Uziel Y et al. Cerebral vein thrombosis in childhood systemic lupus erythematosus. <u>J Pediatr</u> May 1995;126:722-727). (Reprints: ED Silverman MD, Division of Rheumatology, The Hospital for Sick Children, 555 University Ave, Toronto, Ontario, Canada M5G 1X8).

COMMENT. Headache is the chief presenting symptom of cerebral venous thrombosis. These are of the tension or vascular type in 25%, but migraine headache and those associated with increased intracranial pressure also occur. Associated seizures, papilledema, and hemiparesis are also suggestive. A severe, persistent, throbbing headache, unresponsive to analgesics, points to a possible cerebral vein thrombosis, and is an indication for CT examination. -Editor. *Ped Neur Briefs* June 1995.

MIGRAINE AND ISCHEMIC STROKE

The relation between migraine and ischemic stroke in 72 young women aged under 45 and 173 controls was investigated at five hospital in Paris and suburbs. A questionnaire based on the International Headache Society's criteria for headache and migraine was used in telephone interviews. Migraine and ischemic stroke were strongly associated. Migraine was diagnosed in 60% of patients with stroke compared to 30% of controls. Women with migraine had a more than threefold increased risk of ischemic stroke (19 per

100,000 per year) compared with women without migraine (6 per 100,000 per year). The risk of stroke was higher in cases with aura than in those without aura. It was increased for migrainous women who used oral contraceptives or who were heavy smokers (>20 cigarettes/day). (Tzourio C et al. Case-control study of migraine and risk of ischaemic stroke in young women. BMJ 1 April 1995;310:830-833). (Respond: Dr Tzourio, INSERM U 360, Recherches Epidemiol en Neurologie et Psychopathologie, Cedex 94807 Villejuif, France).

COMMENT. The authors concluded that despite a relatively small risk of ischemic stroke, smoking and the use of oral contraceptives should be discouraged or limited in young women with migraine. It was not known whether the increased risk of stroke related to all young migrainous women or only to a subgroup that remains to be defined. -Editor. *Ped Neur Briefs* June 1995.

HEADACHE AND GINSENG-RELATED CEREBRAL ARTERITIS

A 28-year-old woman who had a severe headache after ingesting a large quantity of ethanol-extracted ginseng was diagnosed with cerebral arteritis in the Department of Neurology, Chang Gung Memorial Hospital, Keelung, Taiwan. Ginseng root 25 gm stewed in rice wine was taken for fatigue associated with sore throat. An explosive headache with nausea and vomiting developed 8 hours later and was temporarily relieved by acetaminophen. Smaller quantities of ginseng had never caused headache. CT showed increased density over the falx, suggestive of subarachnoid hemorrhage. Cerebral angiograms revealed multiple areas of alternating focal constriction and dilatation (beading) in anterior and posterior cerebral arteries and superior cerebellar artery, consistent with arteritis. The headache gradually resolved within 10 days. (Ryu S-J, Chien Y-Y. Ginseng-associated cerebral arteritis. Neurology April 1995;45:829-830). (Reprints: Dr Shan-Jin Ryu, Department of

Neurology, Chang Gung Memorial Hospital, 199, Tung Hwa North Road, Taipei 105, Taiwan).

COMMENT. The temporal association between the ingestion of the ethanolic ginseng extract and the onset of a severe headache was strongly suggestive of a causal relationship. The use of cocaine, amphetamine, phenylpropanolamine, and other sympathomimetic drugs was denied. Most ginseng users are not medically supervised, and adolescents and adults may be experimenting with doses larger than those generally recommended in Chinese practice (0.5 to 2 gm). The expected benefits are listed as prevention of aging or tiredness, improved stamina or concentration, and increased resistance to stress or disease. -Editor. *Ped Neur Briefs* June 1995.

NEUROCARDIOGENIC (VASOVAGAL) SYNCOPE

A retrospective analysis of 54 consecutive patients with recurrent syncope, examined with or without tilt table testing, is reported from the Children's Heart Center, Egleston Children's Hospital, Emory University, Atlanta, GA. The group of 27 patients without tilt table tests received a greater number of neurology consultations, EEGs, and CTs, but a positive diagnosis (Wolff-Parkinson-White syndrome, 1; conversion reaction, 2; hyperventilation, 1; migraine, 1) was made in only 5 (18%). In contrast, a diagnosis was made early in all of 27 patients tested by tilt table; 25 had neurocardiogenic syncope and 2 had conversion reaction. (Strieper MJ et al. Evaluation of recurrent pediatric syncope: Role of tilt table testing. <u>Pediatrics</u> April 1994;<u>93</u>:660-662). (Reprints: Dr Margaret J Strieper, 98-1955 Hapaki St, Aiea, HI 96701).

COMMENT. The extensive workup currently employed, including EEG, CT, MRI, ECG, echocardiogram, blood chemistries, and thyroid function, etc, is not routinely indicated in syncopal pediatric patients with a history consistent with neurocardiogenic syncope.

Tilt table testing performed early in the evaluation increases the frequency of a definitive diagnosis, and avoids the inconvenience and expense of further extensive investigations.

Neurocardiogenic syncope, the most common explanation for recurrent syncope in children, is characterized by a prodrome of nausea, pallor, diaphoresis, and blurred vision followed by syncope. Head-up tilt table testing reproduces the effects of gravity during ECG and blood pressure monitoring and uncovers autonomic dysfunction in patients with susceptibility to syncopal episodes. -Editor. *Ped Neur Briefs* April 1994.

CHAPTER 12

CNS TRAUMA

OVERVIEW OF RECENT ADVANCES

Post-head injury functional limitations and complications, eg headaches, hyperactive behavior, are correlated with the severity of the injury and pre-injury health status. Children with a history of chronic ill-health or a loss of consciousness have a greater frequency of post-concussive symptoms. Inappropriate discharge instructions for young athletes hospitalized for concussion are a common occurrence, and guidelines are suggested. Sports injuries include vertebral artery stroke following neck trauma sustained in football and other activities, both in boys and girls. (see Chap 11, pp 448-450 for articles on trauma related vertebral artery dissection).

Infants and toddlers may sustain head injury and serious sequelae, including epidural hematoma, as a result of prenatal maternal trauma, amniocentesis, and falls, especially when placed in car seats on vibrating elevated surfaces, such as washing machines. Fathers, boyfriends, and female baby-sitters are the most common perpetrators of abusive head trauma to infants and children. Non-accidental head injury ("shaken baby syndrome") remains the leading cause of death or long-term disability among child abuse cases. Mild trauma is often mistaken for feeding problems or colic. Long-term outcome after severe brain injury in preschoolers is worse than expected after initial satisfactory recovery. A normal CT after head injury is predictive of a good prognosis and a lack of subsequent deterioration. Laceration and retraction of the dura are the reasons for enlarging, non-healing, skull fractures.

Mild head injury, not sufficient to require admission, may result in cognitive deficits and dyslexia, which is contrary to some previous reports. Hyperactive behavior following head injury may be significant and worthy of careful follow-up. Dyscalculia and dyslexia in adolescence after right hemisphere injury in infancy is explained by an acquired left parietal dysfunction caused by competition for left hemisphere representation between verbal and visuospatial functions. Early interhemispheric transfer of right parietal function and skills to the left parietal lobe may be documented by a functional MRI showing left hemisphere activation during calculation tests. (*see also* Chapter 4).

J. Gordon Millichap, M.D., Editor.

POST-HEAD INJURY FUNCTIONAL DEFICITS

The functional outcome in 95 children (aged 5 to 15) at 1 year after hospitalization for head injury was evaluated at the Johns Hopkins University, School of Hygiene and Public Health, Baltimore, MD. More than half of all injuries were motor vehicle related: 21% pedestrians, 18% passengers, and 17% bicycles. Lower extremity injuries were sustained in 20. Severity of head injury was determined using the Abbreviated

Injury Scale (AIS 2-5) and the Glasgow Coma Scale (GCS 3-15). GCS were highly correlated with AIS severity. Chronic health problems pre-dating the injury were reported in 23%; these were minor in 15%, and major (mental retardation, seizures, lead poisoning) in 8%. After controlling for head injury severity, poorer outcomes were associated with poverty, preinjury chronic health problems, and lower extremity injuries. At 1 year follow-up, 55% had one or more health problems: headaches in 32%, limb or peripheral nerve disorders (13%), weakness or ataxia (7%), and vision, hearing, or speech disorder (6%). The presence of functional limitations in physical activity (31%) or self-care mobility (19%) was associated especially with severe head injuries (AIS 5), but those with AIS 2-4 were not spared at least one limitation. Hyperactive behavior was directly correlated with head injury severity, and head-injured children had a greater number of behavioral problems at 1 year follow-up when compared with a randomly selected sample of children, ages 6 to 16 years. (Greenspan AI, MacKenzie EJ. Functional outcome after pediatric head injury. <u>Pediatrics</u> October 1994;94:425-432). (Reprints: Dr Arlene I Greenspan, National Center for Injury Prevention and Control, Centers for Disease Control and Prevention, 4770 Buford Highway, NE, Mailstop F-41, Chamblee, GA 30341).

COMMENT. In children who sustain head injury, the severity of the injury is correlated with pre-injury health status, and even those with minor injuries have a greater incidence of chronic health problems than the general population. The risk of post-injury functional limitations was increased in children with a history of chronic ill-health and those who sustained lower extremity injuries. Evidence of cognitive, physical, or behavioral dysfunction requires intervention and rehabilitation.

The frequency of postconcussive symptoms in 41 children (ages 6-12) with traumatic brain injury (TBI) was evaluated at the Dept of Psychology, Case Western Reserve University, Cleveland, OH. Compared to 40 controls with orthopedic injuries only, those with TBI had more postconcussive symptoms both at baseline and at 6 month follow-up. The number of symptoms was related to injury severity and initial loss of consciousness (GCS <9), Nonverbal IQ, and the baseline Children's Depression Inventory. (Barry CT, Klein SK, Taylor HG. Validity of postconcussive symptoms in children with traumatic brain injury. <u>Ann Neurol</u> Sept 1994;36:519 [abstr]). -Editor. *Ped Neur Briefs* Oct 1994.

EPIDURAL HEMATOMA AND ACCIDENTAL INJURY

A 7-month-old infant who suffered a fall from a washing machine and sustained a frontal epidural hematoma is reported from the Division of Neurosurgery, Oregon Health Sciences University. The infant had been placed on an engaged washing machine strapped in his car seat and left unattended. Within 2 hours of the fall, the infant became more irritable, vomited, was listless, and had a generalized seizure. CT showed a fracture of the skull and a epidural hematoma. He was discharged on postoperative day 3, and his development at 13 month of age was normal. Awareness of the potential consequences of this apparently popular and physician-endorsed child-consoling practice is important for physicians who must distinguish accident from abuse. (Hulka F, Piatt J. An infant in a car seat on a washing machine: epidural hematoma. <u>Pediatrics</u> October 1994;94:556-557).

COMMENT. Placement of infants in car seats on vibrating elevated surfaces might have a desired soporific effect but the practice carries the risk of falls and serious head injury. More than two-thirds of brain injuries in infants are attributable to falls, and epidural hematomas occur in 3%. (<u>Ped Neur Briefs</u> Sept 1992). The rule that children falling from elevated household surfaces do not sustain serious injuries does not apply when an infant is buckled into a car seat. Righting reflexes are vitiated and the weight of the car seat adds to the impact.

Brain injury due to amniocentesis is reported in 4 children with hemiparesis and porencephalic cysts evaluated at Bowman Gray School of Medicine, Winston-Salem, NC. (Kandt RS, DeLong GR. <u>Ann Neurol</u> Sept 1994;36:516 [abstr]). -Editor. *Ped Neur Briefs* Oct 1994.

MANAGEMENT OF CONCUSSION IN YOUNG ATHLETES

The discharge instructions received by youth athletes hospitalized for a sports-related closed head injury over a 5-year period (1987-1991) were examined at the Children's Hospital and University of Alabama, Birmingham, AL. Injury severity was graded according to Cantu's 1986 guidelines and compared to the Colorado Medical Society guidelines as endorsed by the American Academy of Pediatrics. Concussions were grade 1 (least severe) in 8 patients (24%), grade 2 in 10 (30%), and grade 3 (most severe) in 15 (45%). Discharge instructions were inappropriate and not in compliance with guidelines in 8 of 10 patients with grade 2, and in all of 15 with grade 3 concussions. The majority had uneventful hospital courses, but most received inadequate counseling regarding potential future risk. Of 23 for whom instructions were inadequate, 3 were allowed to return to sports participation too quickly, and no instructions were documented for 20 (87%) patients. (Genuardi FJ, King WD. Inappropriate discharge instructions for youth athletes hospitalized for concussion. <u>Pediatrics</u> February 1995;95:216-218).

(Reprints: Dr FJ Genuardi, University of Florida Health Science Center, Dept of Pediatrics, 653-1 W 8th St, Jacksonville, FL 32209).

COMMENT. Lack of familiarity with guidelines for the management of concussion in sports-related head injuries was one explanation for the frequency of inappropriate discharge instructions. The Colorado Medical Society guidelines are summarized as follows:
• Grade 1. Confusion without amnesia or loss of consciousness. Return to sport permitted after 20 minutes, if no symptoms at rest or on exertion.

• Grade 2. Confusion with amnesia but no loss of consciousness. Observe 24 hours. Return permitted after 1 week without symptoms.
• Grade 3. Any loss of consciousness. Admit if neuro exam abnormal. Return permitted after 1 month, if asymptomatic for past 2 weeks.

Football accounted for 55%, baseball 12%, soccer 6%, and wrestling 3% of injuries in the above study. Documentation of discharge instructions is important for medico-legal reasons. -Editor. *Ped Neur Briefs* Feb 1995.

PERPETRATORS OF ABUSIVE HEAD TRAUMA

The identity of abusers and their relationship to victims was studied by reviewing medical charts of 151 head injured children, aged 24 months or younger, seen at the Children's Hospital, Denver, CO from Jan 1982 - Jan 1994. All infants had documented intracranial bleeding and other injuries. Male infants were abused more frequently than female (60% v 40%); and 23% died. Male perpetrators outnumbered females 2.2:1. Fathers and boyfriends were the most common perpetrators: 37% and 20%, respectively. From 1989 to 1993, the percentage of infants abused by men nearly doubled. Female baby-sitters were a large, previously unrecognized group of perpetrators, accounting for 17%. Mothers were responsible for only 12%. (Starling SP et al. Abusive head trauma: The relationship of perpetrators to their victims. <u>Pediatrics</u> February 1995;95:259-262). (Reprints: Dr SP Starling, The Children's Hospital, B-138, 1056 East 19th Ave, Denver, CO 80218).

COMMENT. These findings should focus attention on baby-sitters as a previously unrecognized group of abusers. Despite an increase in support services and media publicity, non-accidental head injury ("shaken baby syndrome") remains the leading cause of death or long-term disability among child abuse cases. Subtle or mild trauma is particularly difficult to diagnose, often mistaken for viral illness, feeding problems, or infant colic. Shaking injuries are rare after the second year. The most common age for whiplash abuse is 5 months, when the head is large in relation to the body, and the neck muscles and head control are weak. (Brown JK, Minns RA, 1993). See <u>Progress in Pediatric Neurology II</u>, Chicago, PNB Publ, 1994. pp387-396, for an overview of head injury in children by Dr J Keith Brown, Edinburgh, and various recent articles and editorial commentaries. -Editor. *Ped Neur Briefs* Feb 1995.

LONG-TERM OUTCOME AFTER SEVERE BRAIN INJURY

The outcome in adulthood of severe brain injury in 39 preschoolers, aged 7 years or less, was evaluated at the Kauniala Hospital for Disabled War Veterans, the Rehabilitation Centre of Insurance Companies, Kauniainen, and the University of Helsinki, Finland. Twenty three (59%) attended a typical school, 8 (21%) attended a school for the physically disabled, and 7 (18%) attended school for the mentally retarded. In adulthood, 9 patients (23%) worked full-time, 10 (26%) worked at sheltered work-places, 14 (36%) lived independently at home, and 6 (15%) needed physical or psychological support. Of the 23 who attended a normal school in childhood, only 9 were capable of full-time work as adults. A sense of identity was the best indicator of final outcome. (Koskiniemi M et al. Long-term outcome after severe brain injury in preschoolers is worse than expected. <u>Arch Pediatr Adolesc Med</u> March 1995;149:249-254). (Respond: Mr Taina Nybo, Kauniala Hospital for Disabled War Veterans, 02700 Kauniainen, Finland).

COMMENT. The long-term outcome was worse than expected from initial recovery or by school achievement. One-half the patients with severe brain injury in early childhood attended normal school, but only one-fourth could work full-time as adults. The authors stress the importance of providing the brain-injured child with a firm identity. -Editor. *Ped Neur Briefs* April 1995.

CEREBRAL BLOOD FLOW STUDIES IN SEVERE HEAD INJURY

The results of 151 serial measurements of cerebral blood flow, arteriojugular venous oxygen difference, and cerebral metabolic rate for oxygen performed in 21 children with severe head injury are reported from the Bristol Hospital for Sick Children, UK. Cerebral hyperemia was uncommon, occurring in only 10 (7%) of the blood flow measurements. Cerebral blood flow was inversely correlated with intracranial pressure. Cerebral metabolic rate was initially normal in 81% of children, but both metabolic rate and AV oxygen difference fell significantly between the first and third days after injury. Children with head injury are most at risk of sustaining ischemic brain damage in the first few hours after injury when cerebral metabolic rate and cerebral oxygen extraction are maximal. (Sharples PM et al. Cerebral blood flow and metabolism in children with severe head injury. Part 1: relation to age, Glasgow coma score, outcome, intracranial pressure, and time after injury. <u>J Neurol Neurosurg Psychiatry</u> Feb 1995;58:145-152). (Respond: Dr PM Sharples, Institute of Child Health, Bristol Hospital for Sick Children, St Michael's Hill, Bristol BS2 8BJ, UK).

COMMENT. In Part 2 of the above study, the authors measured cerebrovascular resistance in 17 children with severe head injuries. Values were normal or raised in most cases. Cerebrovascular resistance was correlated with cerebral perfusion pressure, except in 4 of 5 most severely injured patients who died or survived with major handicap.

The pathophysiology of traumatic encephalopathy in children is similar to that in adults. Normal autoregulatory mechanisms are preserved in most children with head injury, but pressure autoregulation may be disturbed in those with very severe injury. The adequacy of cerebral blood flow for cerebral metabolic demands should be closely monitored by continuous jugular oxygen saturation measurement in the severely injured patients. (Sharples PM, Matthews DSF, Eyre JA. Cerebral blood flow and metabolism in children with severe head injuries. Part 2: cerebrovascular resistance and its determinants. <u>J Neurol Neurosurg Psychiatry</u> Feb 1995;58:153-159).

A normal CT scan after mild head injury predicts a good prognosis and lack of subsequent deterioration requiring neurosurgical intervention, according to a study of 400 brain injured children reported from the University of Washington, Seattle. (Davis RL et al. The use of cranial CT scans in the triage of pediatric patients with mild head injury. <u>Pediatrics</u> March 1995;95:345-349). -Editor. *Ped Neur Briefs* April 1995.

ENLARGING SKULL FRACTURES

The diagnosis, management, and treatment of large unhealed skull fractures are reported in 10 children, aged 2 weeks to 27 months, seen at the Children's National Medical Center, Washington, DC in a 4 year period. The parietal bone was involved, and an underlying cortical contusion was associated with a contralateral hemiparesis. Five (50%) had post-traumatic seizures, and 4 (40%) had mild hydrocephalus and porencephaly. The fractures enlarged in 8 preoperatively. At surgical repair, 1-11 months after injury, the lacerated dura was retracted beneath the fracture edge and grafted, and a cranioplasty or transposition of adjacent bone with normal dura was performed. A shunt was placed in those with hydrocephalus. None had formed a leptomeningeal cyst at the site of the fracture. Enlargement of the fracture was not caused by erosion but by expansion of the skull to accommodate growing brain or increased pressure. The diagnosis was made clinically, without need for serial skull X-rays. (Johnson DL, Helman T. Enlarging skull fractures in children. <u>Child's Nerv Syst</u> May 1995;11:265-268). (Respond: Dr DL Johnson, Division of Neurosurgery, Milton S Hershey Medical Center, PO Box 850, Hershey, PA 17033).

COMMENT. Laceration and retraction of the dura, the tissue needed for osteoplastic repair, are the reasons for the failure of the fracture to heal. The fracture widens as the skull expands with growth or the result of pressure of the uncontained brain, apparently not because of cyst formation, the most widely accepted theory.

Mortality from head injury. In Geneva, Switzerland, the mortality from head injuries in children has decreased progressively during the last quarter century from 10.4/100,000 to 3.5/100,000 annually, according to a study at the University Hospital (Berney J et al. Head injuries in children: a chronicle of a quarter of a century. <u>Child's Nerv Syst</u> May 1995;11:256-264). Better organization and management and a drop in severe cases due to less traffic accidents accounted for the improved statistics. The number of children handicapped by head injury was unchanged, however, indicating a need for prevention. -Editor. *Ped Neur Briefs* July 1995.

MILD HEAD INJURY AND COGNITIVE DEFICIT

The effect of mild head injury in 78 preschool children on their cognitive performance, especially reading ability, evaluated one year after injury and at 6.5 years of age was investigated at the Department of Neurosurgery, Auckland Hospital, New Zealand. Compared to a control group with minor injury not involving the head, head injured preschoolers showed impairment of interpretation of visual puzzles, a visual closure test, and increased incidence of reading difficulties at 6 and 12 months after injury and at age 6.5 years. Another head injury occurred within 6 months in 14% of the head injured group compared to <1% of the control group. Reading ability was correlated with the scores on visual closure at one year after injury. (Wrightson P et al. Mild head injury in preschool children: evidence that it can be associated with a persisting cognitive defect. <u>J Neurol Neurosurg</u>

<u>Psychiatry</u> October 1995;59:375-380). (Respond: Mr Philip Wrightson, 18 Crocus Place, Remuera, Auckland 1005, New Zealand).

COMMENT. Mild head injury, not sufficient to require admission for observation, may result in cognitive deficits and impairment of reading and school performance. In this study, the development of visual skills necessary for reading appeared to be interrupted by the injury.

In a previous report reviewed in <u>Progress in Pediatric Neurology I</u>, (PNB Publishers, 1991, p408), mild head injury in 114 school aged children did not have an adverse effect on global measures of cognition and achievement at one to five years after injury. Children with head injuries were indistinguishable from uninjured children on all tests except the teachers' report of hyperactivity which was 4/10 of a standard deviation higher. (Bijur PE et al. <u>Pediatrics</u> 1990;86:337). Hyperactivity noted after head injury might be significant and worthy of careful follow-up and management. -Editor. *Ped Neur Briefs* Nov 1995.

BRAIN INJURY IN INFANCY AND LEARNING DISABILITIES

Dyscalculia and dyslexia in a 17-year-old boy after right hemisphere injury in infancy is reported from the Division of Neurosurgery and Department of Pediatrics, University of Maryland, Baltimore; and Cognitive Neuroscience Section, National Institutes of Health, Bethesda, MD. Social behavior was normal, but math and spelling abilities were impaired and his attention span was short. A functional MRI showed predominantly left hemisphere activation involving frontal and posterior parietal regions while the patient performed calculations. In normal subjects this test produced bilateral activation of the supramarginal gyrus. These MRI findings were consistent with early interhemisperic transfer of right parietal visuospatial skills to the left parietal region. Dyscalculia and dyslexia with normal IQ suggest an acquired left parietal dysfunction caused by competition for left hemisphere representation between verbal and visuospatial functions. (Levin HS et al. Dyscalculia and dyslexia after right hemisphere injury in infancy. <u>Arch Neurol</u> Jan 1996;53:88-96). (Reprints: Dr Grafman, Cognitive Neuroscience Section, NIH/NINDS/MNB, Bldg 10, Room 5S 209, 10 Center Dr, MSC 1440, Bethesda, MD 20892).

COMMENT. The authors conclude that interhemispheric reorganization of function and language may be bidirectional and not only a left hemisphere feature of language development. The MRI showed an intact left hemisphere following the injury. Visuospatial functions normally subserved by the right parietal area were probably transferred to the left parietal region, causing a crowding effect and disproportionate impairment of reading and math skills in relation to his other cognitive abilities. -Editor. *Ped Neur Briefs* March 1996.

FETAL CNS DAMAGE WITH MATERNAL PRENATAL TRAUMA

The neurologic findings in nine infants who were exposed to maternal trauma during pregnancy are reported from the University Hospital Essen, Hufelandstr, Germany. Motor-vehicle accidents occurred in 7 and blunt abdominal trauma in 2. One infant required resuscitation and one premature needed assisted ventilation. Movement disorders occurred in 3, hemiparesis in 2, convulsions (1), and 3 were normal. Neuroimaging showed periventricular leukomalacia in 2, localized vascular infarction in 2, hemorrhage (1), hydrocephalus (2), and diffuse brain damage (1). The relation of the cerebral damage to the maternal trauma was certain in one child and probable in the remainder. (Baethmann M, Kahn T, Lenard H-G, Voit T. Fetal CNS damage after exposure to maternal trauma during pregnancy. <u>Acta Paediatr</u> Nov 1996;85:1331-1338). (Respond: Dr Martina Baethmann, Department of Pediatrics, University Hospital Essen, Hufelandstr, 55, 45122, Essen, Germany).

COMMENT. Maternal trauma during pregnancy may result in fetal cerebral damage that manifests with neurologic symptoms in surviving infants. Mothers should be examined carefully for signs of premature labor after trauma, and the newborn infant monitored for neurologic damage. Maternal acidosis is found to correlate with severity of fetal damage and mortality. -Editor. *Ped Neur Briefs* Dec 1996.

CHAPTER **13**

INFECTIOUS DISORDERS

INTRODUCTION

Charles N. Swisher, M.D.
Division of Neurology,
Children's Memorial Hospital,
Northwestern University Medical School, Chicago, IL.

The years 1994 through 1996 have been notable in the area of infectious disease affecting the developing nervous system, primarily by the continuing successes of vaccine prophylaxis for bacterial meningitis and the new promise of antiviral agents against the continuing challenge of CNS AIDS.

Prophylaxis continues to provide a dramatic reduction of bacterial meningitis frequency in infancy, with the considerable effectiveness of early immunization against H. influenzae meningitis. The common occurrence of this meningitis on the pediatric inpatient service is now almost an historical recollection. Pediatric residents are less challenged by the likelihood of meningitis in the febrile, irritable child, although streptococcal, pneumococcal, and other forms of meningitis still are cause for continued concern and vaccine research.

The most exciting infectious disease development occurring in 1996 was clearly the clinical success of the protease inhibitors in the treatment of AIDS. In replication of the AIDS virus, viral RNA is transcribed into DNA via the reverse transcriptase enzyme. Inhibition of this enzyme is achieved by AZT and similar drugs, but the developing resistance of the HIV to this therapeutic approach alone has led to inevitable demise in HIV+ patients.

The recent clinical introduction of the protease inhibitors, which block the effective site of the protease, has resulted in dramatic reductions in AIDS mortality. The protease inhibitor, taken together with two inhibitors of reverse transcriptase, can reduce blood concentrations of HIV to undetectable levels.[1] An earlier development in 1995 was the observation that HIV+ mothers treated with AZT during gestation gave birth to fewer HIV+ infants. Untreated mothers have a 25% incidence of affected children, while treated mothers have an 8% incidence of HIV+ infants. These two developments will do much to reduce the frequency of the devastating progressive encephalopathy of pediatric HIV positive and AIDS patients.

Despite these dramatic improvements in specific prophylaxis and treatment, the world pattern of infectious diseases affecting the developing nervous system reflects the reality of social and economic imbalance amongst the world's children. The incidence of tuberculous meningitis, while a rarity in the western hemisphere, is a major problem of management in India, as described by our colleagues at the International Child Neurology Association meeting in 1994.[2] However, tuberculosis is not a rarity in developed nations. In the United States, reported cases of tuberculosis have risen 20% in the years 1985 to 1992, indicating public health problems unrelated to availability of current knowledge of tuberculosis prophylaxis and treatment.[3]

The improvements in therapy for AIDS encephalopathy have been associated with a greater understanding of the pathophysiology of the infection. There has been a clear recognition of apoptotic neurons present in the brains of children dying of AIDS.[4] Imaging studies have aided in our understanding of the pathophysiology as well. Reports of a large series of CT-scans have clarified criteria for early diagnosis of HIV encephalopathy.[5]

Since its development in 1991, the polymerase chain reaction (PCR) has been established as the best available method for the early diagnosis of herpes simplex encephalitis.[6] PCR is also reported of value in the diagnosis of cytomegalovirus, M. tuberculosis, and Toxoplasma gondii infections. The availability of PCR testing and subsequent early identification and aggressive treatment of neonates with congenital toxoplasmosis has resulted in a much more optimistic outcome, even for those infants with frank neonatal infection with intracranial involvement.[7]

The years 1994 through 1996 have therefore produced exciting developments and sophisticated approaches to the treatment of devastating viral infections. At the same time, however, there is a continuing limited opportunity to utilize well-established prophylaxis and treatment methods world-wide, because of ongoing economic, political and social barriers. *Charles N. Swisher, M.D.*

BIBLIOGRAPHY

1. Balter, M. Breakthrough of the year. Science 1996;274:1987.
2. Cantwell MF et al. JAMA 1994;272:535-539.
3. Udani PM. Tuberculosis in the 1990s. ICNS Meeting, 1994.
4. Gelbard HA et al. Ann Neurol CNS Meeting Abstr. Oct 1994.
5. DeCarli C et al. Ann Neurol 1993:34:198-205.
6. Schlesinger Y et al. J Pediatr 1995;126:234.
7. Swisher CN et al. Seminars in Pediatr Neurol. 1994;1:4-25.

LYME DISEASE NEUROLOGIC SYNDROMES

The neurologic manifestations and syndromes associated with Lyme disease are reported in 96 patients, ages 3 to 19 years, living on Long Island and referred to University Hospital, Stony Brook, New York. All were seropositive for anti-*B burgdorferi* antibodies. One-third had no prior history of extraneural manifestations of Lyme disease (erythema migrans, arthritis, flulike symptoms, and arthralgias/myalgias), and 90% had no memory of a tick bite. The most frequent neurologic symptom was headache (in 71%), and the most common sign was facial palsy (14%). Sleep disturbance was reported in 7%, papilledema was present in 6%, diplopia in 2%, and 1 had a Guillain-Barre-like syndrome with a CSF protein of 231 mg/dL. Elevations in CSF protein (32-58 mg/dL) were found in 25 of 53 patients examined, and a mild lymphocytic pleocytosis in 15. Neurologic syndromes included encephalopathy, lymphocytic meningitis, cranial neuropathy, and pseudotumor cerebri. (Belman AL et al. Neurologic manifestations in children with North American Lyme disease. <u>Neurology</u> Dec 1993;<u>43</u>:2609-2614). (Reprints: Dr AL Belman, Department of Neurology, HSC T-12-020, SUNY at Stony Brook, Stony Brook, NY 11794).

COMMENT. The clinical course of Lyme disease in most children in this study was milder and shorter than that reported for adults, and meningoradiculitis (Bannwarth's syndrome) and peripheral neuropathy syndromes were rare. A pseudotumor cerebri syndrome appears to be unique to childhood Lyme disease. A first report of stroke caused by Lyme disease in North America involved a woman of 56 years (Reik L, Jr. <u>Neurology</u> Dec 1993;<u>43</u>:2705-2707). -Editor. *Ped Neur Briefs* Jan 1994.

NEUROLOGIC SIGNS OF LYME DISEASE

Clinical manifestations of Lyme disease (LD) in 97 seropositive children were reviewed at the Children's Hospital of Philadelphia, with particular attention to neurologic symptoms and signs. Of 69 children with LD, 22 (32%) had new neurologic abnormalities, mainly facial palsy and aseptic meningitis. Only 27% of children with neurologic abnormalities due to LD had a history of erythema migrans or arthritis. Seropositivity for LD and neurologic symptoms usually indicates an active neuroborreliosis. (Bingham PM et al. Neurologic manifestations in children with Lyme disease. <u>Pediatrics</u> Dec 1995;96:1053-1056). (Respond: Dr Peter M Bingham, Division of Neurology, Children's Hospital of Philadelphia, 34th Street and Civic Center Blvd, Philadelphia, PA 19104).

COMMENT. Definite evidence for neuroborreliosis requires characteristic neurologic abnormalities and either erythema migrans, arthritis or heart involvement, positive spinal fluid serology, or seroconversion. Peripheral neuropathy is infrequent in children compared to adults. Facial palsy and aseptic meningitis are the most frequent neurologic manifestations of LD in children. In the approaching summer months, children presenting with these disorders should be checked for possible Lyme disease. -Editor. *Ped Neur Briefs* May 1996.

SHIGELLOSIS FEBRILE STATUS EPILEPTICUS

A 4-year-old boy who became blind, deaf and mute after status epilepticus caused by hyperpyrexia from shigellosis is reported from the Sophia Children's Hospital, Rotterdam, The Netherlands. Hyperpyrexia and diarrhea developed 2 days after eating tainted Chinese food at a family feast. Stool cultures grew *Shigella flexneri*. CT showed cerebral swelling. He had several generalized tonic clonic seizures followed by status and prolonged coma. On day 9 he opened his eyes and localized painful stimuli. He was blind, deaf and mute. Vision and hearing recovered within 6 months but expressive language impairment was more persistent. At 4 year follow-up he could repeat simple sentences and speech was more fluent. A "disconnection syndrome" was proposed to explain the language deficit. (van Dongen HR et al. Blind, deaf and mute after a status epilepticus caused by hyperpyrexia from shigellosis - a case report with a four-year follow-up. <u>Neuropediatrics</u> Dec 1993;<u>24</u>:343-345). (Respond: Dr HR van Dongen, Dept of Child Neurology, Sophia Children's Hospital, 40 Dr Molewaterplein, 3015 GD Rotterdam, The Netherlands).

COMMENT. Shigellae are chiefly waterborne, and foods were incriminated in only 8 of 366 outbreaks in one report, the organism spread by fecal contamination and improper food handling. (<u>Environmental Poisons in Our Food.</u> Millichap JG, PNB Publishers, 1993). Children under 10 years of age are at greatest risk, and a neurotoxin produced by *Shigella shiga* has been implicated as a possible convulsive agent. The incidence of febrile convulsions with shigellosis is as high as 45% in some reports, whereas shigella-negative diarrheas cause convulsions in less than 2%. The incidence is independent of the species of Shigella that include Flexner and Sonne, dysenteries not associated with neurotoxin formation. (Millichap JG. <u>Febrile Convulsions.</u> New York, Macmillan, 1968).

Kluver-Bucy syndrome with Shigella encephalopathy. A reversible case of Kluver-Bucy syndrome in a 7-year-old child suffering from *Shigella flexneri* encephalopathy is reported from the Hebrew Univ of Jerusalem, Israel. (Guedalia JSB et al. <u>J Child Neurol</u> 1993;<u>8</u>:313-315). He was apathetic, his affect was dull, he did not recognize common objects or his relatives, he touched and placed objects in his mouth impulsively, and he exhibited an insatiable appetite and signs of bulimia. Hypermetamorphosis, a tendency to be distracted by minute visual stimuli, was questionable, and abnormal sexual behavior was absent. The patient showed 4 of the 6 classical signs of the K-B syndrome, a rare occurrence in children, and recovery was previously unreported. -Editor. *Ped Neur ⬚Briefs* Feb 1994.

HERPESVIRUS-6 INFECTION AND FEBRILE SEIZURES

For articles on herpesvirus-6 infection, roseola infantum, and febrile seizures, *see* Chapter 1, pp 24-28.

CAMPYLOBACTER JEJUNI INFECTION AND GUILLAIN-BARRE SYNDROME

For articles on the role of *Campylobacter jejuni* infection in Guillain-Barre syndrome and Chinese paralytic syndrome, *see* Chapter 6, pp 353-4.

HELICOBACTER PYLORI INFECTION AND BRAIN DYSFUNCTION

Helicobacter pylori infection was identified in 5 children with severe neurologic impairment who underwent upper gi endoscopy at the Alfred I duPont Institute, Wilmington, De, and Jefferson Medical College, Philadelphia. Subsequently, patients with severe neurologic impairments, such as cerebral palsy and head trauma, who had endoscopies because of gastrointestinal symptoms were examined for *H. pylori* infection in gastric antral mucosa biopsies. Of 61 examined, 7 (11%) were positive for infection and had gastritis. Institutionalized patients were at much greater risk of infection than those seen as outpatients (75% cf 7%). Resolution of gi symptoms (emesis, guiac-positive stools, refusal to eat, and irritability during feedings) was complete in 6 of the 12 infected patients and partial in 4 after antibiotic treatment. (Proujansky R et al. Symptomatic *Helicobacter pylori* infection in young patients with severe neurologic impairment. <u>J Pediatr</u> Nov 1994;125:750-752). (Reprints: Roy Proujansky MD, Alfred I duPont Institute, 1600 Rockland Rd, Wilmington, DE 19899).

COMMENT. All neurologically impaired, and especially institutionalized, children with persistent gastrointestinal symptoms should be examined and treated when positive for *H. pylori* infection.

A possible *H. pylori* infection should be considered in children with epilepsy who develop gastritis and feeding difficulties after long-term treatment with valproic acid, divalproex sodium, and other antiepileptic drugs. (see <u>Progress in Pediatric Neurology I</u>, PNB Publishers, 1991). Gastritis and gastric ulceration attributed to the antiepileptic drugs may be due primarily to infection in the gastric mucosa. -Editor. *Ped Neur Briefs* Dec 1994.

E. COLI HEMOLYTIC-UREMIC SYNDROME

A retrospective analysis of 37 children with *Escherichia coli* O157:H7-associated hemolytic-uremic syndrome (HUS) traced to contaminated hamburger meat is reported from the University of Washington, Children's Hospital, Seattle. The majority (95%) had severe hemorrhagic colitis, 19 (51%) had multisystem disease, and 6 (16%) had neurological complications. Seizures occurred in 3, stroke in 3, and 3 became comatose. Three (8%) died, 1 en route to the hospital after a seizure and cardiorespiratory arrest. A poor outcome was seen in all 3 with coma, 2 of 3 with seizures, and 1 of 3 with focal neurologic abnormalities. (Brandt JR et al. *Escherichia coli* O157:H7-associated hemolytic-uremic syndrome after ingestion of contaminated hamburgers. <u>J Pediatr</u> Oct 1994;125:519-526). (Reprints: Ellis D Avner MD, Department of Nephrology, CH-46, Children's Hospital and Medical Center, 4800 Sandpoint Way NE, PO Box 5371, Seattle, WA 98105).

COMMENT. Neurologic complications of the HUS occur in 14% to 83% of previously published outbreaks.They were the most common cause of death in one report. The outbreak of E coli HUS in Seattle was a tragic reflection of the hazards of "Environmental Poisons in Our Food" (Millichap JG, PNB Publ, 1993). The importance of this topic in neurologic practice is emphasized by the inclusion of neurotoxicology symposia at the recent meeting of the Child Neurology Society and at the May 1995 annual meeting of the American Academy of Neurology in Seattle. -Editor. *Ped*

Neur Briefs Nov 1994.

PERINATAL HIV AND NEURODEVELOPMENT

The natural history of HIV disease and neurodevelopmental disorders in 21 perinatally infected children were examined in a collaborative prospective study sponsored by the National Institute of Child Health & Human Development, Rockville, MD. Bayley Scales were compared during the first 24 months of life in the infected group, in 65 seroreverted children born to HIV-infected mothers, and 95 non-HIV-infected children of non-HIV-infected mothers. Mental and motor impairments (<50) in all functional areas were present predominantly in HIV-infected children who developed AIDS in the first 2 years. These children also had small head circumferences and neurologic abnormalities. Children with AIDS manifesting only lymphoid interstitial pneumonitis showed inconsistent, mild, developmental impairments delayed in onset. HIV-infected children without AIDS and uninfected children were not developmentally impaired. (Nozyce M et al. Effect of perinatally acquired human immunodeficiency virus infection on neurodevelopment in children during the first two years of life. <u>Pediatrics</u> December 1994;94:883-891). (Reprints: Dr Anne Willoughby, Pediatric AIDS Branch, National Institute of Child Health & Human Development, National Institutes of Health, 6100 Executive Blvd, Rm 4B11, Rockville, MD 20852).

COMMENT. Children of HIV-infected mothers who develop AIDS are at very high risk for serious neurodevelopmental disorders. Those without symptoms of AIDS may develop normally but require frequent monitoring to determine need for therapy. Uninfected children of HIV-infected mothers are not affected by the viral exposure. - Editor. *Ped Neur Briefs* Dec 1994.

PERINATAL HIV ENCEPHALOPATHY

The characteristics and survival of 178 children with perinatally acquired human immunodeficiency virus (HIV) infection and encephalopathy are reported from the Centers for Disease Control and Prevention, Public Health Service, US Department of Health and Human Services, Atlanta, GA. Ten percent of HIV-infected children and 23% of children with AIDS had HIV encephalopathy that was diagnosed at a median age of 19 months. The estimated risk of HIV encephalopathy by age 1 year was 4%, and by age 4 years it was 14%. HIV encephalopathy correlated with an increased risk of cardiomyopathy, more hospitalizations, and with severe immunodeficiency. Estimated median survival after diagnosis was 22 months. (Lobato MN et al. Encephalopathy in children with perinatally acquired human immunodeficiency virus infection. <u>J Pediatr</u> May 1995;126:710-715). (Reprints: M Blake Caldwell MD, MPH, Division of HIV/AIDS, Centers for Disease Control and Prevention, 1600 Clifton Rd, MS E-45, Atlanta, GA 30333).

COMMENT. A recent American Academy of Neurology AIDS Task Force consensus report on nomenclature suggested that the term "HIV associated progressive encephalopathy of childhood" be adopted to replace AIDS encephalopathy and other terms used to describe the CNS abnormalities directly related to HIV-1 infection. (<u>Neurology</u> 1991;41:778-785). Belman AL reviews the recent advances in AIDS and the nervous system in <u>Progress in Pediatric Neurology II</u> (Millichap JG, Ed. PNB Publishers, 1994, pp397-400). -Editor. *Ped Neur Briefs* June 1995.

EFFECTS OF HIV ON COGNITIVE AND MOTOR DEVELOPMENT

The cognitive and motor development of 126 infants born to nondrug-using,HIV-seropositive Haitian women, assessed at 3-month intervals from birth to 24 months, is reported from the University of Miami School of Medicine, FL. By 18 months of age, 28 were HIV-infected, and these infants were compared to 98 uninfected infants used as controls. The mean mental and motor scores on the Bayley Scales of Infant Development were significantly lower for infected compared to uninfected controls. Initial differences between the two groups, noted at 3 months, increased over time. Cognitive development was within normal levels in one third of infected infants, despite low mean scores for the group, and motor development was normal in one half. (Gay CL, Armstrong FD et al. The effects of HIV on cognitive and motor development in children born to HIV-seropositive women with no reported drug use: Birth to 24 months. <u>Pediatrics</u> Dec 1995;96:1078-1082). (Respond: Dr F Daniel Armstrong, Department of Pediatrics-R131, Box 016960, Miami, FL 33101).

COMMENT. Infants perinatally infected with HIV are at risk of cognitive and motor delays in the first two years of life. Visual-motor integration, processing speed, verbal memory, and other neuropsychological measures, not tested in infants and toddlers, may be uncovered at later follow-up.

Cytomegalovirus encephalitis with AIDS has been studied in 7 adults treated at the Department of Neurology, Northwestern University Medical School, Chicago (Cohen BA. <u>Neurology</u> Feb 1996;46:444-450). Retrospective series showed a poor prognosis with rapid mortality, whereas 4 of the 7 patients diagnosed and treated responded to therapy. Polymerase chain reaction amplification of cytomegalovirus DNA allowed detection in CSF, specific for CNS infection. -Editor. *Ped Neur Briefs* May 1996.

For further articles on HIV infection, learning, and neurodevelopment, *see* Chapter 4, pp 282-286.

CONGENITAL TOXOPLASMOSIS: TREATMENT AND OUTCOME

Neurologic, cognitive, and motor outcomes for 36 children with congenital toxoplasmosis treated with pyrimethamine and sulfadiazine for 1 year are reported from Michael Reese Hospital, Chicago, IL, and other Centers. Active infection, seizures, and motor abnormalities resolved in most during therapy. Of 29 infants evaluated at 1 year of age, 23 (79%) had a

Mental Developmental Index of 102, and 6 had scores
<50. Sibling controls had higher scores than patients,
but sequential IQ testing showed no deterioration over
time. Six of eight children with obstructive
hydrocephalus relieved by shunts had normal
neurologic and developmental outcomes. In contrast, of
10 with hydrocephalus ex vacuo from birth, eight had
severe disabilities. Nine of 34 (26%) children had
microcephaly. Of those presenting with chorioretinal
lesions (69%), the majority had residual visual loss after
therapy. Risk factors for poor outcome included
diabetes insipidus, hypoxia, hydrocephalus with high
CSF protein, and delay in medical treatment. These
results compared to previous reports for untreated
children were thought to justify treatment of pregnant
women with acute gestational Toxoplasma infection and
young infants with congenital toxoplasmosis. (Roizen
N, Swisher CN et al. Neurologic and developmental
outcome in treated congenital toxoplasmosis. <u>Pediatrics</u>
January 1995;95:11-20). (Reprints: Dr Rima McLeod, 114
Baumgarten, Department of Medicine, Michael Reese Hospital,
2929 South Ellis Ave, Chicago, IL 60616).

COMMENT. One third of the treated patients were
severely impaired neurologically, and two thirds of
those with normal developmental outcomes had retinal
lesions and visual problems. The need for prevention
and improved therapies was emphasized. -Editor. *Ped
Neur Briefs* Jan 1995.

BACTERIAL MENINGITIS OUTCOME

The neurologic, psychological, and educational
outcomes of bacterial meningitis in 130 children
evaluated at a mean age of 8 years, and 6 years after
their meningitis, are reported from the Department of
Paediatrics and Clinical Epidemiology and Biostatistics
Unit, University of Melbourne, and the Royal Children's
Hospital, Victoria, Australia. Compared to controls,
children with meningitis as a group were at greater
risk (26.9%) for abnormal neurologic and audiologic
sequelae, had lower IQs and neuropsychologic

performance, and behavior and adaptive difficulties at school. Eleven (8.5%) had major deficits (IQ <70, seizures, hydrocephalus, spasticity, blindness, or severe to profound hearing loss); and 24 (18.5%) patients compared to 14 (10.8%) controls had minor deficits (IQ 70-80, inability to read, some hearing loss, speech problems, and behavior disorders). Those who suffered acute neurologic symptoms with the meningitis had a poorer outcome than those with uncomplicated meningitis or controls (39% vs 18% vs 11%). (Grimwood K, et al. Adverse outcomes of bacterial meningitis in school-age survivors. <u>Pediatrics</u> May 1995;95:646-656). (Reprints: Dr Keith Grimwood, Royal Children's Hospital, Parkville, Victoria 3052, Australia).

COMMENT. Even with optimal treatment, one in four children who recover from meningitis may have severe or functionally significant disabilities which affect academic performance. The poor outcome is not restricted to those having acute neurologic complications. All children recovering from meningitis should be followed carefully until school age to exclude learning, hearing, and neurologic disorders that may require treatment. -Editor. *Ped Neur Briefs* June 1995.

ACUTE NECROTIZING ENCEPHALOPATHY

The clinicopathological features of an acute necrotizing encephalopathy are described in a review of 13 consecutive children treated and 28 previously reported cases seen at various institutions in Japan. The onset was preceded by an upper respiratory infection, frequently treated with antipyretics and antibiotics. Aspirin was taken by only 2 patients. Symptoms of brain dysfunction, including impaired consciousness, convulsions, and vomiting, developed rapidly within 1 to 3 days. One third had hematemesis, one half had diarrhea, and all had liver enlargement without clinical jaundice. Hyperpyrexia, hyperventilation, and decorticate or decerebrate posturing occurred at the comatose stage. Twenty eight per cent died. In survivors, recovery of consciousness and neural function beginning after 6 to 10 days was slow, and serious sequelae such as spasticity, mental retardation, and seizures were common. Laboratory findings showed liver dysfunction, uremia, and hypoproteinemia. Liver histology was nonspecific and distinguished from Reye's syndrome. CSF protein was increased. CT and MRI revealed symmetric, multifocal areas of necrosis in the thalamus, white matter, brainstem, and cerebellum. The etiology of this previously unrecognized type of acute encephalopathy was not determined. (Mizuguchi M et al. Acute necrotizing encephalopathy of childhood: a new syndrome presenting with multifocal, symmetric brain lesions. <u>J Neurol Neurosurg Psychiatry</u> May 1995;58:555-561). (Respond: Dr M Mizuguchi, Department of Mental Retardation and Birth Defect Research, National Institute of Neuroscience, NCNP, 4-1-1 Ogawahigashi-cho. Kodaira, 187, Japan).

COMMENT. In addition to Reye's syndrome, the differential diagnosis included Wernicke's and Leigh's encephalopathies, carbon monoxide poisoning, acute disseminated encephalomyelitis, and acute hemorrhagic leukoencephalitis. The patients reported here appear to show some characteristics that differentiate this form of "acute toxic encephalopathy" from those already recognized. It is of interest that several patients (16%) were retarded, and 16% had congenital anomalies, including ventricular septal defect, radial agenesis, and polydactyly. Evidence of recent viral infections (influenza A and B, coxackie A9, Rotavirus) was detected in 10 patients, and one patient had 3 paternal aunts who had died of Ekiri, a fulminant form of acute encephalopathy secondary to *Shigella dysenteriae* infection, prevalent in Japan up to the 1950s. -Editor. *Ped Neur Briefs* July 1995.

MMR VACCINE AND TRANSVERSE MYELITIS

Postvaccination transverse myelitis developed within 5 days following measles, mumps, and rubella vaccine in a 20 year old man diagnosed and treated at the Hurstwood Park Neurological Centre, Haywards Heath, West Sussex, England. The combined vaccine had been substituted for the rubella vaccine required for employment at a children's facility in the United States. Fever, malaise, sore throat and rash fluctuated over 2 weeks and were followed by urinary retention, ascending paresthesia, and flaccid paraplegia. Cerebrospinal fluid contained $370x10^6$ white cells (80% lymphocytes), 1.8 mg/l protein, and 3 mmol/l glucose. Serological tests showed a significant rise only in rubella antibody titers. MRI was normal. Treatment with IV steroids provided limited improvement and paralysis persisted below T6. (Joyce KA, Rees JE. Transverse myelitis after measles, mumps, and rubella vaccine. <u>BMJ</u> 12 August 1995;311:422).

COMMENT. The authors cite 3 previous reports of rubella postvaccinal transverse myelitis. They caution that antibody status be checked before immunization and only the required vaccine be used.

My mentors, W.G. Wyllie and Randolph K. Byers, were convinced of the potential neurological complications of immunization. My own clinical bias, though based on case studies, is in agreement with their views and teachings. Today, the tendency is to minimize the dangers of vaccines as only temporally related, probably coincidental, and unproven by statistics. It was Thomas Carlyle who said "one can prove anything with figures." The tragic consequence of a seemingly simple and innocuous injection in a young person on the threshold of a new life and occupation as an immigrant to the US, as reported above, should be a reason for pause and moderation of the enthusiasm of some for universal immunization, including the new varicella vaccine.

Non-specific benefits from measles immunization are reported from the Epidemiology Research Unit, Copenhagen, Denmark. (Aaby P et al. <u>BMJ</u> 19 August 1995;311:481-5). Analysis of mortality studies from developing countries showed that protective efficacy against death after measles immunization ranged from 30% to 86%, much higher than the proportion of deaths that could be attributed to acute measles. DTP and polio vaccinations were not associated with mortality reduction. The prevention of measles did not explain the reduced mortality among immunized children. Child survival might benefit from standard titre measles immunization before 9 months of age and by reimmunization. -Editor. *Ped Neur Briefs* Sept 1995.

PERTUSSIS VACCINE CNS SEQUELAE REASSESSMENT

The role of whole-cell pertussis vaccine as a cause of permanent neurologic damage has been reassessed by the American Academy of Pediatrics, Committee on Infectious Diseases, in light of new 10-year follow-up findings of the National Childhood Encephalopathy Study (NCES) in Great Britain. Although causal relationship is not definitely acknowledged, the committee now concludes that DTP vaccination can be associated with chronic neurologic dysfunction in children who had severe acute neurologic illnesses after DTP vaccination. The immunization guidelines in the 1994 *Red Book* continue to be recommended, but specific guidelines for acellular pertussis vaccines will be revised after FDA approval of new products. (AAP Committee on Infectious Diseases Report. The relationship between pertussis vaccine and central nervous system sequelae: continuing assessment. <u>Pediatrics</u> February 1996;97:279-281).

COMMENT. Pediatric neurologists caring for patients with increased susceptibility to precipitation or exacerbation of neurologic disorders such as seizures, behavior disorders, or language and developmental delays should use caution in advising parents concerning risks of immunizations. The AAP committee is careful to qualify their recommendations by a disclaimer rider.

Varicella vaccine-induced acute cerebellar ataxia is reported for the first time, affecting a 2-year-old boy who developed vomiting and ataxia 10 days after vaccination. MRI showed multiple demyelinating lesions. Recovery followed in 3 weeks. (Sunaga Y et al. Pediatr Neurol 1995;13:340-342). -Editor. *Ped Neur Briefs* Feb 1996.

BENIGN NEUROLOGIC COMPLICATIONS OF PERTUSSIS

The neurologic complications of pertussis infection among 340 unvaccinated patients admitted to hospital between 1979-1994 are reported from the Pediatric Clinic of the University of Catania, Sicily. Fourteen (4.1%) developed neurologic complications: Seizures occurred in all cases, 4 with fever, and 3 with signs of acute encephalopathy, including obtundation and vomiting which lasted only 12 to 24 hours. None of the patients developed epilepsy, all attend regular schools in appropriate grades, and at 14-18 year follow-up, only one has a mild behavioral disorder as a possible sequel of encephalopathy. No serious neurologic complications or permanent sequelae were observed in this series of children hospitalized for pertussis infection. (Incorpora G et al. Neurological complications in hospitalized patients with pertussis: a 15-year Sicilian experience. Child's Nerv System June 1996;12:332-335). (Respond: Dr G Incorpora, Clinica Pediatrica, Universita di Catania, Viale Andrea Doria, 6, I-95125 Catania, Italy).

COMMENT. The relatively mild and benign nature of the neurologic complications of pertussis infection reported in this study contrast with the severity and permanent sequelae of some reported cases of pertussis vaccine encephalopathy. Seizures were not associated with anoxic episodes and coughing bouts and were not complicated by epilepsy. -Editor. *Ped Neur Briefs* July 1996.

CHANGING PATTERNS OF REYE'S SYNDROME

Trends in the clinical pattern of Reye's syndrome in the British Isles between 1982 and 1990, and their relation to the June 1986 warnings against the use of aspirin in children, were analysed at the PHLS Communicable Disease Surveillance Centre, London, and other Centres in the UK. Of 445 cases reported, 354 had confirmed diagnoses and received scores of severity ranging from non-classical "Reye-like" (low scorers) to classical Reye's syndrome (high scorers). Classical cases occurred more frequently in the 4 1/2 year period before June 1986 compared with the subsequent period of surveillance. After June 1986, non-classical cases declined by 50% and classical by 79%. Classical, high scorers had received aspirin more frequently and were older than low scorers. (Hardie RM et al. Changing clinical pattern of Reye's syndrome. <u>Arch Dis Child</u> May 1996;74:400-405). (Respond: Dr Susan Hall, Floor C, Stephenson Building, Children's Hospital, Western Bank, Sheffield S10 2TH, UK).

COMMENT. Reports of Reye's syndrome declined in the surveillance period between 1982 and 1990, with a greater reduction in the number of classical Reye's syndrome cases than non-classical Reye-like cases after aspirin was withheld in 1986. Cases of classical Reye's syndrome were older and were more likely to have received aspirin. The authors conclude that their findings support a subset of Reye's syndrome but not all cases etiologically associated with aspirin. An inherited metabolic disorder is more likely in the Reye-like, non classical cases. -Editor. *Ped Neur Briefs* July 1996.

VIRAL-RELATED ACUTE CEREBELLAR ATAXIA: COURSE AND OUTCOME

A study of 73 consecutive children with acute cerebellar ataxia seen over a 23 year-period is reported from the Departments of Pediatrics and Neurology, Washington University School of Medicine and St Louis Children's Hospital. Mean age at onset was 5 years (range, 1 to 21 years); 60% were 2 to 4 years at onset.

Prodromal illnesses identified in 57 children included chicken pox in 26%, other presumed viral illness in 52% and immunization related in 3%. No prodrome was recognized in 19%. Epstein-Barr virus was identified in 2 children. Gait ataxia was most severe in patients with varicella, EBV, and vaccination. Other neurologic abnormalities included dysmetria, nystagmus, cranial nerve palsies, and corticospinal tract signs. WBC counts were elevated in half the postviral ataxia cases and normal in the remainder. CSF protein averaged 24 mcg/dl and the mean WBC count was 10 (range, 0-107/mm^3). Pleocytosis >5 was present in one half. Brain scans were normal with one temporary exception. Recovery was complete in 91% of 60 followed for 4 months or longer; 100% in post-varicella cases and 89% in children with non-varicella-related ataxia. Transient behavioral or intellectual difficulties occurred in 20%, and learning problems persisted in 5 (8%). Four children had recurrences of acute ataxia, usually after another presumed viral illness. (Connolly AM, Dodson WE, Prensky AL, Rust RS. Course and outcome of acute cerebellar ataxia. <u>Ann Neurol</u> June 1994;35:673-679). (Respond: Dr Rust, University of Wisconsin School of Medicine, Department of Neurology-H6/546, 600 Highland Avenue, Madison, WI 53792).

COMMENT. The prognosis for non-varicella cases in this study was superior to that reported by Weiss and Carter (<u>Neurology</u> 1959;9:711) who found 33% of 18 cases with persistent gait disturbance at follow-up. Findings in the above St Louis study previously unreported include the following: 1) boys are affected more frequently than girls (57%/43%), have more severe ataxia, and more frequent cranial nerve palsies and nystagmus; 2) varicella related cases have worse ataxia but more rapid and complete recovery than non-varicella cases; 3) recurrences are not rare and may affect 5% of patients. -Editor. *Ped Neur Briefs* July 1994.

CHAPTER 14

TOXIC DISORDERS

OVERVIEW OF RECENT ADVANCES

In the three year period, 1994 through 1996, several articles pertain to lead poisoning and risk assessment. The value of routine survey questionnaires is controversial, and blood tests in high risk patients is preferred in many centers. Environmental lead abatement should take precedence over the use of children as lead detectors. Other environmental hazards with adverse effects on cognitive function and neurodevelopment include polychlorinated biphenyls (PCBs), methylmercury, and diazinon.

The neurologic complications of fetal cocaine exposure are discussed in at least four articles. Affected offspring may show decreased developmental scores in infancy and ADHD in childhood. Fetal alcohol syndrome and toluene embryopathy have a common mechanism. Toluene is an underrecognized form of substance abuse with serious acute and chronic toxicities.

Toxins, drugs, and food supplements with

reported neurotoxic effects include thallium poisoning, isoniazid, amphotericin B, manganese, and vitamin A. Gastrointestinal symptoms followed closely by painful paresthesiae of extremities are early diagnostic manifestations of thallium poisoning. Thallium is radiopaque, and abdominal radiographs may demonstrate metallic densities. In children receiving prophylactic treatment for tuberculosis who present with an acute onset of seizures refractory to anticonvulsants, isoniazid toxicity should be suspected and pyridoxine administered intravenously.

Manganese poisoning presenting with dystonia is a risk in children receiving long-term parenteral nutrition, especially when complicated by cholestatic liver disease. Encephalopathy with Parkinsonian features, in addition to seizures, may complicate bone marrow transplants and treatment with amphoteracin B for leukemia. Infants receiving vitamin A supplements together with routine DPT/OPV immunization have a 10% incidence of bulging fontanelle. The effects of the vitamin A and immunization appear to be synergistic or additive, since both can be complicated by increased intracranial pressure. *J. Gordon Millichap, M.D.,* Editor.

LEAD POISONING RISK ASSESSMENT: BLOOD LEAD SCREENING

The Centers for Disease Control and Prevention (CDC) lowered the blood lead level (BPb) considered a toxic risk to children from 25 mcg/dL to 10 mcg/dL in Oct 1991. A five-item questionnaire is now completed at regular office visits for all children from 6 months to 6 years of age to identify those at high risk of lead exposure. In some States, including Illinois, all children are required to have BPb testing at 12 months of age or before entering a state-licensed day care, preschool, or kindergarten. High risk infants must be tested at 6 months and biannually.

A study to determine the efficacy of the questionnaire and prevalence of elevated BPb in 1393 suburban children at 12 and 24 months of age is reported from the Department of Pediatrics, Children's Memorial Hospital, Northwestern University, Chicago, Illinois. A venous BPb =/> 10 mcg/dL was found in 2.1%, and none was >30 mcg/dL. CDC and Illinois screening tests failed to predict high risk exposure in 9 of 29 (31%) children with elevated BPb. Living in a pre-1960 house, a question not included in CDC or Illinois screening, was most predictive, with positive correlation in 24 of 29 (83%) children with elevated BPb levels. The authors point out that optimal risk assessment questions may vary in different areas and populations. (Binns HJ et al. Is there lead in the suburbs? Risk assessment in Chicago suburban pediatric practices. <u>Pediatrics</u> Feb 1994;<u>93</u>164-171). (Reprints: Helen J Binns MD, Children's Memorial Hospital, 2300 Children's Plaza, Chicago, IL 60614).

COMMENT. Questions about the home environment were the most sensitive indicators of elevated lead levels in a similar study reported from the California Pacific Medical Center, San Francisco, CA. (Tejeda DM et al. Do questions about lead exposure predict elevated lead levels? <u>Pediatrics</u> Feb 1994;<u>93</u>:192-194). An abbreviated screening using only the first three items was as effective as the complete CDC questionnaire in a study at the University of Rochester, NY.(Schaffer SJ et al. Lead poisoning risk determination in an urban population through the use of a standardized questionnaire. <u>Pediatrics</u> Feb 1994;<u>93</u>:159-163).

Selective screening with a community-specific questionnaire is proposed following a study at the Gunderson Clinic, La Crosse, WI, which found a great variability in prevalence of elevated BPb between clinics even within a homogeneous community. (Rooney BL et al. Development of a screening tool for prediction of children at risk for lead exposure in a Midwestern clinical setting. <u>Pediatrics</u> Feb 1994;<u>93</u>:183-187).

A survey of 556 pediatricians in Virginia revealed an overall deficiency in physicians' knowledge of lead poisoning with specific deficiencies in knowledge of the literature. Subspecialists scored lower than primary care pediatricians. (Baron ME, Boyle RM. Are pediatricians ready for the new guidelines on lead poisoning? <u>Pediatrics</u> Feb 1994;<u>93</u>:178-182). Since 17% of all children < 7 years in the USA are reported to have elevated BPb levels known to increase the risk of cognitive and behavioral deficits, both physician and parent awareness of the environmental sources, symptoms, and long-term hazards of lead is an urgent priority. -Editor. *Ped Neur Briefs* Feb 1994.

LEAD EXPOSURE: INAPPROPRIATE SCREENING PRACTICES?

Physician screening practices at a hospital-based, university-affiliated pediatric primary care center serving an urban high-risk population in Rochester, NY were evaluated to determine the feasibility of the 1991 Centers for Disease Control guidelines. Among 632 children aged 9 to 25 months who attended the center between 1989 and 1991, screening was deficient in 55%, 34%, and 29% at ages 9-13 months, 14-19 months, and 20-25 months, respectively. Many high-risk children living in houses built before 1950, including those making well-child visits, were not appropriately screened for lead toxic effects, and opportunities for testing were frequently missed. (Campbell JR, McConnochie KM, Weitzman M. Lead screening among high-risk urban children. Are the 1991 Centers for Disease Control and Prevention Guidelines feasible? <u>Arch Pediatr Adolesc Med</u> July 1994;148:688-693). (Reprints: Dr Campbell, Department of Pediatrics, Rochester General Hospital, 1425 Portland Ave, Rochester, NY 14621).

COMMENT. The authors believe that the new CDC guidelines for biannual screening and retesting can be achieved with a modest increase in tests, if sick visits are also utilized for retesting. Proper cleansing of the fingertip or alternatively, venipuncture should decrease the proportion of false-positive results and reduce the need for additional visits. At this urban PC Center, 30% of the screened high-risk children had lead levels of 10 mcg/dL or higher, now considered to be toxic. In contrast, only 4.7% of children screened from a suburban, middle class private practice in Cherry Hill, NJ, were found to have elevated blood lead levels, and no child had a level of 25 mcg/dL or higher requiring treatment. (Taubman B et al. Arch Pediatr Adolesc Med July 1994;148:757-760).

Who Bears the Burden? Wical BS, of the Departments of Neurology and Pediatrics, University of New Mexico, Albuquerque, addresses the dilemmas and burdens of blood lead testing of 22 million children in the US from 6 to 72 months of age. (Arch Pediatr Adolesc Med July 1994;148:760-761). In Milwaukee, private physicians play a major role in lead poisoning screening and case identification. In 1992, the number of cases of poisoning identified (BPb 25 mcg/dL or higher) in the private sector increased by over 600% in a 2 year period, a higher number than in public centers. Physicians voluntarily changed their practice patterns in accordance with 1991 CDC recommendations, partly as a result of physician education by the Milwaukee Health Department and the Children's Hospital of Wisconsin. (Schlenker TL et al. Arch Pediatr Adolesc Med July 1994;148:761-764).

The Child Neurologist's Role. Pediatric neurologists may need to take some responsibility in the blood lead screening of their patients, particularly those in high-risk categories. No child is exempt from risk, however; one infant, a pediatric surgeon's child, living in a high-rise co-op apartment, the first to be built in Chicago in 1924, and another, a house master's child at a renown boarding school in Massachusetts, were exposed to lead containing paint in the homes. Blood lead levels, in both cases prompted by the mothers and found to be elevated, responded to a temporary change of residence and lead abatement measures.

Declining Lead Levels. Despite the dramatic overall decrease in blood lead levels in the US population in recent years to 2.8 mcg/dL, national estimates for children 1 to 5 years of age show that 8.9%, or 1.7 million children, have BPb levels of 10 mcg/dL or greater, high enough to be of concern. (Brody DJ, Pirkle JL et al. Blood lead levels in the US population. Phase 1 of the third National Health and Nutrition Examination Survey (NHANES III, 1988 to 1991). <u>JAMA</u> July 27, 1994;272:277-283). Pirkle JL, Brody DJ et al, commenting on the decline in blood lead levels in the US, attribute the fall to the removal of lead from gasoline and soldered cans. Lead in paint, dust and soil needs to be addressed before the decline can continue, especially in children in low income, urban areas. (<u>JAMA</u> July 27, 1994;272:284-291). Goldman LR and Carra J, from the Office of Prevention, Pesticides, and Toxic Substances, US Environmental Protection Agency, Washington, DC, emphasize the need for both targeted screening efforts and improvements in screening methods in high-risk children.(Childhood lead poisoning in 1994. <u>JAMA</u> July 27, 1994;272:315-316).

Public Lead Awareness and Responsibility.
Since current compliance with CDC recommended guidelines for blood lead screening is not universally appropriate, an increased public and parent awareness of the hazards and the symptoms and signs of lead poisoning, especially in children, should be encouraged. (Millichap JG. <u>Environmental Poisons in Our Food</u>. Chicago, PNB Publ, 1993). -Editor. *Ped Neur Briefs* Aug 1994.

LEAD NEUROTOXICITY: COGNITIVE EFFECTS

The interpretation of the literature on lead and child development is presented with open peer commentary from the Neuroepidemiology Unit, Children's Hospital, Harvard Medical School, Boston, and other centers. Discussions about association between lead and IQ have focussed on determinants of accuracy of estimation, with insufficient consideration of the influence of the experimental system on estimation. Inconsistencies in findings and controversy over the effect of lead on cognition could be due to differences in environmental characteristics, dose, timing, age, and genetic susceptibility, and may explain the failure to identify a lead-associated "behavioral signature." A clinical "process" approach to assessment should be modelled after studies of behavioral toxicity in animals. Neuropsychological tests conveying information about the process of a child's learning would be more sensitive and revealing than IQ test scores. Lead exposure may have attentional or motivational effects that reduce ability to accumulate knowledge tapped by IQ tests. (Bellinger DC. Interpreting the literature on lead and child development: The neglected role of the "experimental system." <u>Neurotoxicol Teratol</u> 1995;17:201-212).

COMMENT. Among the 10 commentaries appearing in the same issue, one from Columbia University, New York, stresses the need to consider behavior that may be affected by lead, in addition to IQ. Clinical reports suggest that lead-exposed children may be distractible and/or hyperactive, but few studies have examined the effects of lead on behavior using statistical controls. Lawsuits correlating a child's disability with a blood lead level are often lacking in proof of cause and effect. Conditions such as Pervasive Development Disorder, or speech articulation problems, offered as indications of lead effects, are unrelated to lead exposure. (Wasserman GA. Effects of early lead exposure: Time to integrate and broaden our efforts. <u>Neurotoxicol Teratol</u> 1995;17:243-244).

Fingerstick screening for lead poisoning was a reasonable alternative to venous testing in private practice, as evaluated at the Yale Study Center, New Haven, Conn, provided that specimen contamination was avoided, and medical and environmental interventions were based on confirmatory venous testing. (Schonfeld DJ et al. <u>Arch Pediatr Adolesc Med</u> Apr 1995;149:447-450).

Venous blood lead screening was offered to children 1 to 6 years of age attending the Emergency Departments of St Christopher's Hospital for Children and Children's Hospital of Philadelphia. Of 254 children attending these two centers, 65% had no record of previous lead screening in the previous 30 months, and 71% and 50%, respectively, had blood lead levels >10mcg/dL. (Wiley JF II et al. Lead poisoning: Low rates of screening and high prevalence among children seen in inner-city emergency departments. <u>J Pediatr</u> March 1995;126:392-5). The emergency department is an appropriate resource for lead screening of selected inner-city children, but preliminary fingerstick may be a more practical and less costly method.

Lead in soil and paint in well-maintained homes contributed little to the lead exposure of children in an urban population surrounding a closed lead smelter in Granite City, Illinois, and reported from the Institute for Evaluating Health Risks, Washington, DC, and the Illinois Department of Public Health, Edwardsville, IL. (Kimbrough R et al. <u>Pediatrics</u> April 1995;95:550-554). Indiscriminate removal of leaded paint and soil in residential areas should be discouraged, and the education of parents concerning removal of house dust, personal hygiene and good nutrition is of more practical benefit. -Editor. *Ped Neur Briefs* June 1995.

LEAD EXPOSURE IN DAY CARE CENTERS

The risk of lead poisoning among 155 of 234 eligible children (mean age, 4.8 years) enrolled in university affiliated day care centers with elevated environmental lead sources was determined at the Department of Pediatrics and University Hygienic Laboratory, The University of Iowa, Iowa City. Elevated levels of lead in paint (2.4% - 40% lead) were found in all six centers tested. Three centers were found to have elevated lead levels in windowsill dust (62000-180000 g Pb/sqM) or soil (530-1100 mg Pb/kgm). Questionnaires completed by parents showed low risk of lead exposure in the homes. Blood lead levels were less than 10 mcg/dL in all but one child. (Weismann DN et al. Elevated environmental lead levels in a day care setting. <u>Arch Pediatr Adolesc Med</u> August 1995;149:878-881). (Respond: Dr Weismann, Department of Pediatrics, University of Iowa Hospitals and Clinics, 200 Hawkins Dr, Iowa City, IA 52242).

COMMENT. The lead-safe home environment, careful supervision, and good personal hygiene of these children would explain the relatively low blood lead levels despite elevated environmental lead levels in the day care centers. Major, costly lead abatement efforts would have been unwarranted in this situation.

Pediatric neurologists evaluating children with ADHD are cognizant of the role of lead exposure in the etiology of learning and behavior problems. The home and play environment questionnaire is important in determining the need for blood lead level determinations. Treatment guidelines for lead exposure in children are outlined in an American Academy of Pediatrics Committee on Drugs report. (Berlin CM Jr et al. <u>Pediatrics</u> July 1995;96:155-160). Chelation therapy is indicated in patients with blood lead levels of 45 mcg/dL and above, and sometimes in those with persistent levels of 25-45 mcg/dL, despite environmental abatement. Chelation is not indicated for levels less than 25 mcg/dL. -Editor. *Ped Neur Briefs* Aug 1995.

ATAXIA AND EARLY LEAD EXPOSURE

The effect of chronic exposure to lead on postural balance was studied in 162 six-year-old children examined in the Department of Environmental Health, and Children's Hospital Medical Center, University of Cincinnati Medical School, Cincinnati, OH. The five-year geometric mean blood lead concentration was 11.9 mcg/dL (range 4-28 mcg/dL). Most children reached peak PbB concentrations by 18-24 months. Increases in blood lead in CDC Class III category (<20mcg/dL) were significantly associated with increase in postural sway and poor postural balance, indicative of damage to vestibular/proprioceptive systems. Postural balance was measured with eyes open and eyes closed using a microprocessor-based strain gauge-type force platform system. (Bhattacharya A, Berger O et al. Effect of early lead exposure on children's postural balance. <u>Dev Med Child Neurol</u> 1995;37:861-878). ((Respond: Dr Amit Bhattacharya, Department of Environmental Health, University of Cincinnati Medical School, Cincinnati, OH 45267).

COMMENT. Because of the epidemiological nature of the study, the authors note that the results imply an association between elevated lead levels and impaired postural balance rather than a cause. However, because other neurotoxin exposures such as methylmercury and organochlorines were excluded, the association between lead exposure and ataxia most likely reflects an adverse effect of the lead on the developing nervous system. This postural balance measurement may be useful in assessing gross motor function of children at or below the CDC Class III category (<20mcg/dL) of lead exposure. -Editor. *Ped Neur Briefs* Jan 1996.

LEAD INTOXICATION IN CHILDREN WITH AUTISM

The incidence of reexposure to lead poisoning in 17 children with pervasive developmental disorders (PDD), including autism, compared to a randomly selected group of 30 children without PDD who were treated for plumbism over the same six year period, was evaluated by a retrospective chart review at the lead treatment program, Children's Hospital, Harvard Medical School, Massachusetts Poison Control System, Boston, MA. Despite close monitoring, inspection and lead hazard reduction or alternative housing, 75% of children with PDD were reexposed to lead compared to 23% without PDD. Those with PDD were older at diagnosis (46 vs 30 months) and had a longer period of elevated lead (39 vs 14 months) during management. (Shannon M, Graef JW. Lead intoxication in children with pervasive developmental disorders. <u>Clin</u>

<u>Toxicology</u> March 1996;34:177-181). (Respond: Dr Michael Shannon, Children's Hospital, 300 Longwood Ave, Boston, MA 02115).

COMMENT. Children with developmental delays and PDD are at increased risk of lead poisoning beyond 3 years of age. Children with PDD and other behavior disorders should be tested for lead at regular intervals beyond 4 years of age. More importantly, primary preventive measures designed to abate lead from the environment before lead intoxication occurs may be the only successful method of management. -Editor. *Ped Neur Briefs* May 1996.

PREDICTIVE VALUE OF LEAD SCREENING PRACTICES

The prevalence of elevated blood lead levels and the accuracy of a lead screening questionnaire in an urban pediatric population were evaluated in the primary care clinics of 10 community health centers in the city and county of Denver, CO. Of approx 3000 low-income children tested, only 0.3% had blood lead levels >20 mcg/dL. The predictive value of the CDC questionnaire was 3%, little better than chance, and the cost of identifying a child with a lead level > 20 mcg/dL was approx $5000. (France EK, Gitterman BA, Melinkovich P, Wright RA. The accuracy of a lead questionnaire in predicting elevated pediatric blood lead levels. <u>Arch Pediatr Adolesc Med</u> Sept 1996;150:958-963). (Respond: Eric K France MDCM, Department of Preventive Medicine, Kaiser Permanente, 10350 E Dakota Ave, Denver, CO 80231).

COMMENT. The Editor, Dr Catherine D DeAngelis, notes that "when a survey questionnaire is only slightly better than chance, it's better to take the chance and save the money for the blood tests." The Denver Health and Hospitals chose to screen all low-income children between 12 and 30 months of age and to forgo the use of the questionnaire. Universal screening may be omitted in low-prevalence communities, according to current CDC guidelines.

A recent survey of a nationally representative sample of pediatricians found that 53% screen all their patients aged 9 to 36 months, 96% using a blood lead assay. Most of the remainder report screening of high-risk patients only. (Campbell JR, Schaffer SJ, Szilagyi PG et al. Blood lead screening practices among US pediatricians. <u>Pediatrics</u> Sept 1996;98:372-377). In pediatric neurology practice, a blood lead level may be indicated in high-risk children who present with neurodevelopmental delay, ADHD, seizures, or signs of encephalopathy or neuropathy. -Editor. *Ped Neur Briefs* Oct 1996.

ASYMPTOMATIC HEAVY LEAD EXPOSURE

Three asymptomatic children, ages 34, 23, and 26 months, with blood lead levels >100 mcg/dL on routine screening are reported from the Kennedy Krieger Institute and Department of Pediatrics, Johns Hopkins, Baltimore, MD. All suffered from pica and one was described as "hyper." Screening appears to be essential in at risk children if lead poisoning is to be detected and eradicated. (Davoli CT, Serwint JR, Chisolm JJ Jr. Asymptomatic children with venous lead levels >100 mcg/dL. <u>Pediatrics</u> Nov 1996;98:965-968). (Reprints: Cecilia T Davoli MD, Kennedy Krieger Institute, 707 North Broadway, Baltimore, MD 21205).

COMMENT. It is unfortunate that children must be used as "lead detectors" before lead violations in homes and schools are corrected and lead abatement instituted. Critics of routine screening at 6 months to 6 years must be impressed by this report and conclude that in certain populations, screening is the only way to prevent childhood morbidity and mortality from lead exposure. -Editor. *Ped Neur Briefs* Dec 1996.

PRENATAL PCB EXPOSURE AND COGNITIVE DYSFUNCTION

The neuropsychological effects of in utero exposure to PCBs and their related compounds were evaluated in 27 'Yu-Cheng' ('oil disease') children (ages 7 to 12 years) at the Departments of Pediatrics and Psychiatry, National Cheng Kung University, Tainan, Taiwan. Full-scale IQ scores on the WISC-R were significantly lower than in the 27 controls. Mean P300 latencies of auditory event-related potentials were significantly longer and the amplitudes reduced. Pattern visual evoked potentials and somatosensory evoked potentials were unaffected. Apart from a slight increase in soft signs, the neurologic examinations of the exposed children were not different from controls. (Chen Y-J, Hsu C-C. Effects of prenatal exposure to PCBs on the neurological function of children: A neuropsychological and neurophysiological study. <u>Dev Med & Child Neurol</u> April 1994;<u>36</u>:312-320). (Respond: Dr Yung-Jung Chen, Dept of Pediatrics, Medical College, National Cheng Kung University, 138 Sheng-Li Road, Tainan 70428, Taiwan, R.O.C.).

COMMENT. PCBs affect cognitive function of children exposed in utero. Evoked potentials are useful in examining the neurotoxicity of environmental pollutants in the young child. The P300 wave latency is related to the solving of cognitive tasks and the amplitude of P300 reflects concentration abilities. A significantly greater difference in P300 latencies was found for exposed children with lower IQ scores compared to controls. Delayed effects of PCBs on newborns whose mothers consumed contaminated Lake Michigan fish during pregnancy have been reported; smaller head circumference and growth retardation persisted beyond infancy and short-term memory and behavioral deficits occurred at later follow-up (see <u>Ped Neur Briefs</u> Jan 1990, and March 1993). -Editor. *Ped Neur Briefs* May 1994.

POLYCHLORINATED BIPHENYLS AND ATTENTION DEFICITS

The effects of in utero exposure to polychlorinated biphenyls (PCBs) on cognitive function in 212 children at 11 years of age were tested at Wayne State University, Detroit, MI. Prenatal exposure to PCBs from maternal ingestion of contaminated Lake Michigan fish was associated with significantly lower full-scale and verbal IQ scores. Concentrations of PCBs in maternal serum and milk at delivery, only slightly higher than in the general population, caused long-term intellectual impairment, especially affecting memory, attention, and reading comprehension. (Jacobson JL, Jacobson SW. Intellectual impairment in children exposed to polychlorinated biphenyls in utero. <u>N Eng J Med</u> Sept 12 1996;335:783-9). (Reprints: Dr Joseph L Jacobson, Department of Psychology, Wayne State University, Detroit, MI 48202).

COMMENT. Deficits in short-term memory and developmental delays, previously noted in infants and at 4 years of age in children exposed to PCBs in utero, have now been demonstrated in children tested at 11 years of age. PCBs may have a long-term adverse effect on cognitive function, and prenatal exposure to these environmental toxins should be included among potential causes of attention deficit disorders in children. -Editor. *Ped Neur Briefs* Oct 1996.

DIAZINON EXPOSURE AND INFANTILE HYPERTONIA

A 12-week-old infant girl who developed persistent hypertonicity 5 weeks following exposure to the organophosphate insecticide diazinon (Knox-Out 2FM) in the home is reported from Oregon State University, Corvallis, OR. The infant's urine contained alkylphosphate metabolites of diazinon (60 ppb diethylphosphate and 20 ppb diethylthiophosphate). Serum cholinesterase was normal. Diazinon levels in the home (floor, vacuum cleaner dust, and air) were excessive even at 6 months after application. Six weeks after evacuating the home, the infant's muscle tone returned to normal, ankle clonus had resolved, and subsequent development was normal. (Wagner SL, Orwick DL. Chronic organophosphate exposure associated with transient hypertonia in an infant.

<u>Pediatrics</u> July 1994;94:94-97). (Reprints: Dr Sheldon L Wagner, Agricultural Chemistry, Oregon State University, Agricultural & Life Sciences 1007, Corvalllis, OR 97331).

COMMENT. None of the typical muscarinic or nicotinic symptoms of organophosphate intoxication was present in this infant. Organophosphates can cause a delayed neurobehavioral toxicity, characterized by neuritis, paralysis, and psychological changes, the result of degeneration of myelin and nerve axons and effects on neurotransmitters. A relationship between Parkinson's disease and exposure to pesticide chemicals has been demonstrated in agricultural workers. Children presenting with unexplained neuro-behavioral symptoms should be investigated for possible exposure to insecticide environmental toxins. -Editor. *Ped Neur Briefs* Aug 1994.

LONG-TERM EFFECTS OF METHYLMERCURY POISONING

The clinical, neuropsychological, and radiological features of a family, and the toxicological and neuropathological findings of one family member, who were acutely and severely intoxicated with methylmercury are reported after a 22-year follow-up from the Albuquerque Veterans Affairs Medical Center, the University of New Mexico School of Medicine, and the Environmental Health Sciences Center, the University of Rochester School of Medicine, NY. In 1969 a family in New Mexico had consumed pork containing methylmercury. Three children and a neonate developed severe neurological signs. At 22-year follow-up, the 2 oldest patients, ages 42 and 35 years, had cortical blindness, impaired stereognosis and graphesthesia, poor hand coordination, ataxia, choreoathetosis, dysarthria, and attentional deficits. MRIs showed loss of tissue in calcarine cortices, parietal lobes, and cerebellar folia. The 2 youngest were quadriplegic, blind, and mentally retarded and they died at ages 29 and 21 years. The brain of the patient poisoned at 8 years and dying at 29 showed cortical atrophy, neuronal loss and gliosis. Total mercury level in the occipital cortex was 1,974 ng/gm, 50 times that of a control; the Hg was mainly inorganic. Hair and systemic organs had Hg levels comparable to controls. (Davis LE et al. Methylmercury poisoning: Long-term clinical, radiological, toxicological, and pathological studies of an affected family. <u>Ann Neurol</u> June 1994;35:680-688). (Respond: Dr Davis, Chief, Neurology Service (127), Albuquerque VA Hospital, 2100 Ridgecrest Drive SE, Albuquerque, NM 87108).

COMMENT. Methylmercury crosses the blood-brain barrier easily while inorganic mercury does not. Biotransformation to inorganic Hg over time may account for the high level of inorganic Hg and absence of methyl Hg in the patient's brain at autopsy. The possible role of inorganic Hg in the brain damage is debatable; it is usually considered to be inert and nontoxic. See <u>Environmental Poisons in Food</u> , Chicago, PNB Publishers, 1993, for an account of the sources, metabolism, epidemiology, clinical manifestations, treatment, and prevention of mercury poisoning.

Accidental exposure to mercury vapor is a persisting hazard in nurseries with broken thermometers and in school science labs. The symptoms of mild exposure, *micromercurialism*, are subtle and difficult to diagnose without a high index of suspicion. Acrodynia, or Pink disease, is a relatively rare occurrence, but a diagnosis which should be familiar to the pediatric neurologist and pediatrician. -Editor. *Ped Neur Briefs* July 1994.

NEUROLOGIC COMPLICATIONS OF FETAL COCAINE EXPOSURE

Cocaine-positive urine toxicology at birth in 51 newborns was associated with hypertonia during infancy in 21(41%) studied at the Harlem Hospital Center, New York. Cocaine-positive infants were four times more likely to show hypertonic tetraparesis than cocaine-negative infants. Hypertonia diminished over time and resolved by 24 months. Those with early hypertonia showed significantly lower developmental scores at 6 and 12 months than infants without hypertonia. (Chiriboga CA et al. Neurological correlates of fetal cocaine exposure: Transient hypertonia of infancy and early childhood. <u>Pediatrics</u> December 1995;96:1070-1077). (Reprints: Dr CC Chiriboga, Division of Pediatric Neurology, College of Physicians and Surgeons, Columbia University, 710 West 168th St, New York, NY 10032).

COMMENT. In our clinic for children with Attention Deficit Disorders at Children's Memorial Hospital, Chicago, I have observed an unusual incidence of a history of fetal cocaine exposure in those placed in foster homes soon after birth. Other complications of cocaine exposure in utero are small head circumference, cerebral infarction or hemorrhage, seizures, and SIDS. Disturbances in corticogenesis have been demonstrated in experiments on laboratory animals (see <u>Progress in Pediatric Neurology I and II, PNB Publishers,</u> 1991, pp452-3, and 1994, pp439-41). -Editor. *Ped Neur Briefs* Feb 1996.

COCAINE-INDUCED HORMONAL AND BEHAVIORAL CHANGES

Behavioral and hormonal responses in 30 preterm cocaine-exposed infants were compared with a cohort of 30 non-cocaine-exposed preterm infants at the Touch Research Institute, University of Miami School of Medicine, FL. Cocaine-exposed infants had smaller head circumference at birth, longer stays in the intensive care unit, a higher incidence of intraventricular hemorrhage, inferior performance on the Brazelton Neonatal Behavioral Assessment Scale (range of state, regulation of state, and depression clusters), decreased periods of quiet sleep, and increased levels of agitated behavior, including tremulousness, limb movements, and clenched fists. They also had higher urinary norepinephrine, dopamine, and cortisol levels and lower plasma insulin levels than controls. Epinephrine and glucose levels were unchanged. (Scafidi FA, Field TM et al. Cocaine-exposed preterm nenates show behavioral and hormonal differences. Pediatrics June 1996;97:851-855). (Reprints: Dr Tiffany M Field, Touch Research Institute, University of Miami School of Medicine, PO Box 016820, Miami, FL 33101).

COMMENT. Cocaine-exposed infants require careful follow-up for early diagnosis and therapy of neurobehavioral complications. A frequent history of prenatal cocaine exposure in foster children with attention deficit hyperactivity disorders is of interest in relation to the changes in catecholamine metabolism noted in the above study. For reference to neurological correlates of fetal cocaine exposure, see Ped Neur Briefs Feb 1996;10:9-10; and Progress in Pediatric Neurology I and II PNB Publishers, 1991 and 1994.

Other prenatal toxic factors that may underly cognitive, behavioral, and attentional deficits in childhood include alcohol, PCBs, and nicotine.

Fetal alcohol syndrome and ophthalmological abnormalities are reported in 25 children examined at Children's Hospital, Goteberg, Sweden. (Stromland K, Hellstrom A. Pediatrics June 1996;97:845-850). The fundus was abnormal in 23, of whom 19 had optic nerve hypoplasia. Concomitant strabismus occurred in 13. Other abnormalities included microphthalmos, coloboma, cataract, and nystagmus. Mental retardation required special school placement for 16, and only 3 attended normal schools without extra assistance. The finding of ocular abnormalities in a child suspected of having FAS should strengthen the diagnosis.

Developmental neurotoxicity of PCBs in humans is reviewed from the Institute of Environmental studies, University of Illinois at Urbana-Champaign, Urbana, IL. (Schantz SL. Neurotoxicol and Teratology May/June 1996;18:217-227). Studies included those in Yusho, Japan; Yucheng, Taiwan; Michigan; North Carolina; Oswego, NY; New Bedford, MA; on Inuit people in the Arctic regions of Quebec; and in Faroe Islanders. Concurrent methylmercury poisoning may be an issue in interpretation of some studies. Children born to mothers exposed to PCBs showed abnormalities in behavior and development, including higher activity levels, behavior problems, lower IQ scores, decreased birth weight and head circumference, lowered scores on the Brazelton Neonatal Battery, deficits in memory at 4 years, and delays in psychomotor development. Although the deficits in cognition were often small, the public health implications of low-level PCB exposure was compared to that of lead exposure. At a population level, a decrease of 4 points on the Bayley Scales is estimated to result in a 50% increase in the number of children with subnormal scores. Subtle alterations in neuropsychological functioning caused by exposure to these environmental toxins were proposed as explanations for some cases of ADHD, either by a direct effect on the brain in the prenatal period or secondary to effects on thyroid function. The potential impact of postnatal exposure to PCBs via breast milk was also reviewed.

Maternal smoking is a preventable cause of mental retardation according to a study at the Rollins School of Public Health of Emory University, Atlanta, GA. (Drews CD et al. <u>Pediatrics</u> April 1996;97:547-553). Children whose mothers smoked one pack a day during pregnancy had more than a 75% increase in mental retardation. Maternal smoking has also been linked to lesser impairments of cognitive function and academic achievement, auditory deficits, and behavioral problems in children.

Environmental factors should be considered more frequently as potential causes of attention deficits and learning disabilities. -Editor. *Ped Neur Briefs* June 1996.

IN UTERO COCAINE EXPOSURE AND INFANT BEHAVIOR

The effects on neurobehavior in 20 infants with prenatal exposure to cocaine, alcohol, marijuana, and cigarettes, compared to 17 infants exposed to alcohol and/or marijuana and cigarettes without cocaine and 20 drug-free infants, were assessed using the Neonatal Intensive Care Unit Network Neurobehavioral Scale at Brown University School of Medicine, Women and Infants Hospital, Providence, RI. Cocaine-exposed infants showed increased tone and motor activity, more jerky movements, startles, tremors, back arching, and signs of central nervous system and visual stress than unexposed infants. Visual and auditory following responses, and birth weight and length of cocaine-exposed infants were also reduced. (Napiorkowski B, Lester BM et al. Effects of in utero substance exposure on infant neurobehavior. <u>Pediatrics</u> July 1996;98:71-75). (Reprints: Barry M Lester PhD, Women and Infant's Hospital, 101 Dudley St, Providence, RI 02905).

COMMENT. Meconium testing was used to confirm lack of illicit drug use in the unexposed group. Positive meconium or urine assays were found in 5 women who had denied prenatal drug use. Urine toxicology can detect cocaine within 1 to 4 days of last use. Cocaine-exposed infants had neurobehavioral changes especially involving increased tone and motor activity. Synergistic effects of cocaine with alcohol and marijuana could not be ruled out.

Dose-related effects of cocaine on 3-week neurobehavior were demonstrated in a study at Children's Hospital, Boston, MA. Comparing 38 heavily exposed infants, 73 lightly exposed, and 94 unexposed, after controlling for covariates, a significant dose effect was observed, heavily exposed infants showing poorer regulation of arousal and greater excitability at 3-week examination but not in the first few days of life. (Tronick EZ et al. Late dose-response effects of prenatal cocaine exposure on newborn neurobehavioral performance. <u>Pediatrics</u> July 1996;98:76-83). (Reprints: Edward Z Tronick PhD, Children's Hospital, 300 Longwood Ave, Boston, MA 02115).

Since regulation of arousal and attention are important to learning, infants exposed to cocaine in utero may be expected to show decreased developmental scores and to have attention deficit disorders in childhood. (<u>Ped Neur Briefs</u> Feb 1996;10:9-10). -Editor. *Ped Neur Briefs* July 1996.

PRENATAL COCAINE AND INFANT BEHAVIOR

The Brazelton Neonatal Behavioral Assessment Scales (BNBAS) were administered to 23 infants exposed to cocaine in utero and 29 nonexposed infants recruited from the low-risk nursery, Wayne State University Hospital, Detroit. Cocaine exposure was determined by quantitative analysis of the infant's meconium stool. Exposed infants performed less well than controls on 6 of the 7 BNBAS clusters, particularly in tests for autonomic stability. A dose-response relationship was evident, with a negative effect of meconium cocaine concentration on motor, orientation, and regulation of state. (Delaney-Black V, Covington C, Ostrea E Jr et al. Prenatal cocaine and neonatal outcome: evaluation of dose-response relationship. <u>Pediatrics</u> Oct 1996;98:735-740). (Reprints: Virginia Delaney-Black MD, Children's Hospital of Michigan, 3901 Beaubien, Detroit, MI 48201).

COMMENT. Significant adverse behavioral effects may be demonstrated in neonates born to cocaine addicted mothers. Quantitative determination of cocaine exposure by meconium analysis is essential, since screening by history alone is found to be inadequate.

Three additional studies of the effects of prenatal cocaine on neurobehavior are summarized as follows. The Brazelton NBAScale, used at the Western Psychiatric Institute, University of Pittsburgh, showed impaired scores in motor maturity and tone, autonomic instability, and an increased number of abnormal reflexes on the 2nd day postpartum, but not at day 3. (Richardson GA et al. The effects of prenatal cocaine use on neonatal neurobehavioral status. <u>Neurotoxicol Teratol</u> Sept/Oct 1996;18:519-528). Heavy cocaine exposure early in pregnancy was related to faster responsiveness on an infant visual expectancy test but poorer recognition memory and information processing in 464 inner-city, black infants tested at 6, 12, and 13 months in the Psychology Department, Wayne State University, Detroit, MI. (Jacobson SW et al. New evidence for neurobehavioral effects of in utero cocaine exposure. <u>J Pediatr</u> Oct 1996;129:581-590). The motor development of 28 infants exposed to cocaine in utero compared to that of an unexposed group followed from birth through 15 months at Boston University, Department of Physical Therapy and Child Development Unit, Children's Hospital, Boston, showed impairments in performance at 4 and 7 months of age but not at 15 months. However, all infants, both exposed and unexposed, were motor impaired when compared to norms, a reflection of the effects of poverty and malnutrition in inner-city infants. (Fetters L, Tronick EZ. Neuromotor development of cocaine-exposed and control infants from birth through 15 months: poor and poorer performance. <u>Pediatrics</u> Nov 1996;98:938-943). The combination of cocaine exposure and poor nutrition is a cumulative risk factor for impaired infantile motor performance in minority subjects and potentially detrimental to later neurocognitive development. -Editor. *Ped Neur Briefs* Dec 1996.

TOLUENE EMBRYOPATHY

The clinical manifestations of toluene embryopathy in 18 infants with a history of in utero exposure are reported from the Department of Pediatrics, University of Arizona College of Medicine, Tucson, and Maricopa Medical Center, Phoenix, AZ. Mothers were regular abusers of solvents and the fetus was exposed to toluene by maternal spray paint sniffing. Nine of the infants had been exposed to alcohol in addition, but except for an increased incidence of prenatal microcephaly, the resultant phenotype was unchanged. Premature birth occurred in 39%, and 9% died, 54% were small for gestational age, 52% had postnatal growth deficiency, 33% prenatal microcephaly, 67% postnatal microcephaly, 80% developmental delay, and 83% had craniofacial features similar to the fetal alcohol syndrome. Micrognathia, small palpebral fissures, and abnormal ears were most frequent with toluene, whereas the thin upper lip, smooth philtrum, and small nose were more common with alcohol exposure. Other less prominent features common to both toluene and alcohol embryopathies were nail hypoplasia, abnormal muscle tone, hemangiomata, renal anomalies, and altered palmar creases. (Pearson MA et al. Toluene embryopathy: Delineation of the phenotype and comparison with fetal alcohol syndrome. <u>Pediatrics</u> Feb 1994;<u>93</u>:211-215). (Reprints: H Eugene Hoyme MD, Section of Genetics, Dept of Pediatrics, Arizona Health Sciences Center, Tucson, AZ 85724).

COMMENT. It is estimated that 3 to 4% of teenagers engage in paint or glue sniffing. Toluene is the active organic solvent. It is an underrecognized form of substance abuse with serious acute and chronic toxicities. Acute symptoms of toluene toxicity include dizziness, euphoria, headache, vomiting, vertigo, convulsions, and loss of consciousness, sometimes preceded by delirium. Chronic toluene abuse causes headache, muscle weakness, peripheral neuropathy, nervousness, anemia, petechiae, abnormal bleeding, bone marrow aplasia, irreversible encephalopathy, and renal tubular acidosis. Following an initial report of a "Fetal solvents syndrome"(Toutant C, Lippman S. <u>Lancet</u> 1979;<u>1</u>:1356), the effects of toluene on the fetus have been described infrequently. This Arizona University study of a fetal toluene syndrome compares findings in their 18 patients with others in the literature and with the fetal alcohol syndrome. The authors conclude that the craniofacial teratogenetic effects of toluene and alcohol have a common mechanism.

An additional 6 cases of toluene embryopathy are reported from the Denver General Hospital, Colorado (Arnold GL et al. <u>Pediatrics</u> Feb 1994;<u>93</u>:216). Only one was exposed to alcohol as well as toluene. -Editor. *Ped Neur Briefs* Feb 1994.

ALCOHOL-RELATED PERINATAL BRAIN INJURY IN PREMATURES

The relation between maternal alcohol use and intraventricular hemorrhage in 349 prematures weighing 2000 g or less was examined by the Neonatal Brain Hemorrhage Study Team at the Epidemiology Department, Michigan State University, East Lansing, MI; National Institute of Environmental Health Sciences, Research Triangle Park, N Carolina; and the Dept of Pediatrics and Clinical Epidemiology, University of Pennsylvania School of Medicine, Philadelphia, PA. Infants of women reporting "high" alcohol use (7 or more drinks per week and/or 3 or more per occasion) during preganancy were at increased risk of developing brain hemorrhage and white matter damage. (Holzman C et al. Perinatal brain injury in premature infants born to mothers using alcohol in pregnancy. <u>Pediatrics</u> January 1995;95:66-73).

COMMENT. Premature infants of mothers who are high alcohol consumers during pregnancy have an increased risk of brain damage. Mothers' alcohol use before pregnancy had no observed adverse effect on the infant. However, alcohol taken during breast feeding may cause delay in motor development. (see <u>Progress in Pediatric Neurology I</u>, Chicago, PNB Publ, 1991, pp448-50).

The fetal alcohol syndrome (FAS) in adolescence was studied in 44 patients followed for 10-14 years at the Department of Pediatrics, Rittberg Hospital of the German Red Cross, Berlin, Germany, and the Department of Child and Adolescent Psychiatry, University of Zurich, Switzerland. (Spohr HL et al. <u>Acta Paediatr</u> Nov 1994;404:19-26). Although the pronounced growth retardation and dysmorphism of the early childhood FAS diminishes in the older child, a characteristic syndrome remains. The "juvenile" pattern of FAS showed the following features: microcephaly, growth retardation, cognitive deficits, behavioral problems, and craniofacial dysmorphism consisting of short palpebral fissures, thin upper lip, prominent nasal bridge, maxillary hypoplasia, strabismus, and malaligned teeth.

In a study of 64 families with alcoholism at the Karolinska Institute, Stockholm, Sweden, children had retarded development and more behavioral problems than controls until 4 years of age. Boys were more vulnerable than girls. Behavioral disorders were more pronounced when both parents were alcoholic. (Nordberg L et al. <u>Acta Paediatr</u> Nov 1994;Suppl 404:14-18). -Editor. *Ped Neur Briefs* Jan 1995.

MANGANESE SUPPLEMENTS AND DYSTONIA

A 7 month old girl who developed dystonic movements of the arms after a 3 month period of parental nutrition for jejunal atresia and bowel resection is reported from Great Ormond Street Hospital, London, UK. Development and head growth stopped at 12 months. Liver function tests showed cholestatic liver disease, a complication of parenteral nutrition. MRI showed basal ganglia changes in T1 weighted images compatible with trace metal deposition. A high blood manganese of 1740 nmol/L (ref. 73-210 nmol/L) was diagnosed at 17 months. She died 1 month later with neurological deterioration.

A subsequent investigation of 53 children who had been on parenteral nutrition for more than 6 weeks showed that all those with cholestatic liver disease (35/53), and consequent impairment of biliary excretion of manganese, had whole blood manganese levels of >360 nmol/L. The parenteral supplement in the UK contained 55 times more manganese than that recommended by the American Society for Clinical Nutrition. This product has now been replaced with one containing 1 mcg/kg manganese, in line with the American guidelines. (Reynolds AP, Kiely E, Meadows N. Manganese in long term paediatric parental nutrition. <u>Arch Dis Child</u> Dec 1994;71:527-528). (Respond: Dr Reynolds, Department of Chemical Pathology, Great Ormond Street Hospital, Great Ormond St, London WC1N 3JH, UK).

COMMENT. Blood manganese should be monitored

in patients on parenteral nutrition, especially those who develop cholestatic liver disease. MRI is recommended if blood manganese is >360 nmol/L and/or if patient develops dystonia.

Manganese poisoning with dystonia in an 8 year old girl with Alagille's syndrome (hepatic duct hypoplasia, chronic cholestasis, facial dysmorphism, vertebral malformations, retarded development, and cardiac murmur) responded to treatment with ursodeoxycholic acid (see Progress in Pediatric Neurology II, Chicago, PNB Publ, 1994, pp438-9). Toxicity from dietary sources of manganese appears to require a prolonged period of exposure before neurologic symptoms develop. -Editor. *Ped Neur Briefs* Jan 1995.

THALLIUM POISONING

Four young adults poisoned with thallium contained in maliciously contaminated marzipan ball candy are reported from the New York City Poison Center, and East Carolina University School of Medicine, Greenville, NC. Gastrointestinal symptoms, including diarrhea, vomiting, abdominal cramps, and constipation, and pleuritic chest pains developed on the second day, and painful paresthesiae of hands and feet on the third day. Weight bearing caused pain in the soles of the feet, so that walking was avoided. Stroking the back of the hands elicited severe pain. Radiographs of the candies showed metallic densities, and atomic absorption spectroscopy measurement of thallium content was 4 g/100g candy. Radiographs of the abdomen on the third day were negative for radiopaque thallium. Hypertension and tachycardia developed on day 4 to 8, and alopecia onset began on day 8 to 15. Treatment consisted of prussian blue (2 g 3x/d orally) to bind enteric thallium, activated charcoal orally, potassium chloride infusion, and iv morphine for pain. All patients recovered without sequelae within one month. (Meggs WJ et al. Thallium poisoning from maliciously contaminated food. Clin Toxicol Nov 1994;32:723-730). (Reprints: Dr William J Meggs, New York

City Poison Control Center, 455 First Avenue, Room 123, New York, NY 10016).

COMMENT. Gastrointestinal symptoms followed closely by painful paresthesiae of extremities are the early diagnostic manifestations of thallium poisoning. Alopecia is a late sign. The authors advocate early treatment with prussian blue. Thallium is radiopaque and radiographs of poisoned food may demonstrate metallic densities. -Editor. *Ped Neur Briefs* Jan 1995.

ACUTE ISONIAZID NEUROTOXICITY

An increased incidence of acute isoniazid (INH) neurotoxicity correlating with a resurgence of tuberculosis (TB) in New York City is reported from the Children's Medical Center of Brooklyn and the Department of Emergency Medicine, State University of New York, Health Science Center at Brooklyn. Nine patients receiving INH prophylaxis for TB between 1991 and 1994 developed refractory seizures, metabolic acidosis, vomiting, and/or coma after accidental or suicidal ingestion of toxic doses of INH (14 - 99 mg/kg). Eight patients were adolescents and one was a 5 day old infant. Symptoms began within 45 - 150 min (aver, 90 min). IV pyridoxine controlled seizures. (Shah BR et al. Acute isoniazid neurotoxicity in an urban hospital. Pediatrics May 1995;95:700-704). (Reprints: Binita R Shah MD, Box 49, Department of Pediatrics, Children's Medical Center of Brooklyn, State University of New York, Health Science Center at Brooklyn, 450 Clarkson Ave, Brooklyn, NY 11203).

COMMENT. In children receiving prophylactic treatment for tuberculosis who present with an acute onset of seizures refractory to anticonvulsants, isoniazid toxicity should be suspected and pyridoxine administered intravenously. Pyridoxine reverses the depletion of GABA caused by INH and restores the balance of inhibitory and excitatory neurotransmitters in the brain. If the amount of INH ingested is known, the dose of pyridoxine is limited to a gram-for-gram replacement, and is given in 15 to 30 minutes. Multiple excessive doses of pyridoxine may result in sensory loss and should be avoided. INH inhibits phenytoin metabolism and may lead to phenytoin toxicity. Diazepam can be used to supplement the specific anticonvulsant effect of the pyridoxine in INH induced seizures that are severe or prolonged. -Editor. *Ped Neur Briefs* June 1995.

CHLORAL HYDRATE: A POTENTIAL CARCINOGEN

The long-term health effects of chloral hydrate are discussed and its carcinogenicity in mice are reported from the University of California, Davis, and the California School of Public Health, Berkeley. In a group of 8 mice receiving 10 mg/kg, 6 developed hepatic adenomas or carcinomas, an incidence significantly greater than that of 2/19 controls with carcinomas. Of 24 mice receiving 166 mg/kg/daily intake of chloral hydrate in drinking water for 104 weeks, 17 developed hepatic adenomas or carcinomas compared to 3 of 20 controls. Other recent studies have shown chloral hydrate to be genotoxic, causing chromosome changes in vivo and in vitro. (Salmon AG, Kizer KW et al. Potential carcinogenicity of chloral hydrate - a review. Clin Toxicol 1995;33:115-121). (Respond: Dr Kenneth Kizer, Department of Community and International Health, School of Medicine, TB-168, University of California, Davis, CA 95616).

COMMENT. Many of us who have stocked chloral hydrate in large quantities for use in sedating children for EEGs and other short procedures may want to reconsider its safety and substitute an alternative. Certainly, its chronic long-term use as a sedative in mentally retarded children should be discouraged until further studies are completed. Chloral hydrate is a metabolite of trichloroethylene, a known carcinogen. -Editor. *Ped Neur Briefs* June 1995.

AMPHOTERICIN B ENCEPHALOPATHY

Three children with refractory leukemia treated

by bone marrow transplantation at the Children's National Medical Center, Washington, DC, developed encephalopathy, leukoencephalopathy, and parkinsonism after receiving high-dose amphotericin B for pulmonary aspergillosis All three had previously been treated with high-dose chemotherapy and total body irradiation. MRIs showed basal ganglia, cerebellar, and cerebral atrophy, and frontal and temporal lobe white matter changes. One died and two recovered after withdrawal of the amphotericin, 1 having intellectual impairment. (Mott SH, Packer RJ et al. Encephalopathy with Parkinsonian features in children following bone marrow transplantations and high-dose amphotericin B. <u>Ann Neurol</u> June 1995;37:810-814). (Respond: Dr Mott, Department of Neurology, Children's National Medical Center, 111 Michigan Ave, NW, Washington, DC 20010).

COMMENT. Neurologic complications of bone marrow transplantation in children with leukemia are a common occurrence. These have included seizures, infections, and encephalopathies, but Parkinsonian symptoms associated with amphotericin B appear to be unique. -Editor. *Ped Neur Briefs* July 1995.

HEMORRHAGIC SHOCK AND INFANTILE ENCEPHALOPATHY

The clinical characteristics, treatment and possible causes of hemorrhagic shock and encephalopathy in infants are described and a 5-month-old patient is reported from the Section of Neurology, The Children's Mercy Hospital, Kansas City, MO. The infant presented with fever and irritability. She developed respiratory distress, requiring endotracheal intubation, followed by cardiorespiratory arrest. Excessive bleeding from puncture sites was associated with a disseminated intravascular coagulopathy. Admission diagnosis was septic shock. Other complications of this encephalopathy are bloody diarrhea and hepatorenal failure. Treatment requires fluids and electrolytes, fresh frozen plasma, and vitamin K. Hyperthermia appeared important in causation. (Chaves-Carballo E. Hemorrhagic shock and encephalopathy: a new neurologic syndrome in infants. <u>Acta Neuropediatr</u> 1995;1:178-184). (Reprints: Dr E Chaves-Carballo, Section of Neurology, Children's Mercy Hospital, 2401 Gillham Road, Kansas City, MO 64108).

COMMENT. The syndrome was first described in Great Britain in 1983 as cited by the author (Levin M et al. <u>Lancet</u> 1983;2:64-67). The differential diagnosis includes septic shock, toxic-shock syndrome, Reye syndrome, and hemolytic-uremic syndrome. Early aggressive therapy was recommended. -Editor. *Ped Neur Briefs* July 1995.

MRI IN KERNICTERUS

The magnetic resonance images (MRI) of three children with athetotic cerebral palsy and severe neonatal jaundice were examined in the Department of Pediatric Neurology, Ohzora-no-iye Hospital and Seirei-Mikatahara General Hospital, Shizuoka, Japan. High intensity areas in the posteromedial border of the globus pallidus on T2-weighted images were found bilaterally in all 3 children. No abnormalities were demonstrated on T1-weighted imaging. (Yokochi K. Magnetic resonance imaging in children with kernicterus. <u>Acta Paediatr</u> August 1995;84:937-9). (Respond: Dr K Yokochi, Ohzora-no-iye Hospital, 7448 Nakagawa, Hosoe, Inasa, Shizuoka 431-13, Japan).

COMMENT. Kernicteric encephalopathy is a rare neonatal disorder since the introduction of phototherapy. Autopsy findings have revealed bilirubin staining of the globus pallidus, subthalamic nucleus, hippocampus, and dentate and olivary nuclei. The posteromedial border of the globus pallidus is the most sensitive region to kernicterus in MR imaging. Perinatal hypoxic-ischemic encephalopathy is distinguished by involvement of the putamen and thalamus on pathological and MR studies. The author lists other diseases with MR lesions in the globus pallidus including Leigh syndrome, Hallervorden-Spatz disease, hemolytic uremic syndrome (associated with E coli 0157:H7 and *Shigella dysenteriae* food poisoning), carbon monoxide intoxication, hepatic encephalopathy, and neurofibromatosis. See <u>Progress in Pediatric Neurology II</u> (PNB Publishers, 1994, pp242-3) for a previous article by the same author and commentary on MRI in 22 athetotic cerebral palsied children. The value of the MRI in the timing of basal ganglia pathology has been alluded to in other reports of dyskinetic and dystonic cerebral palsy (*ibidem.* pp243-4). Of 219 dyskinetic CP cases seen between 1955 and 1986 in the Cheyne CP Centre, Chelsea, London, 25% had been diagnosed with kernicterus. -Editor. *Ped Neur Briefs* Oct 1995.

VITAMIN A SUPPLEMENTS AND BULGING FONTANELLE

Safety of vitamin A supplements in early infancy was investigated by double-blind, randomized, placebo-controlled trial in 167 infants in the Urban Surveillance System area of the International Centre for Diarrhoeal Research, Bangladesh. Three doses of 25000 IU of vitamin A or placebo were given at 6, 12 and 17 weeks of age, and infants were examined by physicians on days 1, 2, 3 and 8 after supplementation. Bulging fontanelle occurred in 9 (10.5%) infants receiving vitamin A compared to 2 (2.5%) in the placebo group (p<0.05). The side effect was not observed after the first dose, 3 infants were affected after the second supplement, and 9 after the third. A cumulative effect of vitamin A was likely. (Baqui AH et al. Bulging fontanelle after supplementation with 25000 IU of vitamin A in infancy using immunization contacts. <u>Acta Paediatr</u> August 1995;84:863-6). (Respond: Dr AH Baqui, Urban MCH-FP Extension Project, ICDDR,B, GPO Box 128, Dhaka 1000, Bangladesh).

COMMENT. The infants in this study received vitamin A supplements together with the routine DPT/OPV immunization. Bulging of the fontanelle has been reported in the US as a side effect of immunization with DTP vaccine and DT vaccine. (Gross TP et al. <u>J Pediatr</u> 1989;114:423-5 [cited in above study]). An additive or synergistic effect of the immunization cannot be excluded. The reliability of the clinical assessment of the fontanelle by observation and palpation is also debated, and a probable underestimation of vitamin A toxicity is suggested by the authors.

With present day enthusiasm for supplemental vitamins and a common attitude of nonchalance toward possible vitamin overdosage, the recognition of early symptoms and signs of vitamin toxicity is important. (Millichap JG. <u>Environmental Poisons in Our Food</u>, Chicago, PNB Publishers, 1993). -Editor. *Ped Neur Briefs* Oct 1995.

MINT TEA (PENNYROYAL) EPILEPTIC ENCEPHALOPATHY

For an interesting report of epileptic encephalopathy and fulminant liver failure in two infants given tea brewed from home-grown mint plant leaves, *see* Chapter 1, pp 14-16. This reports alerts physicians to the potential toxicity of some mint teas which contain pennyroyal oil, a highly neurotoxic and hepatotoxic agent. Herbal remedies are added to the list of causes of infantile generalized seizures and encephalopathy.

CHAPTER **15**

METABOLIC DISORDERS

INTRODUCTION

John H. Menkes, M.D.
Department of Pediatric Neurology,
Cedars-Sinai Medical Center,
University of California, Los Angeles, CA.

The importance of metabolic disorders in the practice of pediatric neurology is overshadowed by the static encephalopathies and by the numerous developmental and seizure disorders. Yet, genetic or acquired disorders of intermediary metabolism are responsible for a significant percentage of neurologic disease, and unless considered in the differential diagnosis and diligently searched for by the clinician they will remain undetected. As I like to tell my students: "The infant or child with an inborn error of metabolism will not come to the clinic with a placard saying: 'I have an inborn error of metabolism'."

In this time of limited health care expenditures, it is important to remember that screening for metabolic disorders is relatively inexpensive and for the greater part is non-invasive. In view of the protean clinical picture of these diseases, they must be considered in the differential diagnosis of neurologic problems whenever other causes are not readily apparent. In particular, the presence of a neurologic disorder or developmental delay in first degree relatives should arouse suspicion of a genetically induced metabolic disorder, as should recurrent episodes of altered consciousness, movement disorders or other neurologic dysfunction, and a progressive cerebral degeneration. A good review of this field is by Hoffmann, GF et al (Neurologic manifestations of organic acid disorders. Eur J Pediatr 1994;153:(Suppl 1), S94-100).

Even the presence of dysmorphic features does not preclude a metabolic disorder. Dysmorphic features have been encountered in glutaric acidemia, type II (Dobyns WB, Truwit, CL. Lissencephaly and other malformations of cortical development: 1995 update. Neuropediatrics 1995;26:132-147), Zellweger syndrome, pyruvic dehydrogenase deficiency, and in the Smith-Lemli-Opitz syndrome, a disorder in cholesterol biosynthesis at the point of conversion of 7-dehydrocholesterol to cholesterol. (Shefer S et al. Markedly inhibited 7-dehydrocholesterol-delta 7-reductase activity in liver microsomes from Smith-Lemli-Opitz homozygotes. J Clin Invest 1995;96:1779-1785). (*see also* Ped Neur Briefs Sept 1996, and Chap 7, p 389).

An outline of the various laboratory tests which should be included in a diagnostic evaluation are presented in my Textbook of Child Neurology, 5th Edition, pp 30-32. In addition to the tests mentioned in the text, two other tests have received recent prominence.

An assay of plasma free and combined carnitine will not only uncover primary carnitine deficiency, an extremely rare disorder, but also a variety of carnitine deficiencies secondary to disorders in fatty acid oxidation, and mitochondrial disorders. These measurements therefore serve as an excellent screening test, (Ped Neur Briefs 1996;10;5-6). In my opinion, the question whether carnitine deficiency acquired by children who are receiving valproate should be corrected has not been resolved. Since carnitine therapy is relatively harmless it is probably best to advise carnitine supplementation in children who are receiving valproate, or who are on multiple anticonvulsants. (Ped Neur Briefs 1996;10:6).

The role of iodine deficiency in the evolution of learning disabilities and attention deficit disorders has been considered in several publications. (Ped Neur Briefs 1996;10:41-42; Ped Neur Briefs 1996;10:69-70). Measurements of T4 and TSH levels are therefore indicated in the clinical evaluation of every child who presents with an attention deficit disorder.

John H. Menkes, M.D.

TESTS FOR SUSPECTED INBORN ERRORS OF METABOLISM

The initial laboratory assessment of infants and children with suspected inborn errors of metabolism (IEM) is reviewed by the Department of Medical Genetics, Mayo Clinic, Rochester, MN. Classes of IEM include organic acidemias, aminoacidopathies, urea cycle defects, glycogen storage diseases, lysosomal storage diseases, B-oxidation defects, and peroxisomal disorders. Signs and symptoms of IEM include failure to thrive, loss of milestones, vomiting, seizures, coma, hepatosplenomegaly, dysmorphic features, sparse or abnormal textured hair, cataract and other eye findings, and urine or body odor. Initial tests suggested include blood gases, glucose, urinary ketones, ammonia, electrolytes, uric acid, liver function, lactate and pyruvate, carnitine, free fatty acids, B-hydoxybutyrate, and acetoacetate. (Lindor NM, Karnes PS. Initial assessment of infants and children with suspected inborn errors of metabolism. <u>Mayo Clin Proc</u> October 1995;70:987-988). (Reprints: Dr NM Lindor, Department of Medical Genetics, Mayo Clinic, 200 First Street SW, Rochester, MN 55905).

COMMENT. Examples of IEM requiring additional preliminary tests include Menkes' kinky-hair disease (serum copper and ceruloplasmin), and molybdenum cofactor deficiency (urine sulfite dipstick). -Editor. *Ped Neur Briefs* Nov 1995.

METABOLIC DISORDERS AND SEIZURES

Metabolic disorders are frequently manifested as seizures refractory to anticonvulsant medications. *See* Chapter 1, pp 93-99, for articles on pyridoxine-dependent epilepsy and complications, and hypocalcemic and hypomagnesemic seizures. Also, biotinidase deficiency and infantile spasms, pp 38-39.

DISTAL VACUOLAR MYOPATHY IN NEPHROPATHIC CYSTINOSIS

See Chapter 6, Neuromuscular Disorders, p 351, for this relatively common late complication of cystinosis. Cysteamine therapy may prove effective.

GENETICS OF MENKES DISEASE

Fibroblast cultures from 12 unrelated patients with classical Menkes disease, an X-linked disorder of copper metabolism, were analyzed for mutations in the MNK gene at the Howard Hughes Medical Institute, University of California, San Francisco. Mutations were observed in 10 patients. Southern blot hybridization and reverse transcription-PCR should identify mutations in the majority of patients. (Das S et al. Diverse mutations in patients with Menkes disease often lead to exon skipping. <u>Am J Hum Genet</u> Nov 1994;55:883-889). (Reprints: Dr Seymour Packman, Department of Pediatrics, Division of Genetics, University of California, San Francisco, CA 94143).

COMMENT. The authors conclude that these studies should help to clarify the role of mutations leading to mild and atypical cases of Menkes disease, X-linked cutis laxa, and classical Menkes disease. Partial gene deletions have been observed in 15 - 20% of patients with Menkes disease. The majority of patients have the severe, classical symptoms of a progressive neurologic degeneration, connective-tissue defects, hypopigmentation, kinky hair, and death in early childhood. A deficiency of copper-containing enzymes results from a defect in copper transport. -Editor. *Ped Neur Briefs* Nov 1994.

CONGENITAL LACTIC ACIDOSIS: PET AND MRS STUDIES

Positron emission tomography (PET) and proton magnetic resonance spectroscopy (MRS) identified an increase in rate of cerebral glycolysis (PET) and cerebral lactate (MRS) in 2 children with defective mitochondrial respiration and congenital lactic acidosis studied at the Universitat zu Koln, Germany, and the University Hospital, Nijmegen, The Netherlands. These changes were not apparent in a child with lactic acidosis and normal respiratory chain activity. Defects of oxidative phosphorylation may cause increases in glycolysis and accumulation of cerebral lactate. (Duncan DB et al. Positron emission tomography and magnetic resonance spectroscopy of cerebral glycolysis in children with congenital lactic acidosis. Ann Neurol March 1995;37:351-358). (Respond: Prof Dr Heiss, Max-Planck-Institut fur neurologische Forschung, Gleueler Str 50, 50931 Koln, Germany).

COMMENT. PET and MRS have been used to demonstrate the metabolic changes associated with defective mitochondrial respiration in the brain without resort to diagnostic muscle biopsy. For further discussion of MRS in mitochondrial disorders, see Progress in Pediatric Neurology II, 1994, p454. -Editor. *Ped Neur Briefs* April 1995.

CARNITINE PT II DEFICIENCY AND CEREBRAL DYSGENESIS

A newborn female infant with neonatal lethal multiorgan carnitine palmitoyltransferase II (CPT II) defiency is reported from the Departments of Medicine and Pathology, Children's Hospital, Boston, MA; and the Department of Pharmacology and Medicine, Case Western Reserve University, VA Medical Center, Cleveland, OH. The infant was referred at 4 days of age because of hyperammonemia and seizures. Pregnancy was complicated by oligohydramnios. Ultrasound on day 1 showed enlarged kidneys with cortical cysts. Cranial ultrasound revealed a periventricular cyst. On day 3, seizures with prolonged apnea were followed by unresponsiveness. Pupils were fixed and dilated. Dysmorphic features included microcephaly, long fingers and toes, extra digital creases, and joint contractures. The liver enlarged, and the infant died at 10 days with cardiac and renal failure. Long-chain acylcarnitines were elevated in blood and multiple tissues, and lipid accumulations and deficiency of CPT II activity were found in heart, liver, muscle, and kidney tissue. (North KN et al. Lethal neonatal deficiency of carnitine palmitoyltransferase II associated with dysgenesis of the brain and kidneys. J Pediatr September 1995;127:414-420). (Reprints: Kathryn N North MD, Department of Neurology, Children's Hospital, Bridge Road, Camperdown, New South Wales 2050, Australia).

COMMENT. The authors cite two previous reports of families with neonatal CPT II deficiency associated with multiple malformations. Autopsy findings include diffuse lipid accumulation, cardiomegaly, dysplastic kidneys, and brain migration defects. They conclude that this metabolic disorder should be included in the differential diagnosis of neonates dying with dysmorphism and multiple organ malformations, along with Zellweger syndrome, other disorders of peroxisomal B-oxidation, and glutaric acidemia type II. -Editor. *Ped Neur Briefs* Jan 1996.

CARNITINE DEFICIENCY SYNDROMES

Carnitine deficiency syndromes are reviewed from the Departments of Neurology and Pediatrics, Columbia Presbyterian Medical Center, New York, NY.

Primary carnitine deficiency is a decrease of intracellular carnitine that impairs fatty acid oxidation and is not associated with another systemic illness. It may be systemic or muscular, presenting as progressive cardiomyopathy, hypoketotic hypoglycemic encephalopathy, or myopathy. Age at onset is 1 month to 7 years, with a mean of 2 years. In encephalopathy, carnitine levels in plasma and tissues are below 10% of normal, and acylcarnitines are proportionately reduced. Acylcarnitine to free carnitine ratio is normal. Treatment is oral carnitine at daily doses of 100 to 200 mg/kg. Intermittent diarrhea and a fishy body odor are described as side effects of carnitine replacement. Muscle carnitine deficiency is characterized by severe reduction in muscle carnitine levels and normal serum carnitine.

Secondary carnitine deficiency is manifested by a decrease in levels of plasma or tissue carnitine, and is associated with genetically determined metabolic errors, acquired medical conditions, or iatrogenic factors. Metabolic errors involve fatty acid oxidation, B-oxidation cycle, aminoacidurias, and mitochondrial disorders. Acquired disorders include cirrhosis, malnutrition, vegetarian diet, celiac disease, extreme prematurity, AIDS, and Fanconi syndrome. Anticonvulsant treatment with valproate has been linked to some carnitine deficiencies. Several mechanisms are proposed for valproic acid-induced carnitine deficiency, some involving an underlying primary metabolic inborn error. The authors recommend prophylactic carnitine in all children under 2 years of age who are treated with valproate. Secondary carnitine deficiencies are managed by high carbohydrate, low fat frequent feedings, and vitamin/cofactor supplements (carnitine, glycine, and riboflavin). (Pons R, De Vivo DC. Primary and secondary carnitine deficiency syndromes. <u>J Child Neurol</u> November 1995;10(Suppl):2S8-2S24). (Respond: Dr Darryl C De Vivo, Neurological Institute, 710 West 168 Street, New York, NY 10032).

COMMENT. In the same issue, Coulter DL, from the Boston City Hospital, discusses the risk factors and treatment of carnitine deficiency in epilepsy. (<u>J Child Neurol</u> 1995;10(Suppl):2S32-2S39). Carnitine deficiency in epilepsy results from metabolic diseases, poor nutrition, and anticonvulsants, especially but not exclusively valproate. Carnitine supplements benefit high-risk, symptomatic patients and those with free carnitine deficiency, but not the low-risk, asymptomatic patients and those with normal carnitine levels. -Editor. *Ped Neur Briefs* Jan 1996.

VISUAL EVOKED POTENTIALS IN PHENYLKETONURIA

Visual evoked potentials (VEPs) were studied in 36 patients with phenylketonuria, and compared with MRI findings, dietary state, and IQ, at the Institute of Neurology, Queen Square, and the Institute of Child Health, Great Ormond Street Hospital, London, UK. Four patients presented with progressive neurological deficits. Twenty six were detected by routine neonatal screening, and 9 were diagnosed with developmental delay at age 5 years. All except one showing no symptoms had received a low phenylalanine diet until age 7 years or later. In 9 patients aged less than 14 years who were still on the diet, VEPs were normal in 8 and the MRI was abnormal in all but only mildly irregular in 6. The one patient with abnormal VEPs had the most pronounced MRI abnormalities and the lowest IQ score (74 compared to 90-119 in the remaining 8). Of 27 patients aged 14-31 years, >80% had abnormal VEPs, showing reduction of amplitude and prolonged latencies, whereas neuro-ophthalmological examination was normal. VEP amplitude was inversely correlated with MRI abnormalities and severity of white matter lesions in the parieto-occipital region, and with IQ. VEP abnormalities were marginally correlated with plasma phenylalanine concentrations but were not dependent on a sustained low phenylalanine diet. (Jones SJ et al. Visual evoked potentials in phenylketonuria: association with brain

MRI, dietary state, and IQ. <u>J Neurol Neurosurg Psychiatry</u> September 1995;59:260-265). (Respond: Dr SJ Jones, Department of Clinical Neurophysiology, National Hospital for Neurology and Neurosurgery, Queen Square, London WC1N 2BG, UK).

COMMENT. This study confirms reports of the frequency of abnormal VEPs in patients with phenylketonuria, even in those diagnosed and treated early. VEP decreased amplitude and prolonged latency are correlated to some extent with subcortical myelin defects revealed by MRI. A striking increase in incidence of VEP and MRI abnormalities in older patients coincided with relaxed dietary management, plasma phenylalanine concentrations, and intellectual performance. -Editor. *Ped Neur Briefs* Oct 1995.

FUCOSIDOSIS WITH DYSTONIA

A Canadian male child with fucosidosis and dystonia is reported from the Department of Biochemical Genetics, University of Western Ontario, London, Ontario, Canada. All milestones were delayed, he crawled at 14 months, walked by 18 months, and his developmental quotient at 27 months was 50. At 46 months the quotient had dropped to 35. At 5 years, dystonic posturing of the left leg began, and 6 months later, he had episodes of choking, staring spells, and nocturnal apnea. At 7 years,he could not walk or talk, and the dystonia was bilateral. An angiokeratomatous rash became generalized. Cultured lymphoblasts showed absent a-fucosidase activity and protein. He was homozygous for the Q422X mutation. (Gordon BA et al. Fucosidosis with dystonia. <u>Neuropediatrics</u> 1995;26:325-327). (Respond: Dr BA Gordon, Department of Biochemical Genetics, CPRI, 600 Sanatorium Road, London, ON, Canada N6H 3W7).

COMMENT. Fucosidosis is a progressive neurodegenerative disease presenting in early childhood and manifested by loss of mental and motor function, with early hypotonia followed by increasing spasticity and seizures. Dystonia evident in this report had not previously been reported. Dysmorphic features and skeletal changes similar to those in mucopolysaccharidoses develop and include dwarfism, dysostosis multiplex, and visceromegaly. A skin rash occurs in those surviving childhood. The disease is caused by an autosomal recessive genetic deficiency of the lysosomal enzyme a-L-fucosidase. Seventy seven patient reports were reviewed in 1991. Menkes JH refers to two forms, type 1 without, and type 2 with angiokeratoma of the skin, particularly of the gingiva and genitalia. (<u>Textbook of Child Neurology</u> 3rd ed, Philadelphia, Lea & Febiger, 19850. -Editor. *Ped Neur Briefs* Jan 1996.

PRESENTING SIGNS OF MITOCHONDRIAL DISEASE

Clinical features of 51 patients confirmed with mitochondrial respiratory chain disease and clinical investigations most helpful in diagnosis of different phenotypes are reported from the Divisions of Clinical Neuroscience and Neurobiology, University of Newcastle upon Tyne, UK. Ages ranged from birth to 55 years, and 21 patients were <16 years. Presenting symptoms in order of frequency included ptosis and ophthalmoplegia (20), lactic acidosis (10), seizures (6), myopathy (6), failure to thrive (6), and ataxia (5). Features other than ptosis and ophthalmoplegia identified as clues to respiratory chain dysfunction were as follows: 1) lactic acidosis with deafness, short stature/failure to thrive, or basal ganglia calcifications on CT; 2) family history of neurological disease with maternal transmission; and 3) proximal myopathy and CNS disease. In addition to well-recognized syndromes (MERRF and MELAS) many had non-specific encephalopathies. The most useful confirmatory diagnostic test was histochemical analysis of muscle. (Jackson MJ, Bindoff LA et al. Presentation and clinical investigation of mitochondrial respiratory chain disease. A study of 51 patients. <u>Brain</u> April 1995;118:339-357). (Respond: Dr LA Bindoff, Division of Clinical

Neuroscience, The Medical School, University of Newcastle upon Tyne, Framlington Place, Newcastle upon Tyne NE2 4HH, UK).

COMMENT. Mitochondrial respiratory chain disease is manifested by a large variety of syndromes, but histological and chemical analysis of skeletal muscle is frequently diagnostic. Succinate dehyrogenase, cytochrome c oxidase activity, and DNA studies in muscle may be performed on a needle biopsy specimen. Elevated CSF lactate is a good indicator of mitochondrial disease in patients with encephalopathic disorders.

The treatment of congenital lactic acidosis is reviewed from the Center for Inherited Disorders of Energy Metabolism, Case Western Reserve University, Cleveland, OH (Kerr DS. Int Pediatr 1995;10:75-81). Treatments have included diet, vitamins, use of enzyme activators, and enzyme replacement. None has been very successful. See Progress in Pediatric Neurology I and II (Millichap JG, Ed. PNB Publ, 1991 and 1994) for further articles on mitochondrial cytopathies. The diagnosis of mitochondrial disorder should be considered with the following: 1) an unexplained association of symptoms; 2) an early onset and rapidly progressive course; and 3) involvement of unrelated organs sharing no common embryologic origin and no common biological functions. -Editor. *Ped Neur Briefs* June 1995.

LESCH-NYHAN SYNDROME: PRENATAL DIAGNOSIS

The results of carrier and prenatal diagnosis for Lesch-Nyhan syndrome by carrier testing of 83 women and prenatal analysis of 26 pregnancies are reported from the Department of Molecular and Human Genetics, Baylor College of Medicine, Houston, TX. Mutation detection and linkage analysis were used for probands and their families and biochemical measurement of HPRT enzyme activity for at-risk pregnancies. Mutations in the HPRT gene of affected males were detected in 100% cases. Forty five (56%) at-risk women were found not to carry their family's HPRT gene mutation. (Alford RL et al. Lesch-Nyhan syndrome: Carrier and prenatal diagnosis. <u>Prenat Diagn</u> April 1995;15:329-338). (Respond: Dr RL Alford, Department of Molecular and Human Genetics T-528, Baylor College of Medicine, One Baylor Plaza, Houston, TX 77030).

COMMENT. Lesch-Nyhan syndrome is an X-linked recessive disorder characterized by hyperuricemia, choreoathetosis, mental retardation, self-mutilatory behavior, and a deficiency of the enzyme hypoxanthine guanine phosphoribosyltransferase (HPRT). Molecular diagnostic studies of affected males and carrier testing prior to pregnancy have been shown to demonstrate genetic risks, and unnecessary prenatal tests may be avoided. *Editor. Ped Neur Briefs* June 1995.

CHAPTER **16**

HEREDO-DEGENERATIVE AND DEMYELINATING DISORDERS

INTRODUCTION
Paul Richard Dyken, M.D.
Institute for Research in Childhood Neurodegenerative
Diseases, Mobile, Alabama

The heredo-degenerative and demyelinating disorders are the terms used to describe a group of diseases and syndromes which are characterized by progressive neurological symptomatology. Such disorders are also called the neurodegenerative diseases, or less often, the progressive encephalomyelomyopathies. The diseases included in this chapter represent a large portion of the practice of pediatric neurology. Dyken P (Semin Pediatr Neurol 1996;3(4):251-253) estimated that the frequency of such disorders varied between 10 and 28% of ones practice in the United States and exceeded 50% in certain more genetically cloistered populations such as found in the Kingdom of Saudi Arabia. The nosology of these disorders has been of importance in the understanding of the epidemiology and demographics and, therefore, the mechanisms of these disorders, such as recognition, pathogenesis, etiology and therapy.

The chapter to follow is organized, with some chronological outline, to emphasize what is believed to be the major advances in the field in the last few years, with an emphasis on clinical aspects. The recent medical literature is nicely summarized and presented in a succinct fashion. Descriptions are given of several new or previously unrecognized syndromes which fit into this category. There are reviews of articles on hereditary, degenerative, and demyelinating conditions, reviews of the recent advances in previously established neurodegenerative diseases as they affect children, treatments of selected neurodegenerative diseases and establishment of diagnostic criteria for these diseases.

Although the heredo-degenerative and demyelinating disorders represent a sizable proportion of the practice of child neurology, much of the recent progress in the field, at least in the past few years, has been in the descriptions of rare or infrequently encountered forms of these disorders. Included within this chapter are reports on several specific, possibly newly described and unique disorders, documentation of which enrich the entire field. Included are fine reviews and cogent editorial comment on several new or freshly described syndromes on ataxia with idiopathic hypomyelination, sensory ataxia with viatamin E deficiency, cerebellar ataxia and folate deficiency, a variety of childhood forms of what is to be considered multiple sclerosis, infantile leukoencephalopathy of mild course, the harp syndrome (i.e. hypoprebetolipoproteinemia, acanthocytosis, retinitis pigmentosa and pallidal degeneration), Friedreich ataxia with retained reflexes (Farr syndrome), and primary lateral sclerosis with gaze paralysis. The recent literature on these entities has been thoroughly reviewed and related to past literature when the need has arisen.

Additionally, the chapter deals with other new advances concerning these heredodegenerative and demyelinating disorders, ranging from the descriptions of the neuropathological and pathogenetic mechanisms of the sudden infantile death syndrome (SIDS), multiple sclerosis in children, progressive multifocal leukoencephalopathy in children, late onset Krabbe disease and many aspects of the pediatric events in the fascinating entity, Machado-Joseph disease.

Simply listing new diseases or descriptions is not the primary basis for the inclusion of this chapter. Rather it is intended as a review of some of the unique advances in the field. Included in the chapter, therefore, is a section summarizing the treatment of typical Friedreich ataxia with 5 hydroxytryptophan. This represents an important review since, even in these modern times, there remains a generally false misconception that these diseases are not always "treatable." Another interesting review deals with the diagnosis of Hallervorden-Spatz disease by neuroimaging.

In summary, the chapter to follow is of importance in covering most of the recent advances in this sometimes perplexing field of pediatric neurology. It is especially of value to the practicing neurologist to have the literature reviewed and interpreted under the classification of neurodegenerative diseases of childhood. *Paul R Dyken, M.D.*

PROGRESSIVE ATAXIA WITH IDIOPATHIC HYPOMYELINATION

A progressive ataxic diplegia syndrome of unknown etiology is reported in 4 unrelated girls evaluated at the National Institutes of Health, Bethesda, MD; Johns Hopkins University, Baltimore, MD; and Tufts, New England Medical Center, Boston, MA. Following normal early milestones, clumsiness and then progressive ataxia developed at 2 to 5 years of age. Seizures occurred in 3 of the 4 patients, some with fever. The ability to walk or sit independently was lost within one year of onset of ataxia. Other symptoms included progressive dysarthria and painful leg cramps. Two had optic atrophy. Deep tendon reflexes were markedly increased, plantar responses were extensor, and ankle clonus was elicited. Cognition was normal in two and mildly delayed in two. Early CTs and MRIs showed diffuse hypodensity of cerebral and cerebellar white matter, and later studies after clinical deterioration showed no progressive change or atrophy. Known metabolic and degenerative diseases were excluded. Open-brain biopsy specimens from two patients showed white matter hypomyelination, demyelination, and gliosis. Myelin-specific proteins and lipid analyses revealed decreased levels. Magnetic resonance spectroscopic imaging showed decrease of N-acetylaspartic acid, choline, and creatine in white matter, a diagnostic feature of the syndrome. (Schiffmann R et al. Childhood ataxia with diffuse central nervous system hypomyelination. <u>Ann Neurol</u> March 1994;<u>35</u>:331-340). (Respond: Dr Schiffmann, National Institutes of Health, Bldg 10, Rm 3D03, 9000 Rockville Pike, Bethesda, MD 20892).

COMMENT. The MRSI findings appear to be unique to this childhood ataxic syndrome. The degree of white matter hypomyelination, found early and before clinical deterioration, and the absence of further white matter changes despite worsening of ataxia are remarkable findings. -Editor. *Ped Neur Briefs* April 1994.

SENSORY ATAXIA AND VITAMIN E DEFICIENCY

A progressive limb and gait ataxia, distal loss of proprioception and vibration sense, and areflexia, caused by a prolonged and severe vitamin E deficiency, are reported in four patients evaluated as adults at King's College, Hammersmith Hospital, and Institutes of Neurology and Child Health, London, UK. Two patients had abetalipoproteinemia and vitamin E was undetectable from birth. One had a familial vitamin E defiency, and had been diagnosed as Friedreich's ataxia at 13 years of age. One had Crohn's disease and fat malabsorption dating back to 16 years. Three had striking head tremor. Impaired nigrostriatal activity in the patients with abetalipoproteinemia, demonstrated by reduced dopa uptake using PET studies, was similar to that seen in Parkinson's disease. (Dexter DT et al. Nigrostriatal function in vitamin E deficiency: Clinical, experimental, and positron emission tomographic studies. <u>Ann Neurol</u> March 1994;<u>35</u>:298-303). (Respond: Prof AE Harding, University Dept of Clinical Neurology, Institute of Neurology, Queen Square, London, WC1N 3BG, UK).

COMMENT. Some children with typical signs of Friedreich's ataxia have familial vitamin E deficiency syndrome, with autosomal recessive inheritance. (<u>Ped Neur Briefs</u> Dec 1993;<u>7</u>:91). Early identification and supplementation with vitamin E may halt progression of the ataxia. A dose of 800 mg/day vitamin E in the 43-year-old male patient with this syndrome reported above had stabilized the neurologic status and his serum level of vitamin E was normal. -Editor. *Ped Neur Briefs* April 1994.

CEREBELLAR ATAXIA AND CSF FOLATE DEFICIENCY

A slowly progressive cerebellar syndrome associated with disturbed folate transfer across the choroid plexus is reported in an 18-year-old male who presented with incoordination of hands and feet at the Institute of Neurology, University Hospital of Nijmegen, The Netherlands. A rapidly progressive bilateral sensorineural hearing loss had preceeded the onset of ataxia which was complicated by dysarthria and dysphagia, and was followed at 21 years, with muscle cramps and at 26 years, with a distal spinal muscular atrophy and pyramidal tract signs of hyperreflexia and Babinski reflexes. Cranial CT showed cerebral and cerebellar atrophy and hypodensities in the basal ganglia. The serum (9.6-10.5 nmol/l) and red cell (371) folate levels were normal while the CSF folate was severely depleted (1.4-2.6 nmol/l; ref normal range 14-42). Analyses of folate binding protein in CSF performed at laboratories in Denmark showed abnormalities that indicate a defective folate transport into the CNS. (Wevers RA et al. Folate deficiency in cerebrospinal fluid associated with a defect in folate binding protein in the central nervous system. <u>J Neurol Neurosurg Psychiatry</u> Feb 1994;<u>57</u>:223-226). (Respond: Dr RA Wevers, Institute of Neurology, University of Nijmegen, PO Box 9101, 6500 HB Nijmegen, The Netherlands).

COMMENT. Folate occurs in higher concentrations in CSF than in plasma, and it enters the CSF against a concentration gradient. Folate binding proteins in the plasma membrane of the choroid plexus are essential in the transport of folate to the CSF and CNS. Low CSF folate has been reported in inborn errors of metabolism, Kearns-Sayre syndrome, and HIV infection. Neurologic manifestations of inherited disorders of folate metabolism include mental and motor retardation, ataxia, and seizures. Consanguinity of the parents of the above patient suggests an autosomal recessive inheritance.

In addition to folate and vitamin E deficiencies, other degenerative ataxias resembling Friedreich's ataxia that may be amenable to dietary supplements or modifications include vitamin B_{12} and biotin deficiencies and Refsum's disease, responsive to a diet low in phytol and phytanic acid.(<u>Progress in Pediatric Neurology</u>, Chicago, PNB Publ, 1991, p 480). -Editor. *Ped Neur Briefs* April 1994.

CEREBELLAR ATAXIA AND MULTIPLE SCLEROSIS

Clinical manifestations and MRI findings in four Japanese children with multiple sclerosis are reported from the Department of Pediatrics, Sapporo Medical University, Japan. Three presented with gait ataxia and one developed cerebellar intention tremor within 2 months of an onset with weakness of the right arm and speech impairment. The age of onset of symptoms was at 7-12 years. All had optic neuritis. MRI showed multiple white matter lesions and demyelinating plaques in cerebral hemispheres, cerebellum and brain stem. CT abnormalities were indefinite or absent.(Wakai S et al. Childhood multiple sclerosis: MR images and clinical variations in four Japanese cases. Brain Dev 1994;16:52-56). (Respond: Dr S Wakai, Dept of Pediatrics, School of Medicine, Sapporo Medical University, South 1 West 16, Chuo-ku, Sapporo 060, Japan).

COMMENT. MRI was more sensitive than CT in diagnosis of demyelination in these patients. One of the 4 children had presented with Devic disease and 2 years later developed chronic inflammatory demyelinating polyradiculoneuropathy. A survey of 55 pediatric patients with MS in Japan by Prof Y Fukuyama and associates (1991) had found peripheral nerve involvement in 10 (17%). -Editor. *Ped Neur Briefs* April 1994.

CHARACTERISTICS OF CHILDHOOD MULTIPLE SCLEROSIS

The clinical manfestations of multiple sclerosis (MS) in 14 children are reported from the Universidade de Sao Paulo, Brazil. Age at onset ranged from 2 to 15 years. Initial symptoms varied from minor motor impairment, visual disturbances, bladder dysfunction and paresthesias, to a diffuse encephalopathy, with impaired consciousness. All had a relapsing-remitting course, and one died 6 months after onset with disseminated demyelinating lesions. CT showed demyelination in 6 of 9 patients. MRI showed white matter lesions in the brainstem or cerebral hemispheres in 5 of 6 patients. CSF pleocytosis occurred in 8 of 23 attacks, and g-globulin levels were increased in 7. Visual evoked potentials (VEP) were abnormal in 7 of 8 patients; BAEP in 4 of 8: and SEP in 4 of 8. The importance of paraclinical examinations in diagnosis is emphasized. (Guilhoto LM de FF, Diament A et al. Pediatric multiple sclerosis report of 14 cases. Brain Dev Jan/Feb 1995;17:9-12). (Respond: Dr Laura Maria de

Figueiredo Ferreira Guilhoto, Departamento de Neurologia do Hospital das Clinicas da Faculdade de Medicina da Universidade de Sao Paulo, Av Dr Eneas Carvalho Aguiar S/N, CEP 05403-900 Sao Paulo, SP, Brazil).

COMMENT. The 14 cases were seen in a period of 12 years. Four presented before 5 years of age, and the youngest was 2 years.

According to a report from the George-August University, Gottingen, Germany, published in the review International MS Journal (Hanefeld FA. Int. MSJ 1995;1:90-97), 24 cases with MS onset before age 5 years have been published since 1969. In 20 of 39 new patients studied over a 5-year period in Gottingen, the onset was before 10 years. The onset or relapse was preceded by a nonspecific infection, usually an URI, in >50%. Of 8 presenting with optic neuritis, 4 developed MS within 2 years. CSF maximal cell count was 900/ml, and protein was increased >100 mg%. Oligoclonal bands were absent in one third. VEPs were more frequently abnormal than BAEP and SEP. MRI sometimes showed new lesions without accompanying symptoms or relapse, and remissions were not always reflected in less MRI changes. Patients with juvenile onset (>10 years) followed a more severe, frequently relapsing, course than those with onset before puberty. -Editor. *Ped Neur Briefs* March 1995.

MULTIPLE SCLEROSIS PRESENTING SYMPTOMS

Clinical and laboratory presentation and course of multiple sclerosis (MS) in 16 children are reported from the Department of Pediatric Neurology, Hacettepe University, Ankara, Turkey. The age of onset was 6 - 17 years (mean 11 yrs; 8 boys, 8 girls). Presenting symptoms and signs in order of frequency were cerebellar, pyramidal, optic neuritis, cranial nerve/brain stem signs, myelopathy, sensory, and increased intracranial pressure. CSF protein was normal in 11/12 patients tested, IgG index or oligoclonal bands were informative in 75%, evoked potentials abnormal in 70%, EEG abnormalities in 83%, MRI showed multiple plaques with increased density in T2-weighted images in 80%, and CT abnormalities in 45%. Moderate to severe disability after the first attack was seen in only 2 patients. (Selcen D, Anlar B, Renda Y. Multiple sclerosis in childhood: Report of 16 cases. Eur Neurol March/April 1996;36:79-84). (Respond: Dr Banu Anlar, Department of Pediatric Neurology, Hacettepe University, TR-06100 Ankara, Turkey).

COMMENT. MRI and CSF oligoclonal bands are the most helpful laboratory methods as adjuncts to the diagnosis of MS in children. Evoked potentials and CT are not of value in the differential diagnosis, and elevated CSF protein is more compatible with degenerative diseases other than MS. Acute disseminated encephalomyelitis and postinfectious encephalomyelitis resemble MS in the acute phase and diagnosis may only be made by follow up. At least 2 years interval was needed to exclude a relapsing MS course.

Diagnosis of multiple sclerosis in 5 childhood cases is reported from the Department of Pediatrics, La Sapienza University, and Department of Neurology, Tor Vergata University, Rome, Italy. (Iannetti P et al. Primary CNS demyelinating diseases in childhood: multiple sclerosis. Child's Nerv Syst March 1996;12:149-154). Initial symptoms in these patients were optic neuritis (2); paresthesia, dysmetria, dysgraphia; dizziness, weakness; and motor and sensory deficits. Time from first symptom to diagnosis varied from 20 days to 4 years. The MRI was most valuable in diagnosis, and elevation of CSF IgG was the best laboratory supportive finding. Neuropsychological tests may uncover cognitive dysfunction involving memory, language, and visual perception. The authors report an increasing number of pediatric cases of MS in the last 10 years.

Temporal variation in MS incidence was examined over the past 4 decades from 1950 to 1991 in More and Romsdal County, Norway, and reported from the University of Bergen, Norway. (Midgard R et al. <u>Brain</u> 1996;119:203-211). The incidence rate by year of onset increased from 2.87/100,000 in 1950-54 to 5.57/100,000 in 1985-91. A two-fold increase in incidence of MS from 1961 to 1985 was reported previously by these authors. The increase was a general trend and was not explained by a change in age distribution. Could environmental factors and water and food pollutants be involved?

Depression and multiple sclerosis was evaluated in 221 patients examined at the Departments of Psychiatry and Medical Genetics, University of British Columbia, Vancouver, Canada. (Sadovnick AD et al. <u>Neurology</u> March 1996;46:628-632). Index cases had a 50% lifetime risk of depression. Data for the first-degree relatives did not support a genetic basis for depression among MS patients. -Editor. *Ped Neur Briefs* April 1996.

MYELIN DEVELOPMENT IN SIDS: MRI FINDINGS

The MRI brain scans of 28 SIDS infants were compared with 14 controls at the Neuropathology Unit, University of Sydney, and the Department of Radiology, Royal Prince Alfred Hospital, New South Wales, Australia. The amount of myelin assessed by densitometer in 21 of 26 sites showed no changes in 15 sites, and a higher rate of myelination in 6 sites, but only in infants older than 8 months. No focal white matter abnormalities were detected. (Lamont P et al. Myelin in SIDS: Assessment of development and damage using MRI. <u>Pediatrics</u> March 1995;95:409-413). (Reprints: Dr Roger Pamphlett, Department of Pathology, University of Sydney, New South Wales 2006, Australia).

COMMENT. This MRI investigation failed to confirm the histopathological evidence of delayed myelination in SIDS victims reported from the University of Toronto (Becker LE. Neural maturational delay as a link in the chain of events leading to SIDS. <u>Can J Neurol Sci</u> Nov 1990;17:361). See <u>Progress in</u>

Pediatric Neurology I, 1991, pp309-310, for a review of mechanisms of SIDS. It was concluded that a central type of respiratory failure or cardiac dysrythmia was involved. A delayed development of the vagus nerve, similar to the finding in an infant with Ondine's curse, was described in the Canadian study.

The Steering Committee of Collaborative Home Infant Monitoring Evaluation reports on a multi-center study aimed at correlating events in infants at increased risk for SIDS, including siblings of prior SIDS victims. (Hunt CE. Sudden infant death syndrome and subsequent siblings. Pediatrics March 1995;95:430-432). It concluded that siblings are at increased risk for SIDS, and monitoring is cost-effective in sibs of prior SIDS infants.

INTERLEUKIN-6 CSF LEVELS were increased in 20 infants dying of SIDS in a study reported from the Institute of Forensic Medicine, National Hospital, Oslo, Norway. (Vege A et al. Acta Paediatr Feb 1995;84:193-6). The authors suggest that immune activation plays a role in SIDS, and cytokines in the CNS may cause respiratory depression in vulnerable infants.

An increased postneonatal mortality in lower social groups was explained by an association with SIDS in a study from the Department of Epidemiology, National Institute of Public Health, Oslo, Norway. (Arntzen A et al. Acta Paediatr Feb 1995;84:188-92).

A series of articles and an editorial in a recent issue of JAMA address the roles of sleeping position and passive smoking and tobacco exposure through breast milk in the etiology of SIDS. A major factor relating to a decline in SIDS in Tasmania was a reduction in the prevalence of prone sleeping position of infants. (Dwyer T et al. JAMA March 8, 1995;273:783-789). In contrast, routine prone sleeping position was not associated with an increased risk of SIDS in a Southern California study population. (Klonoff-Cohen HS, Edelstein SH. JAMA 1995;273:790-794).

Passive smoking in the same room as infants

increased the risk for SIDS in a study at the University of California, San Diego. (Klonoff-Cohen HS, et al. <u>JAMA</u> 1995;273:795-798). An editorial by Willinger M (<u>JAMA</u> 1995;273:818-819) advises that caregivers should follow AAP recommendations, and parents should be counselled that back or side sleep position is one measure to protect their infant from SIDS, but it is not fool-proof. -Editor. *Ped Neur Briefs* March 1995.

MULTIFOCAL LEUKOENCEPHALOPATHY

A 15-year-old boy with Wiskott-Aldrich syndrome complicated by progressive multifocal leukoencephalopathy (PML) is reported from the University of Miami School of Medicine, FL, and the National Institute of Neurological Disorders and Stroke, Bethesda, MD. At age 4 months he developed thrombocytopenic purpura and with subsequent appearance of eczema and frequent pneumonia and otitis media, the diagnosis of Wiskott-Aldrich syndrome was made at age 7 years. At age 12 years he suffered a retroperitoneal hematoma, liver abscesses, followed by frequent infections, including viral pneumonia, herpes labialis, and Candida septicemia. Neuropsychiatric problems occurred at 14 years of age and progressed, with slurred speech, apathy, and right sided weakness. MRI revealed multiple high-intensity signal lesions in brain stem and cerebrum, including thalamus and basal ganglia. Brain biopsy confirmed PML, characterized by abnormal oligodendroglial nuclei, atypical astocytes, and foamy macrophages. Immunostaining with antibody against papovirus capsid antigen was positive. Bone marrow biopsy and peripheral blood lymphocytes were positive for JC virus DNA. At autopsy the brain showed multiple areas of demyelination. intranuclear inclusions, and a large left frontal hemorrhage. Survival from the time of onset of PML was 10 months. (Katz DA et al. Progressive multifocal leukoencephalopathy complicating Wiskott-Aldrich syndrome. <u>Arch Neurol</u> April 1994;<u>51</u>:422-426). (Reprints: Dr Berger, Dept of Neurology, University of Miami School of Medicine, 1501 NW Ninth Ave, Miami, FL 33136).

COMMENT. Wiscott-Aldrich syndrome is an inherited X-linked recessive immunodeficiency disease characterized by severe eczema, thrombocytopenia, and frequent infections. Patients usually die of infection, hemorrhage, or malignant neoplasm. This case report may be the first described with PML complicating the Wiscott-Aldrich syndrome.

PML is an opportunistic infection of the CNS with JC virus characterized by a rapidly progressive degenerative demyelinating disease. Immunodeficient states associated with PML include AIDS, lymphoma, leukemia, tuberculosis, systemic lupus, organ transplant and rarely, Wiskott-Aldrich syndrome. PML is a disease of adults and is very uncommon in children. An MRI of a 40 year-old man with AIDS and PML is presented by Weiss PJ and DeMarco JK under Images in Clinical Medicine, <u>N Engl J Med</u> April 1994;<u>330</u>:1197. PML changes are best seen on the T2-weighted image as high-intensity abnormalities in the white matter. On T1-weighted image, the lesions are low-intensity and not enhanced by gadolinium, which differentiates them from primary lymphoma of the CNS. -Editor. *Ped Neur Briefs* May 1994.

INFANTILE LEUKOENCEPHALOPATHY WITH MILD COURSE

Eight children, including 2 siblings, with infantile onset cerebral leukoencephalopathy and megalencephaly, and mild neurological signs and symptoms, are reported from Free University Hospital, and Academic Medical Center, Amsterdam, The Netherlands. Ataxia and spasticity were slowly progressive, while intellectual functioning was preserved for a few years. MRI showed swelling of supratentorial hemispheral white matter, subcortical cysts, and sparing of corpus callosum and internal capsule. Metabolic studies were negative. (van der Knaap MS, Barth PG et al. Leukoencephalopathy with swelling and a discrepantly mild clinical course in eight children. <u>Ann Neurol</u> March 1995;37:324-334).

(Respond: Dr MS van der Knaap, Department of Child Neurology, Free University Hospital, PO Box 7057. 1007 MB Amsterdam, The Netherlands).

COMMENT. This type of infantile leukoencephalopathy is distinguished from Canavan and Alexander diseases by an MRI showing severe white matter abnormalities which contrasted with a slow clinical progressive course. Lysosomal and other metabolic white matter disorders characterized by megalencephaly were also ruled out biochemically and clinically.

LATE ONSET KRABBE'S DISEASE WITH PRESERVED INTELLECT in a 24-year-old Swedish male patient is reported from the County Hospital of Jonkoping, and the University of Goteborg, Sweden. (Arvidsson J, Hagberg B et al. Late onset globoid cell leukoencephalopathy (Krabbe's disease) - Swedish case with 15 years of follow-up. <u>Acta Paediatr</u> Feb 1995;84:218-21). The disease presented with visual dysfunction at 4 years of age. At 8 years he developed a limp and ataxia and within 6 months he was wheelchair dependent. Epilepsy began at 14 years. Speech became dysarthric on entering school, but he was able to stay in the mainstream educational system. Leukocyte galactosylceramidase activity was reduced. -Editor. *Ped Neur Briefs* April 1995.

MACHADO-JOSEPH DISEASE: GENETICS

A 22-year-old male of Portuguese Azorean descent, presenting at age 16 years with postural instability and falls and developing severe generalized dystonia by age 20 years, is reported from the Center for Research in Neurodegenerative Diseases, University of Toronto, Ontario, Canada. His parents were first cousins and each had a parent clinically affected by Machado-Joseph disease (MJD). Examination demonstrated in addition to dystonia, slurred speech, horizontal nystagmus, limitation of upward-gaze, unsustained ankle clonus, and flexor plantar reflexes.

MRI revealed slight atrophy of the cerebellar vermis. Linkage studies confirmed the recent mapping of the MJD gene to chromosome 14q, and genotyping of the members of this pedigree indicated that this patient was homozygous for the MJD gene. Gene dosage is an important determinant of age at onset and clinical phenotype in MJD. (Lang AE et al. Homozygous inheritance of the Machado-Joseph disease gene. <u>Ann Neurol</u> Sept 1994;36:443-447). (Respond: Dr Lang, Morton and Gloria Shulman Movement Disorder Centre, The Toronto Hospital, Western Division, MP11-306, 399 Bathurst Street, Toronto, Ontario, Canada M5T 2S8).

COMMENT. Three major phenotypes of MJD are described: Type I, Joseph type, with early age of onset and prominent extrapyramidal signs - dystonia, athetosis, rigidity, as well as pyramidal signs; Type III, Machado type, with later onset, cerebellar signs and peripheral neuropathy; and Type II, intermediate type, both with respect to age of onset and clinical features. Juvenile onset of MJD is very uncommon, occurring in only 5 of 143 Portuguese patients cited by these authors. -Editor. *Ped Neur Briefs* Oct 1994.

MACHADO-JOSEPH DISEASE: PATHOLOGY

The frequency, and clinical, molecular, and neuropathological features of spinocerebellar ataxia 3 (SCA3) and Machado-Joseph disease (MJD) in 125 autosomal dominant cerebellar ataxia (ADCA) families were analyzed at the Service de Neuropathologie, Hopital de la Salpetriere, Paris, and Service de Neurologie, Hopital de Haut Leveque, Pessac, France; and Service de Neurologie, Hopital des Specialites, Rabat, Morocco. Thirty four families (126 patients) carried the expanded CAG repeat in the MJD1 gene. The length of the CAG repeat influenced the age at onset and the frequency of clinical signs associated with cerebellar ataxia (abnormal DTRs, decreased vibration sense). The frequency of supranuclear ophthalmoplegia, swallowing difficulties, and amyotrophy was significantly correlated with the disease duration. The age at onset varied from 14 to 70 years, mean 36 yrs, for the SCA3/MJD. One patient with SCA2 had an onset of ataxia at 8 years, whereas the youngest with SCA1 was 21. Neuropathological lesions distinguished the varieties of SCA, eg. basal ganglia lesions were more severe in SCA3/MJD than in SCA1. (Durr A et al. Spinocerebellar ataxia 3 and Machado-Joseph disease: Clinical, molecular, and neuropathological features. <u>Ann Neurol</u> April 1996;39:490-499). (Respond: Dr Durr, INSERM U289, Hopital de la Salpetriere, 4 boulevard de l'Hopital, 75651 Paris Cedex 13, France).

COMMENT. Despite the infrequent occurrence of Machado-Joseph disease in children, three recent reports from different parts of the world, France, Japan, and Australia, prompted commentary. MJD is an autosomal dominant spinocerebellar degeneration, occurring mainly in people of Portuguese descent. An unstable trinucleotide CAG repeat in MJD maps to the same region of chromosome 14 as the SCA3 locus. Two of 3 patients from Japan noted gait unsteadiness at age 18 years, followed 2 years later by involuntary movements, dysarthria, dysphagia, and hand incoordination. (Sakai T et al. A family with Machado-Joseph disease, previously diagnosed as dentatorubral-pallidoluysian atrophy. <u>Neurology</u> April 1996;46:1154-1156). Four families of Australian aboriginal people with MJD exhibited anticipation and an earlier age of onset. (Burt T et al. Machado-Joseph disease in east Arnhem Land, Australia: Chromosome 14q32.1 expanded repeat confirmed in four families. <u>Neurology</u> April 1996;46:1118-1122). MJD should be included in the differential diagnosis of a progressive ataxia with onset in later childhood, adolescence, or adulthood. -Editor. *Ped Neur Briefs* June 1996.

HARP SYNDROME

Harp syndrome, characterized by hypoprebetalipoproteinemia, acanthocytosis, retinitis pigmentosa, and pallidal degeneration, is described in three patients from the National Hospital, Queen Square, London, Newcastle General Hospital, and the Royal Free Hospital, London, UK. An 18-year-old woman presented with intellectual subnormality, night blindness, and dysarthria and dysphagia associated with orobucco-lingual dystonia. T2-weighted MRI showed the "eye-of-the-tiger" sign. This patient's sister and mother had hypoprebetalipoproteinemia but no retinitis pigmentosa or pallidal degeneration. Two patients with a forme-fruste Harp syndrome had the clinical and radiologic features but no lipid abnormality. (Orrell RW et al. Acanthocytosis, retinitis pigmentosa, and pallidal degeneration: A report of three patients, including the second reported case with hypoprebeta-lipoproteinemia (HARP syndrome). <u>Neurology</u> March 1995;45:487-492). (Reprints: Dr R Orrell, Charing Cross Hospital, Fulham Palace Rd, London W6 8RF, UK).

COMMENT. HARP syndrome is distinguished from Hallervorden-Spatz disease (HSD) by acanthocytosis and the abnormality of lipoprotein. The authors note that all cases of HARP syndrome have been sporadic and lack the autosomal recessive feature of HSD. For further reports of HARP syndrome, see <u>Progress in Pediatric Neurology II</u>, PNB Publ, 1994, p477. -Editor. *Ped Neur Briefs* April 1995.

FRIEDREICH'S ATAXIA WITH RETAINED REFLEXES

Genetic linkage analyses in 11 patients from 6 families with Friedreich's ataxia (FA) phenotype, including cardiomyopathy, but retained reflexes (FARR), are reported from the University of Naples and C Besta Neurological Institute, Milan, Italy; and La Fe University Hospital, Spain. Mean age of onset was 13.5 years. Inheritance was autosomal recessive. All patients had progressive ataxia, dysarthria, dysmetria, scoliosis and pes cavus. FARR mapped to the FA locus on chromosome 9q13-21.1, suggesting that FARR is a variant phenotype of FA. (Palau F et al. Early-onset ataxia with cardiomyopathy and retained tendon reflexes maps to the Friedreich's ataxia locus on chromosome 9q. <u>Ann Neurol</u> March 1995;37:359-362). (Respond: Prof Filla, Clinica Neurologica, Universita Frederico II, via Pansini 5, 80131 Napoli, Italy).

COMMENT. The diagnosis of FARR syndrome, a variant of Friedreich's ataxia, should be considered in patients with early onset cerebellar ataxia, cardiomyopathy, and sensory neuropathy. Barbeau found absence of deep tendon reflexes to be a required criterion in the diagnosis of FA (<u>Can J Neurol Sci</u> 1978a;5:57-59), whereas Bell and Carmichael allowed hyperactive reflexes in some cases (<u>Treas Hum Inherit</u> 1939;4:141-281). (Bala V Manyam, personal communication). -Editor. *Ped Neur Briefs* April 1995.

5-HYDROXYTRYPTOPHAN IN FRIEDREICH'S ATAXIA

The effect of the levorotatory form of 5-hydroxytryptophan (approx 1 gm/day/orally) on cerebellar symptoms in 26 patients with Friedreich's ataxia was evaluated in a double-blind drug-placebo study by the Ataxia Research Center, Hopital Neurologique, Lyon and 11 other research hospitals in France. Of 19 completing the study, 11 were treated with 5-hydoxytryptophan and 8 with placebo. A significant decrease of the kinetic score and improvement in coordination was observed in the active treatment group after 6 months but not at 4 months, indicating a progressive drug effect. Five subtests demonstrating improvement included finger-nose test, heel-knee, and Archimedes' spiral. A trend toward acceleration of the speed of speech was also observed. Gastrointestinal symptoms were the main side-effects of treatment. (Trouillas P et al. Levorotatory form of 5-hydroxytryptophan in Friedreich's ataxia. <u>Arch Neurol</u> May 1995;52:456-460). (Reprints: Dr Trouillas, Ataxia Research Center and Cerebrovascular Unit, Faculte Alexis Carrel, Universite Claude Bernard, Hopital Neurologique, 59 Boulevard Pinnel, 69003 Lyons, France).

COMMENT. The effect of 5-hydroxytryptophan was only partial, improving kinetic ataxic symptoms but not the static scores involving posture. In another double-blind crossover study at the Medical University of Lubeck, and other centers in Germany, Wessel K et al reported no significant effect of hydroxytrytophan on cerebellar symptoms in 19 patients with Friedreich's ataxia (<u>Arch Neurol</u> May 1995;52:451-455). Currier RD, in an editorial, concludes that "the levorotatory form of 5-hydoxytryptophan may have an effect that is minimal, selective, and difficult to detect. The question of clinical usefulness is not settled." -Editor. *Ped Neur Briefs* June 1995.

HALLERVORDEN-SPATZ DISEASE: DIAGNOSIS

The *in vivo* diagnosis of Hallervorden-Spatz disease is discussed in relation to the clinical manifestations and MRI findings in two children examined at the Department of Paediatrics, University Hospital of Aarhus, Denmark. Characteristic clinical findings of the late infantile type are a gradual onset with gait disturbance, corticospinal tract signs, rigidity and dystonia, especially oromandibular involvement, and mental deterioration. MRI may be normal at first and will later show hypo-intensity in the globus pallidus in T2-weighted images and an area of hyperintensity in the anteromedial portion, corresponding to the 'eye-of-the-tiger' sign. In some cases, both globus pallidus and substantia nigra are involved, showing hypo-intensities consistent with iron deposition. The diagnostic findings in five additional cases reported in the literature are also tabulated. Age at onset ranged from 1 to 4 years. MRIs were positive when examined at 7 to 12 years. (Ostergaard JR et al. *In vivo* diagnosis of Hallervorden-Spatz disease. <u>Dev Med Child Neurol</u> Sept 1995;37:827-833). (Respond: JR Ostergaard MD PhD, Department of Paediatrics, Aarhus Kommunehospital, University Hospital of Aarhus, DK-8000 Aarhus, Denmark).

COMMENT. Hallervorden-Spatz disease occurs as 1) a classic post-infantile type, with onset between 7 and 15 years; 2) late infantile type, with onset before 6 years of age and leading to death within 10 years; and 3) an adult form, onset between 20 and 60 years, and fatal within 10 years. In addition to the clinical and MRI findings, the diagnosis of Hallervorden-Spatz disease is made by exclusion of other neurodegenerative disorders, some having identical MRI changes, including the 'eye-of-the-tiger' sign. The rare association of Hallervorden-Spatz disease and acanthocytosis has been described by Swisher CN et al (<u>Trans Am Neurol Assoc</u> 1972;97:212), and HARP syndrome, characterized by hypoprebetalipo-proteinemia, acanthocytosis, retinitis pigmentosa, and pallidal degeneration, may include the 'eye-of-the-tiger' sign in the MRI. Reports of HARP syndrome and commentaries are included in <u>Progress in Pediatric Neurology II</u>, PNB Publishers, 1994, p477; and <u>Ped Neur Briefs</u> April 1995;9:26-27). -Editor. *Ped Neur Briefs* Nov 1995.

HALLERVORDEN-SPATZ DISEASE: CLINICOPATHOLOGY

Clinical and pathological features of familial late infantile Hallervorden-Spatz disease (HSD) are reported in two sisters, one of whom died at 11 years, from the Institute for Neurological Sciences, University of Siena, Italy. Clinical diagnosis was confirmed by the classical "eye of the tiger" sign in the MRI. The appearance of the globus pallidus on MRI correlated with the pathological findings, showing pallidal axonal spheroids and iron deposits without involvement of the substantia nigra. Clinically, retinitis pigmentosa, acanthocytosis, and neuromuscular involvement with increased serum creatine kinase were observed in both patients. HSD is classified as a form of neuroacanthocytosis, along with choreo-acanthocytosis, McLeod syndrome, and HARP syndrome. These diseases have the following clinical features in common but variable in frequency: 1) acanthocytosis,

2) extrapyramidal movements, 3) neuromuscular involvement, and 4) retinitis pigmentosa. (Malandrini A et al. Clinicopathological study of familial late infantile Hallervorden-Spatz disease: a particular form of neuroacanthocytosis. Child's Nerv Syst March 1996;12:155-160). (Respond: Dr A Malandrini, Institute for Neurological Sciences, University of Siena, Viale Bracci, 2, I-53100 Siena, Italy).

COMMENT. Hallervorden-Spatz disease is a rare, progressive, and fatal degenerative disorder, with onset in late infancy, childhood or adulthood, characterized by a bizarre gait and speech disturbance, dystonic postures and choreo-athetotic movements, mental deterioration, retinitis pigmentosa, and occasionally, acanthocytosis. The coexistence of HSD and acanthocytosis in 3 sisters was reported by Swisher CN, Menkes JH, Cancilla PA and Dodge PR. Trans Am Neurol Assoc 1972;97:212. An autosomal recessive inheritance is suggested by familial cases. Diagnosis may be confirmed by the MRI and the "eye of the tiger sign" affecting the globus pallidus. For further reviews of IISD and related disorders, see Ped Neur Briefs Nov 1995;9:85, and Progress in Pediatric Neurology II, PNB Publ, 1994, p 477. -Editor. *Ped Neur Briefs* April 1996.

PRIMARY LATERAL SCLEROSIS WITH GAZE PARALYSIS

Three children in a Jordanian family, with consanguinous parents, who met the Stark and Moersch (1945) criteria for the diagnosis of primary lateral sclerosis (PLS) are reported from the King Faisal Specialist Hospital and Research Centre, and King Khalid Eye Specialist Hospital, Riyadh, Saudi Arabia, and Northwestern University Medical School, Chicago, Illinois, USA. In addition they had a diffuse conjugate saccadic gaze paralysis, especially on down-gaze. A chronic progressive weakness beginning in late infancy, associated with spastic quadriplegia and pseudobulbar palsy, led to wheelchair dependence by adolescence and later loss of speech, while intellect was preserved. CT, MRI, EEG, EMG, NCS, and laboratory tests, including enzyme and amino acid assays, were normal. All patients had absent transcranial magnetic motor-evoked potentials in abductor pollicis and anterior tibial brevis muscles. Molecular testing, using DNA blood extracts, showed no linkage to chromosome 2q33 juvenile amyotrophic lateral sclerosis locus, the 8q recessive familial spastic paraplegia locus, or the 5q13 spinal muscular atrophy locus. The clinical course and absence of specific neuropathological etiologies support the diagnosis of familial, autosomal recessive, primary lateral sclerosis. (Gascon GG, Siddique T et al. Familial childhood primary lateral sclerosis with associated gaze paralysis. Neuropediatrics 1995;26:313-319). (Respond: Dr Generoso G Gascon, Division of Pediatric Neurology, Rhode Island Hospital/Brown University, Physicians Office Building, Suite 438, 110 Lockwood Ave, Providence, RI 02903).

COMMENT. All three of these patients were referred with a diagnosis of cerebral palsy, despite the familial and progressive nature of the disorder. The authors cite only one other case of childhood primary lateral sclerosis in the literature. The present report is presented as the first of familial cases. Ford FR refers to cases of hereditary spastic paraplegia in children with degeneration confined to the pyramidal tracts. (Diseases of the Nervous System 4th ed, Springfield, CC Thomas, 1960, p 379). -Editor. *Ped Neur Briefs* Jan 1996.

CHAPTER **17**

RETT SYNDROME

INTRODUCTION
John Wilson, Ph.D., F.R.C.P.
Formerly Senior Consultant Neurologist,
Great Ormond Street Children's Hospital, London, U.K.

In the past year there have been several further case reports of Rett syndrome, mostly single, in small-circulation journals. They serve as a reminder of the world-wide distribution of the condition. There has, however, been a disappointing lack of major contributions to further understanding of the condition. This does not reflect lack of interest or of endeavour, but is an indication of the lack of inspiration, and an increasing suspicion that the presumed mechanism of inheritance is novel. It is tantalizing that, given the pace of advances in molecular genetics and given the unusual heritable characteristics of Rett syndrome, the mystery of this disease remains unsolved.

It has been suggested that sex limitation in this,

and generally in apparently X-linked dominant conditions could be explained by a high rate of de novo dominant-X mutations in males (Thomas GH. High male:female ratio of germ-line mutations: an alternative explanation for postulated gestational lethality in males in X-linked dominant disorders. Am J Hum Genet 1996;58:1364-1368), but the status of apparently affected males remains uncertain (Christen HJ, Hanefeld F. Male Rett variant. Neuropediatrics 1995;26:81-82). The most enigmatic neurobiological feature of all - age-specific decelerating head growth - is also unexplained. Perhaps it is an apoptotic phenomenon. *John Wilson, Ph.D., F.R.C.P.*

ACYL-COA DEHYDROGENASE DEFICIENCY AND RETT SYNDROME

A female infant with medium-chain acyl-CoA dehyrogenase (MCAD) deficiency who was diagnosed with Rett syndrome at 3.5 years is reported from Twenteborg Hospital, Almelo, and Wilhelmina Kinderziekenhuis, Utrecht, The Netherlands. At 13 months her development was normal. By 20 months she could not walk, her language development had ceased, and tremor with loss of purposeful hand movements was noted. At 30 months she had hypotonia, increased tremor and "handwashing" movements. At 3 years she was mentally retarded with autistic features, and the EEG showed bilateral spikes and spike wave activity and a slow waking background rhythm. The head circumference was at the 98th percentile from birth to 17 months and 50th percentile at 52 months. Four additional Rett syndrome patients had normal lymphocyte MCAD assays. (Beekman RP et al. Rett syndrome in a patient with medium chain acyl-CoA dehydrogenase deficiency. Eur J Pediatr April 1994;153:264-266). (Respond: Dr RP Beekman, Wilhelmina Kinderziekenhuis, PO Box 18009, 3501 CA Utrecht, The Netherlands).

COMMENT. The authors found no reason to propose a causal relationship between MCAD deficiency and Rett syndrome.

Naltrexone therapy for Rett syndrome.
A controlled study of an oral opiate antagonist, Naltrexone, in 25 patients with Rett syndrome at the University of Alabama, Birmingham, AL, and other centers, showed a beneficial effect on respiratory irregularities and improved oxygenation but negative effects on development measured by Bayley scales. (Percy AK et al. <u>Ann Neurol</u> April 1994;<u>35</u>:464-470). The hypothesis that naltrexone may be beneficial in Rett syndrome followed from reports of elevated levels of B-endorphins in the CSF of Rett syndrome patients. Further, the intraventicular administration of endorphins in animals produces naloxone-reversible signs similar to those of Rett syndrome. -Editor. *Ped Neur Briefs* May 1994.

POLYSOMNOGRAPHY IN RETT SYNDROME

Respiratory patterns, awake and asleep, were investigated by polysomnography in 30 female patients with Rett syndrome and compared with 30 controls at the Eudowood Division of Pediatric Respiratory Sciences, Johns Hopkins University, and the Department of Neurology, Kennedy Krieger Institute, Baltimore, MD. The median age was 7 years (range, 1 to 32 years). During wakefulness, 67% of RS patients had a characteristic pattern of disordered breathing (hyperventilation followed by central apnea and desaturation). Breathing was normal during sleep. Arterial oxygen saturation during REM sleep was slightly lower in RS cf controls but within normal range. The authors postulate a normal brain-stem control of ventilation in RS and an abnormality or loss of the normal cortical influence on ventilation during wakefulness. The precise cause of the cortical dysfunction is unknown. (Marcus CL, Naidu S et al. Polysomnographic characteristics of patients with Rett syndrome. <u>J Pediatr</u> Aug 1994;125:218-24). (Reprints: Dr Marcus, Johns Hopkins Hospital, Div Pediatric Pulmonology, Park 316, 600 North Wolfe St, Baltimore, MD 21287).

COMMENT. Patients with Rett syndrome have normal respiration during non-REM sleep, slightly abnormal breathing in REM sleep, and markedly disturbed breathing during wakefulness. The hyperventilation is attributed to a cortical dysfunction. -Editor. *Ped Neur Briefs* Sept 1994.

RETT VARIANTS: A WIDENING SYMPTOM COMPLEX

In a collaborative Swedish-Norwegian project, at Goteborg Sweden and Oslo, Norway, a model for the clinical delineation of atypical cases of Rett syndrome was applied to a pilot series of 16 mentally retarded females, aged 11 to 47 years (median: 23). The atypical variants included forme fruste cases (8), late regression (6), and congenital variants (2). The model was based on age >10 years, 3 of 6 primary inclusion criteria for RS (eg. hand stereotypies, decelerated head growth, stages of regression and recovery of contact), and 5 of 11 supportive characteristics (eg. breathing irregularities, air swallowing, teeth grinding, gait dyspraxia, scoliosis). The model identified RS variants and distinguished them from other disorders, eg. Angelman's syndrome that fulfilled 3 supportive criteria. (Hagberg BA, Skjeldal OH. Rett variants: a suggested model for inclusion criteria. <u>Pediatr Neurol</u> July 1994;11:5-11). (Respond: Dr Hagberg, Dept of Pediatrics, Ostra Sjukhuset, S-416 85 Goteborg, Sweden).

COMMENT. For a review of recent international research on RS, see "Rett syndrome: from gene to gesture." <u>J R Soc Med</u> Sept 1994;87:562-566). -Editor. *Ped Neur Briefs* Sept 1994.

PURINE METABOLISM IN RETT SYNDROME

Levels of purine and pyridine nucleotides and their metabolites were determined in erythrocytes and plasma of 31 Rett pattients and 17 age-matched controls at the Departments of Molecular Biology and Child Psychiatry, University of Siena, Children's Hospital, Siena, Italy. No difference was found in erythrocyte nucleotide concentrations, but plasma nicotinamide levels were significantly lower in Rett syndrome patients compared to controls. Erythrocyte activities of hypoxanthine phosphoribosyl transferase, adenine pbt and pbpp synthetase were also lower. The production rate of pyridine nucleotides from nicotinic acid by erythrocytes was increased in Rett patients. The significance of these metabolic changes was not determined. (Rocchigiani M et al. Purine and pyridine nucleotide metabolism in the erythrocytes of patients with Rett syndrome. <u>Neuropediatrics</u> 1995;26:288-292).

COMMENT. Despite frequent reports of various and diverse metabolic changes in patients with Rett syndrome, no consistent and diagnostic biochemical test has been identified for this disorder. The diagnosis is based on agreed clinical criteria. (*see* DSM-IV, 1994). Alterations in nucleotide metabolism are an interesting addition to the search for a specific cause. -Editor. *Ped Neur Briefs* Jan 1996.

COMMUNICATION DEVELOPMENT IN RETT SYNDROME

The development of linguistic communication in 17 children with Rett syndrome was investigated by a parent questionnaire based on the Clinical Linguistic Auditory Milestone Scale in a study at the Department of Speech Pathology and Audiology, University of Alberta, Edmonton, Canada. From birth to 24 months, no child exceeded the stage of single word utterances, with a maximum of 4-6 single words, such as mama/dada. This milestone represents the transition from babbling to real words, normally occurring before the end of the first year. Gesture milestones involving pointing or showing and the beginning of communication were largely absent. Onset of regression had occurred for 14 of the 17 children. Sixteen children exhibited hand movement symptoms, generally during the second year of life. (Tams-Little S, Holdgrafer G. Early communication development in children with Rett syndrome. <u>Brain Dev</u> Sept/Oct 1996;18:376-378). (Respond:

Fax: (1) (403) 492-1626).

COMMENT. These findings contradict the observation that communication development in Rett syndrome before one year is essentially normal. Children with Rett syndrome may develop language to the mama/dada and other single word stage, but limited intentional gestural communication and lack of finger pointing is a potential early predictor of Rett syndrome. -Editor. *Ped Neur Briefs* Jan 1997.

My colleague, Dr Terry Finn, Clinical Neuropsychologist, has drawn my attention to an excellent review of Rett syndrome, including clinical manifestations, diagnostic criteria and differential diagnosis, epidemiology, etiology, pathophysiology, therapeutic intervention, educational intervention, and 90 references to the literature. It is written as an extension of a doctoral dissertation from the perspective of an educator, and the sections on therapeutic and educational intervention are of particular value to the pediatric neurologist with a bent for rehabilitative medicine. (Van Acker R. Rett Syndrome. A Review of Current Knowledge. In: ME Hertzig and E Farber (Eds), Annual Progress in Child Psychiatry and Child Development. New York, Brunner & Mazel, 1993, pp 358-383),(Respond: Rick Van Acker, Ed.D., University of Illinois at Chicago, College of Education M/C 147, Box 4348, Chicago, IL 60680). -Editor.

CHAPTER **18**

NUTRITION, DIET AND NERVOUS SYSTEM DISORDERS

INTRODUCTION

The role of nutrition and diet in the etiology and treatment of neurological disorders of childhood is emphasized in several articles that involve learning and behavior, seizures, headache, ataxia, and peripheral neuropathies. The food additive and artificial sweetener, aspartame, continues to be suspect as a precipitating factor in the cause of migraine, and a recent study links this ubiquitous substance to an increased incidence of brain tumors (*Ped Neur Briefs* Jan 1997). The relation of aspartame ingestion to cognitive and behavioral disorders and to epilepsy is undetermined; some studies negate a causative role while other equally well designed and controlled observations have suggested an exacerbation effect. The need for further investigations is indicated.

In Australia, the Feingold hypothesis is still alive. Investigators at the University of Melbourne have demonstrated a dose response effect of synthetic food coloring on behavior. Also, the role of sugar in behavior cannot be discounted, according to a study at Yale University. Obviously, the demonstration of statistically significant adverse effects of dietary items is difficult in children because of many variables. Studies that fail to confirm a positive correlation between diet and behavior do not rule out a possible link.

Other dietary items important to the nervous system include various vitamins, especially pyridoxine, biotin (*see* Chapter 1, pp 38, 93-98), and vitamin E, gluten in wheat, and fatty acids. Whereas fat overload may induce seizures, a high fat/low carbohydrate, ketogenic diet has anticonvulsant properties. The mechanism of the antiepileptic effect of the ketogenic diet still stimulates discussion and investigation. The possible value of certain fatty acids in the treatment of dyslexia and ADHD is covered in Chapter 4, p 277.

J. Gordon Millichap, M.D., Editor.

ASPARTAME: BEHAVIOR AND COGNITION IN ADHD

The effects of aspartame (34 mg/kg/day for 2 weeks) on the cognition, behavior, and monoamine metabolism of 15 children with a history of ADD were evaluated at the Yale University School of Medicine, using a randomized, double-blind, placebo-controlled crossover study design. Various measures including Conners Behavior ratings, Children's Checking Task, Airplane Test, and Wisconsin Card Sorting Test revealed no significant differences between aspartame and placebo. The Multigrade Inventory for Teachers showed a significant increase in activity level following aspartame treatments. Phenylalanine and tyrosine levels in plasma were significantly elevated at 1 and 2 hours after aspartame ingestion. (Shaywitz BA et al. Aspartame, behavior, and cognitive function in children with attention deficit disorder. <u>Pediatrics</u> Jan 1994;<u>93</u>:70-75). (Reprints: B A Shaywitz MD, Dept of Pediatrics, Yale University Sch of Med, New Haven, CT 06510).

COMMENT. The authors conclude from this study of 15 ADD children receiving single morning doses before school for 2 weeks that aspartame has no clinically significant effect on behavior and cognition, and does not affect urinary excretion rates of monoamines and metabolites. Studies of aspartame in children with neuropsychiatric problems are limited, but one well controlled evaluation in 10 children with absence seizures has shown that aspartame exacerbates EEG spike-wave discharges. (Camfield PR et al. <u>Neurology</u> 1992;<u>42</u>:1000). The ingestion of aspartame in children with seizures should be limited or avoided until effects on seizure control are investigated further.(<u>Ped Neur Briefs</u> June 1992;<u>6</u>:46-47). Migraine has been exacerbated by aspartame in controlled studies of adult patients. -Editor. *Ped Neur Briefs* Jan 1994.

ASPARTAME-INDUCED HEADACHE

A double-blind crossover study in 32 subjects with self-identified aspartame-induced headache is reported from the University of Washington School of Medicine, Seattle, WA. Volunteers were randomized to receive aspartame (30 mg/kg/d) and placebo in a 2-treatment, 4-period crossover design. Each period was 7 days. Subjects reported significantly more headaches during aspartame treatment (on 33% of the days) compared with placebo (24%). Headache triggered by aspartame was particularly frequent [p < 0.001] in subjects who were "very sure" that aspartame had caused them headaches previously. One-fourth of the subjects withdrew from the study, complaining of too frequent or severe headaches or sleep disturbance. A number of individuals had declined inclusion in the study because of the severity of their reaction to aspartame. (Van Den Eeden SK et al. Aspartame ingestion and headaches: A randomized crossover trial. <u>Neurology</u> Oct 1994;44:1787-1793). (Dr SK Van Den Eeden, Division of Research, Kaiser Permanente Medical Care Program, 3505 Broadway, Oakland, CA 94611).

COMMENT. The authors conclude that aspartame causes headaches in a subset of adults with self-identified aspartame-induced headaches. An underestimation of the adverse effect of aspartame in some studies may reflect differences in subject susceptibility, exclusion of specific responders, and concomitant ingestion of other food or drink. Children with migraine may be more responsive to dietary triggers than adults. (<u>Progress in Pediatric Neurology I & II</u>, Chicago, PNB Publ, 1991, 1994). -Editor. *Ped Neur Briefs* Nov 1994.

FOOD COLORING AND BEHAVIOR

The association between the ingestion of tartrazine synthetic food coloring and behavioral change in children referred for assessment of hyperactivity was investigated at the Royal Children's Hospital, University of Melbourne, Australia. Two hundred hyperactive children whose parents had noted changes in behavior with diet were included in a 6-week open trial of a diet free of synthetic colorings. The parents of 150 reported behavioral improvement with the diet, and deterioration when foods containing synthetic colorings were introduced. A 30-item inventory with 5 behavior clusters (irritability, sleeplessness, restlessness, aggression, and inattention) discriminated between dye ingestion and placebo. A double-blind, placebo-controlled, 21-day study of 34 reactive children, using each child as his or her own control, identified 24 atopic children as clear reactors to tartrazine at all six dose levels, between 1 and 50 mg. They were irritable and restless and had sleep disturbance. A dose response was obtained and the effect was prolonged with doses >10 mg. (Rowe KS, Rowe KJ. Synthetic food coloring and behavior: a dose response effect in a double-blind, placebo-controlled, repeated-measures study. <u>J Pediatr</u> Nov 1994;125:691-698). (Reprints: Katherine S Rowe MBBS, Department of Pediatrics, University of Melbourne, Royal Children's Hospital, Parkville, Victoria 3052, Australia).

COMMENT. The authors appear to have demonstrated a relation between tartrazine ingestion and behavior in 24 atopic children,aged 2 to 14 years. Parents were found to be reliable observers and raters of their children's behavior. The strict criteria of ADDH, and a score of >15 on the Conners Abbreviated Parent-Teacher Questionnaire, required for inclusion in many previous studies of diet and hyperactivity may have missed some reactors, accounting for inconclusive results. Further, the Conner's scale places little emphasis on irritability and sleeplessness, symptoms that were prominent in the reactors in the University of Melbourne study. The number of reactors to tartrazine identified in this study contrasts markedly with those of previous studies, and may have been related to the method used for selection of subjects. In Australia, the Feingold hypothesis is still alive. -Editor. *Ped Neur Briefs* Dec 1994.

SENSORY ATAXIA AND VITAMIN E DEFICIENCY

Some children with typical signs of Friedreich's ataxia have familial vitamin E deficiency syndrome, with autosomal recessive inheritance. (<u>Ped Neur Briefs</u> Dec 1993;<u>7</u>:91). *See* Chapter 16, pp 548-549, for a report of progressive ataxia in four patients with vitamin E deficiency, only one having familial involvement. Early identification and supplementation with vitamin E may halt progression of the ataxia. -Editor. *Ped Neur Briefs* April 1994.

CEREBELLAR ATAXIA AND CSF FOLATE DEFICIENCY

See Chapter 16, pp 549-550, for a report of progressive cerebellar ataxia associated with folate deficiency in an 18-year-old male. Low CSF folate has also been reported in inborn errors of metabolism, Kearns-Sayre syndrome, and HIV infection. Neurologic manifestations of inherited disorders of folate metabolism include mental and motor retardation, ataxia, and seizures. Consanguinity of the parents of the above patient suggests an autosomal recessive inheritance.

In addition to folate and vitamin E deficiencies, other degenerative ataxias resembling Friedreich's ataxia that may be amenable to dietary supplements or modifications include vitamin B_{12} and biotin deficiencies and Refsum's disease, responsive to a diet low in phytol and phytanic acid.(<u>Progress in Pediatric Neurology</u>, Chicago, PNB Publ, 1991, p 480). -Editor. *Ped Neur Briefs* April 1994.

FAT OVERLOAD FOCAL SEIZURES

Two 9-year-old patients receiving fat emulsion therapy presented with focal seizures and other neurologic complications (*see* Chapter 1, p 98). Both patients died of pneumonia. Autopsy findings included cerebral endothelial and intravascular lipid deposition, and multiple areas of necrosis and hemorrhage. Early recognition of the fat overload syndrome may allow prompt withdrawal of fat emulsion therapy and reversal of neurologic symptoms. -Editor. *Ped Neur Briefs* June 1994.

KETOGENIC DIET MECHANISM OF ACTION

The intracellular pH of the cerebral cortex was studied by the neutral red method in 15 adult rats maintained on ketogenic and control diets for 5-6 weeks Rats fed the ketogenic diet had more than a 10-fold increase in plasma ketones, but no significant differences in cerebral pH or in cerebral metabolites and GABA levels were noted. The antiepileptic effect of the ketogenic diet was probably not mediated by cerebral acidosis or changes in cerebral GABA levels. (Al-Mudallal AS, Harik SI et al. Diet-induced ketosis does not cause cerebral acidosis. <u>Epilepsia</u> April 1996;37:258-261). (Reprints: Dr SI Harik, Department of Neurology, University of Arkansas, 4301 W Markham, Slot 500, Little Rock, AR 72205).

COMMENT. The ketogenic diet used in the treatment of some forms of epilepsy in childhood was originally introduced at the Mayo Clinic (Wilder RM. <u>Mayo Clin Bull</u> 1921;2:307), not at Johns Hopkins University, as some recent media publicity would have us believe. Furthermore, some of the earlier work relating to the mechanism of action of the ketogenic diet, not cited in the above paper, also originated at the Mayo Clinic (Millichap JG, Jones JD, Rudis BP. Mechanism of anticonvulsant action of ketogenic diet. <u>Amer J Dis Child</u> 1962;104:506, and 1964;107:593-604). Seizure susceptibility was not modified by a fat diet in normal animals, but an anticonvulsant effect was demonstrated in mice with a seizure threshold lowered by water intoxication and hypoelectrolytemia. In animals and in patients with absence seizures, the anticonvulsant effect of the ketogenic diet was unrelated to diuresis, independent of acidosis and ketosis, similar to the effects of acetazolamide, and correlated most closely with a negative balance of sodium and potassium. -Editor. *Ped Neur Briefs* April 1996.

MECHANISM OF SUGAR-INDUCED BEHAVIORAL EFFECTS

The adrenomedullary response to a standard oral glucose load (1.75 gm/kg; maximum, 120 gm) and susceptibility to neuroglycopenia (assessed by the hypoglycemic clamp and measurements of P300 auditory evoked potentials [AEP]) were studied in 25 healthy children (8 - 16 years of age) compared to 23 young adults at the Children's Clinical Research Center, Yale University School of Medicine, New Haven, CT. Baseline and oral glucose-stimulated plasma glucose and insulin levels were similar in children and adult groups. A late fall in plasma glucose level at 3 - 5 hours after glucose ingestion stimulated a rise in plasma epinephrine, twice as high in children compared to adults. Hypoglycemic symptoms (shaky, sweaty, weak, or tachycardia) increased in children but not in adults, in association with the late fall in plasma glucose. P300 amplitude, a measure of cognitive function, was significantly reduced when glucose concentration was lowered to 75 mg/dl in children, but was preserved until the level fell to 54 mg/dl in adults. Children are more vulnerable to effects of hypoglycemia on cognitive function than are adults. (Jones TW et al. Enhanced adrenomedullary response and increased susceptibility to neuroglycopenia: Mechanisms underlying the adverse effects of sugar ingestion in healthy children. <u>J Pediatr</u> February 1995;126:171-7). (Reprints: William V Tamborlane MD, Department of Pediatrics, Yale University School of Medicine, 333 Cedar St, New Haven, CT 06510).

COMMENT. This study shows that consumption of glucose by healthy children may be followed by a fall in plasma glucose sufficient to induce hormonal changes and adverse behavioral and cognitive effects. The authors stress that their data do not prove a causative role for dietary sugar in children with hyperactivity. However, a balanced diet of protein, fat, and complex carbohydrate, to limit postprandial falls in glucose levels, should avoid symptoms associated with the enhanced adrenomedullary responsiveness demonstrated in healthy children.

Mild hypoglycemia (60 mg/dl) caused a significant decline in performance on a battery of cognitive tests in a study of adolescents with insulin-dependent diabetes mellitus at the University of Pittsburgh School of Medicine. Neither hyperglycemia, nor the rapid drop from acute hyperglycemia to euglycemia, affected symptoms, cognitive function, or counterregulatory hormone secretion. (Gschwend S et al. Effects of acute hyperglycemia on mental efficiency and counterregulatory hormones in adolescents with insulin-dependent diabetes mellitus. <u>J Pediatr</u> Feb 1995;126:178-84). -Editor. *Ped Neur Briefs* Feb 1995.

GLUTEN SENSITIVITY AND NEUROLOGICAL ILLNESS

The frequency of IgG and IgA antigliadin

antibodies, a measure of cryptic gluten sensitivity, and celiac disease was studied using ELISA in 147 adult patients admitted to the Royal Hallamshire Hospital, Sheffield, UK, for neurologic investigation. Of 53 patients with neurological dysfunction of unknown cause, including 25 with ataxia and 20 with peripheral neuropathy, 30 (57%) had positive antigliadin antibody titers, compared to only 5% of 94 patients with specific diagnoses, such as stroke, MS, and Parkinsonism, and 12% of 50 healthy blood donors. In antigliadin-positive patients with ataxia or neuropathy of unknown cause, duodenal biopsies revealed histological evidence of celiac disease in 35% and non-specific duodenitis in 38%. Only one had low vitamin B12 levels and the biopsy was normal. Gluten sensitivity was a common finding in this group of adult patients with ataxia and peripheral neuropathy of unknown cause. (Hadjivassiliou M et al. Does cryptic gluten sensitivity play a part in neurological illness? <u>Lancet</u> February 10, 1996;347:369-71). (Respond: Dr M Hadjivassiliou, Department of Clinical Neurology, Royal Hallamshire Hospital, Sheffield S10 2JF, UK).

COMMENT. This investigation underscores the importance of nutrition and diet in some neurological disorders of undetermined etiology. Antigliadin antibody estimation should be considered in the investigation of patients with neurological dysfunction of unknown cause, including those with refractory seizures, and especially if associated with occipital calcifications. Patients with histological evidence of celiac disease are treated with a gluten-free diet. However, those celiac patients with seizure complications and occipital calcifications are not always benefited by diet, and surgical resection of the involved occipital cortex may be required. (see <u>Progress in Pediatric Neurology II</u>, PNB Publishers, 1994, pp71-73). -Editor. *Ped Neur Briefs* Feb 1996.

JOURNAL INDEX

Clinical Pediatrics
Clinical Toxicology
Current Problems in Pediatrics

D
Developmental Medicine and Child Neurology
Developmental Review

E
Electroencephalography and Clinical Neurophysiology
Epilepsia
European Journal of Pediatrics
European Neurology

H
Headache

I
International Journal of Neurology
International Multiple Sclerosis Journal
International Pediatrics (Miami)

J
Journal of Abnormal Child Psychology
Journal of the American Academy of Child and Adolescent Psychiatry
Journal of the American Medical Association
Journal of Child Neurology
Journal of Child Psychology and Psychiatry and Allied Disciplines
Journal of Clinical Epidemiology
Journal of Clinical Investigation
Journal of Clinical Neurophysiology
Journal of Clinical Psychiatry
Journal of Developmental Behavior and Pediatrics
Journal of Medical Genetics
Journal of Nervous and Mental Disease
Journal of the Neurological Sciences
Journal of Neurology, Neurosurgery and Psychiatry
Journal of Neuropathology and Experimental Neurology
Journal of Neurophysiology
Journal of Neurosurgery
Journal of Nutrition
Journal of Pediatrics
Journal of Pediatrics and Child Health
Journal of the Royal Society of Medicine
Journal of Toxicology and Environmental Health

L
Lancet

M
Mayo Clinic Proceedings
Muscle and Nerve

N
Nature
Neurology
Neuron
Neuropathology and Applied Neurobiology

Neuropediatrics
Neurosurgery
Neurotoxicology and Teratology
New England Journal of Medicine

P
Pediatrics
Pediatric Neurology
Pediatric Neurology Briefs (Chicago)
Prenatal Diagnosis
Progress in Pediatric Neurology (Chicago)

R
Research Publications - Association for Research in Nervous and Mental Disease

S
Science
Seminars in Neurology
Seminars in Pediatric Neurology
Surgical Neurology
Survey of Ophthalmology

T
Thyroid
Transactions of the American Neurological Association